Advancing Frontiers of
PSYCHIATRIC THERAPEUTICS

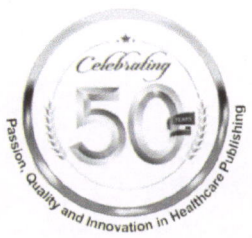

Advancing Frontiers of
PSYCHIATRIC THERAPEUTICS

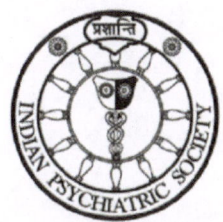

Indian Psychiatric Society Publication

Editor

PK Singh

MBBS (AIIMS) MD (PGIMER)
Professor and Head
Department of Psychiatry
Patna Medical College
Patna, Bihar, India

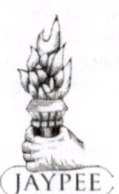

JAYPEE BROTHERS MEDICAL PUBLISHERS
The Health Sciences Publisher
New Delhi | London

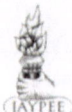
Jaypee Brothers Medical Publishers (P) Ltd

Headquarters
Jaypee Brothers Medical Publishers (P) Ltd
4838/24, Ansari Road, Daryaganj
New Delhi 110 002, India
Phone: +91-11-43574357
Fax: +91-11-43574314
Email: jaypee@jaypeebrothers.com

Overseas Office
J.P. Medical Ltd
83 Victoria Street, London
SW1H 0HW (UK)
Phone: +44 20 3170 8910
Fax: +44 (0)20 3008 6180
Email: info@jpmedpub.com

Website: www.jaypeebrothers.com
Website: www.jaypeedigital.com

© 2020, Jaypee Brothers Medical Publishers and Indian Psychiatric Society

The views and opinions expressed in this book are solely those of the original contributor(s)/author(s) and do not necessarily represent those of editor(s) of the book.

All rights reserved. No part of this publication may be reproduced, stored or transmitted in any form or by any means, electronic, mechanical, photocopying, recording or otherwise, without the prior permission in writing of the publishers.

All brand names and product names used in this book are trade names, service marks, trademarks or registered trademarks of their respective owners. The publisher is not associated with any product or vendor mentioned in this book.

Medical knowledge and practice change constantly. This book is designed to provide accurate, authoritative information about the subject matter in question. However, readers are advised to check the most current information available on procedures included and check information from the manufacturer of each product to be administered, to verify the recommended dose, formula, method and duration of administration, adverse effects and contraindications. It is the responsibility of the practitioner to take all appropriate safety precautions. Neither the publisher nor the author(s)/editor(s) assume any liability for any injury and/or damage to persons or property arising from or related to use of material in this book.

This book is sold on the understanding that the publisher is not engaged in providing professional medical services. If such advice or services are required, the services of a competent medical professional should be sought.

Every effort has been made where necessary to contact holders of copyright to obtain permission to reproduce copyright material. If any have been inadvertently overlooked, the publisher will be pleased to make the necessary arrangements at the first opportunity. The **CD/DVD-ROM** (if any) provided in the sealed envelope with this book is complimentary and free of cost. **Not meant for sale.**

Inquiries for bulk sales may be solicited at: jaypee@jaypeebrothers.com

Advancing Frontiers of Psychiatric Therapeutics

First Edition: **2020**

ISBN: 978-93-89776-56-0

Printed at Repro India Limited

CONTRIBUTORS

Anil Kakunje DPM MD
Professor and head
Department of Psychiatry
Yenepoya Medical College
Mangaluru, Karnataka, India

AQ Jilani
MD DNB DM (Geriatric Mental Health)
Assistant Professor
Department of Psychiatry
Era's Lucknow Medical College
Lucknow, Uttar Pradesh, India

Ashlesha Bagadia MRCPsych FRANZCP
Perinatal Psychiatrist and
Psychotherapist
The Green Oak Initiative Community
Mental Health Centre
Bengaluru, Karnataka, India

Aswin Krishnan Ajit MD
Director and Consultant Psychiatrist
Dhanya Doctors Chamber
Centre for Neurobehavioral Disorders
Kochi, Kerala, India

Bikash R Behera MS MCh FSFN
Fellow (Stereotactic and Functional
Neurosurgery)
Jaslok Hospital and Research Centre
Mumbai, Maharashtra, India

BN Gangadhar MBBS MD
Professor of Psychiatry
Director
National Institute of Mental Health and
Neurosciences (NIMHANS)
Bengaluru, Karnataka, India

Chethan Basavarajappa DNB
Assistant Professor
Department of Psychiatry
National Institute of Mental Health and
Neurosciences (NIMHANS)
Bengaluru, Karnataka, India

Debasish Sanyal MD
Professor and Head
Department of Psychiatry
KPC Medical College
Kolkata, West Bengal, India

Hemant Bhargav
MBBS Diploma in Community Mental Health MD
(Yoga and Rehabilitation) PhD (Yoga)
Assistant Professor of Yoga
Department of Integrative Medicine
National Institute of Mental Health and
Neurosciences (NIMHANS)
Bengaluru, Karnataka, India

Indla Ramasubba Reddy MD DPM
Director
Vijayawada Institute of Mental Health
and Neurosciences
Vijayawada, Andhra Pradesh, India

Jahnavi Kedare MBBS MD
Associate Professor
TNMC and BYL Nair Charitable Hospital
Mumbai, Maharashtra, India

Jitender Jakhar MBBS MD
Senior Resident
Department of Psychiatry
National Institute of Mental Health and
Neurosciences (NIMHANS)
Bengaluru, Karnataka, India

Kabir Garg MD MRCPsych
Highly Specialized OCD/BDD
services and Community Eating
Disorder Services
Hertfordshire Partnership University
NHS Foundation Trust, UK

Kaustav Chakraborty MD DNB
Associate Professor and Head
Department of Psychiatry
College of Medicine and
JNM Hospital, WBUHS
Nadia, West Bengal, India

Konasale M Prasad MD
Department of Psychiatry
University of Pittsburgh
School of Medicine
Pittsburgh, Pennsylvania, USA

Manoj Shettar MD
Assistant Professor
Department of Psychiatry
SDM Medical College
Dharwad, Karnataka, India

Meha Jain MPhil (Clinical Psychology)
Child Psychologist
Department of Pediatrics
All India Institute of Medical Sciences
Patna, Bihar, India

Mohd Aleem Siddiqui MD DPM
Professor
Department of Psychiatry
Era's Lucknow Medical College and Hospital
Lucknow, Uttar Pradesh, India

Nand Kumar MD
Professor and In-charge
Department of Psychiatry
Neuromodulation
All India Institute of Medical Sciences
New Delhi, India

Naresh Nebhinani MD DNB
Associate Professor
All India Institute of Medical Sciences
Jodhpur, Rajasthan, India

Nishitha Jasti BNYS MSc (Yoga)
Research Associate
Department of Integrative Medicine
National Institute of Mental Health and Neurosciences (NIMHANS)
Bengaluru, Karnataka, India

Pankaj Kumar MD
Associate Professor and Head
Department of Psychiatry
All India Institute of Medical Sciences
Patna, Bihar, India

Paresh K Doshi MS MCh
Director
Department of Neurosurgery
Jaslok Hospital and Research Centre
Mumbai, Maharashtra, India

PK Singh MBBS (AIIMS) MD (PGIMER)
Professor and Head
Department of Psychiatry
Patna Medical College
Patna, Bihar, India

Pooja Patnaik Kuppili
Assistant Professor
Department of Psychiatry
Sri Venkateshwaraa Medical College Hospital and Research Centre
Puducherry, India

Rajeev Ranjan MD
Assistant Professor
Department of Psychiatry
All India Institute of Medical Sciences
Patna, Bihar, India

Rakesh K Chadda
MBBS MD FAMS FRCPsych DFAPA
Professor and Head
Department of Psychiatry
Chief, National Drug Dependence Treatment Centre
All India Institute of Medical Sciences
New Delhi, India

Rashmi Arsappa MBBS MD
Assistant Professor
Department of Psychiatry
National Institute of Mental Health and Neurosciences (NIMHANS)
Bengaluru, Karnataka, India

Ravi Gupta MD PhD
Certified Sleep Physician (WSF)
Additional Professor
Department of Psychiatry
All India Institute of Medical Sciences
Rishikesh, Uttarakhand India

Contributors

Rishi Gupta MD
Senior Resident
Department of Psychiatry
Chief, National Drug Dependence
Treatment Centre
All India Institute of Medical Sciences
New Delhi, India

Ruksheda Syeda MBBS DPM
Psychiatrist
Trellis Family Centre
Mumbai, Maharashtra, India

Sai Krishna Tikka MD DPM
Assistant Professor
Department of Psychiatry
All India Institute of Medical Sciences
Raipur, Chhattisgarh, India

Sai Spoorthy Mamidipalli MD
Senior Resident
Department of Psychiatry
All India Institute of Medical Sciences
Raipur, Chhattisgarh, India

Santosh Kumar MD DNB Fellowship in Geriatric Mental Health
Associate Professor
Department of Psychiatry
Nalanda Medical College
Patna, Bihar, India

Saurabh Kumar MD
Assistant Professor
Department of Psychiatry
Patna Medical College
Patna, Bihar, India

Shahul Ameen MD
Consultant Psychiatrist
St Thomas Hospital
Changanassery, Kerala, India

Shivarama Varambally MBBS MD
Professor of Psychiatry and Head
Department of Integrative Medicine
National Institute of Mental Health and Neurosciences (NIMHANS)
Bengaluru, Karnataka, India

Smita N Deshpande MD DPM
Senior Consultant and Professor
Department of Psychiatry
De-Addiction Services and
Resource Center for Tobacco Control
Centre of Excellence in Mental health
Atal Bihari Vajpayee Institute of
Medical Sciences and
Dr Ram Manohar Lohia Hospital
New Delhi, India

Varun S Mehta MD DNB MRCPsych
Associate Professor
Department of Psychiatry
Central Institute of Psychiatry
Ranchi, Jharkhand, India

Vijendra Nath Jha MD
Assistant Professor
Department of Psychiatry
Darbhanga Medical College
Darbhanga, Bihar, India

Vishal Indla MD DNB
Director
Vijayawada Institute of Mental Health and Neurosciences
Vijayawada, Andhra Pradesh, India

Vishwajit L Nimgaonkar MD
Professor of Psychiatry and
Human Genetics
Director
Program for Genetics and Psychosis
University of Pittsburgh
Pittsburgh, Pennsylvania, USA

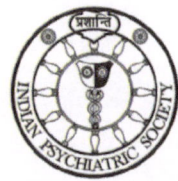

Health professionals are known for their healing touch. Their identity, authority, respectability and livelihood, all revolves around this healing touch. There used to be a time when healing touch was a simple touch, but advances of civilization and burgeoning power of science, this touch has evolved to include almost the universe. It has become more remote, multifaceted and complex. Despite all this the personal touch, however, have to be maintained.

The chapters embodied in this book *Advancing Frontiers of Psychiatric Therapeutics* are diverse and cover almost all aspects of current psychiatric therapeutics comprehensively. Our learned authors have tried intelligently and diligently to explore the different facets and interfaces of varied psychiatric therapeutics that have emerged in recent times. These newer paradigms and strategies will definitely empower mental health professional to become a more effective therapist. It is revealing to go through various chapters of this book to get a glimpse of the possibilities that are yet to be fully utilized for the care and help of people who are afflicted with mental disorders. This is of great practical and everyday importance. We are sure that all you will find it of great value.

The Publication Committee, especially Professor PK Singh needs to be appreciated for this novel update. We must put on record that his contributions as Chair of this committee are historic. The book has been beautifully produced and for this M/s Jaypee Brothers Medical Publishers (P) Ltd, New Delhi, India, deserves a big thank you.

Long live Indian Psychiatric Society (IPS).

Mrugesh Vaishnav **PK Dalal** **Vinay Kumar**
President, IPS *President-elect, IPS* *Hon General Secretary, IPS*

PREFACE

We, the mental health professionals, are constantly engaged in providing freedom from pain and suffering to all seekers of help for mental health issues through our armoury of varied therapeutic tools. This skill of inducting therapy is in fact the ultimate arbiter of our acceptance, respect and power in society as well as our source of livelihood. Different therapeutic paradigms are actually weapons in our hands for our adaptive struggle against all diseases and disorders that are integral part of our life. There immediate aim is freedom from suffering but larger aim is to increase the survival potential of human race as a member of the biosphere. Simultaneously, it also influences their quality of living as well as their productive and creative potentials. It is this linkage of therapy with life that provides justification and meaningfulness to all our related scientific and para-scientific activities, be it hard-core research or their applications in the community.

All systems in the universe, which includes our own species, have a natural tendency to move towards disorderliness. Even though there are naturally occurring, inbuilt homeostatic regulatory mechanisms to take care of this tendency, but often they prove to be inadequate and require to be supplemented by externally introduced, man-made interventions which require constant investment of time, energy and various other resources. There is a constant race and struggle between the order and the disorder. Therapeutic sciences play the role of tilting the balance in favor of orderliness.

The phenomenon of mind itself has hitherto remained inadequately unexplored and continues to remain a perpetual mystery. Mental disorders can be understood properly only when we are able to make some headway in understanding the true nature of mind. Complexity of human mind is reflected in the equally complex nature of its disorders which require varied inputs of a very wide spectrum to reclaim orderliness. Despite our ignorance about the primary order, the disorders of mind continue to be felt in everyday life because of the distress and dysfunctions associated with it and therefore need to be rectified. In fact, the insights gained through our attempts at successfully treating mental disorders, allow us to retrospectively extrapolate them in trying to understand the true nature of mind.

For last several years Indian Psychiatric Society (IPS) has been publishing a series of books annually under a generic heading of "Different Strokes" with varied themes and topics for internal circulation. Last year it was decided to focus on the theme of therapeutics where all knowledge seems to converge. In the book, we had tried to bring together some completely new and innovative therapeutic strategies along with the newer versions of older established treatment strategies. This ranges from spirituality to psychosurgery, from recent drugs to drug-assisted psychotherapy, from pharmacogenomics to stem-cell therapy, from cognitive enhancers to antiviral therapy, from issues related to integration of pharmacotherapy and psychotherapy to issues of polypharmacy, from nutraceuticals to psychobiotic therapy, from cosmetic psychopharmacology to therapeutic role of sleep and exercise, from management of resistant auditory hallucination to non-pharmacological management of psychotic disorders. There are a few more topics from the cutting edge interface of advancing frontier that has been included in the book. We are extremely thankful to all our esteemed and erudite authors for having spared enough time out of their extremely busy schedules, to write outstanding chapters on topics which are mostly unconventional.

Seeing the warm reception and also relevance of this theme, we decided to go for larger circulation of this book to a much wider audience. We are thankful to Jaypee Brothers Medical Publisher, a recognized and established name in the field of medical publishing in India and abroad, to come to our help for this venture. Without their forth-right cooperation and positive interest, this book in its present form would not have seen the light of the day. We express our gratitude to them for the same. Our colleagues at Publication Subcommittee of IPS, Dr Shahul Ameen and Dr Naresh Nebhinani have always been very supportive, helpful and encouraging. Higher leadership of Indian Psychiatric Society, the President, the President-elect, and the Hon General Secretary have been a constant source of strength and support. Especially Dr Vinay Kumar, the present Hon General Secretary, who also happens to be the immediate-past Chairperson of the Publication Subcommittee, has always been a great source of help, support, encouragement, and guidance. With his exemplary dynamism and resourcefulness, he has proved to be a great problem-buster at all stages of this project. At the end, having gone through the ordeal, we have been able to come up with a rich bouquet of rare flowers in the form of this unique book, which we are confident, shall prove a great asset for all, the researchers as well as the practitioners of science of mental health.

Long live Indian Psychiatric Society.

PK Singh

ACKNOWLEDGMENTS

I would like to thank Shri Jitendar P Vij (Group Chairman), Mr Ankit Vij (Managing Director), Mr MS Mani (Group President), Ms Chetna Malhotra Vohra (Associate Director—Content Strategy), Ms Pooja Bhandari (Production Head), Ms Nedup Denka Bhutia (Development Editor) and the publishing staff at M/s Jaypee Brothers Medical Publishers (P) Ltd, New Delhi, India, for their work in completing this book.

CONTENTS

1. **The March of Advancing Frontiers: An Overview** 1
   PK Singh

2. **Artificial Intelligence-based Therapies** 8
   Debasish Sanyal

3. **Recent Advances in Biofeedback Therapy** 14
   Vijendra Nath Jha

4. **Current Status of Yoga and Other Spiritual Therapies in Psychiatry** 23
   Hemant Bhargav, Jitender Jakhar, Nishitha Jasti, Rashmi Arsappa, Shivarama Varambally, BN Gangadhar

5. **The Interface of Psychopharmacology and Psychotherapy** 37
   Rakesh K Chadda, Rishi Gupta

6. **Update on Drug-assisted Psychotherapies** 48
   Pankaj Kumar, Rajeev Ranjan, Meha Jain

7. **Current State of Management for Residual and Resistant Auditory Hallucinations and Delusions** 61
   Varun S Mehta, Smita N Deshpande

8. **Antiviral Therapy in Schizophrenia: Does It Work?** 69
   Smita N Deshpande, Konasale M Prasad, Vishwajit L Nimgaonkar

9. **Nonpharmacological Therapies for Psychotic Disorders** 79
   Jahnavi Kedare, Ruksheda Syeda

10. **Interventions for Personality Disorders** 97
    Ashlesha Bagadia

11. **Critical Overview of Polypharmacy Debate** 109
    Sai Spoorthy Mamidipalli, Sai Krishna Tikka, Mohd Aleem Siddiqui

12. **Cosmetic Psychopharmacology** 123
    Vishal Indla, Chethan Basavarajappa, Indla Ramasubba Reddy

13. **Nutraceuticals in Psychiatry** 131
    Kabir Garg

14. **Therapeutic Role of Sleep and Exercise in Management of Health**   144
    Ravi Gupta

15. **Recent Advances in Drug Treatment of Chronic Depression**   155
    Kaustav Chakraborty

16. **Current Status of Cognitive Enhancers**   169
    AQ Jilani, Santosh Kumar

17. **Pharmacogenomics in Psychiatry**   178
    Anil Kakunje, Manoj Shettar

18. **Stem Cell Therapy for Psychiatric Disorders**   189
    Naresh Nebhinani, Pooja Patnaik Kuppili

19. **Psychobiotic Therapy**   199
    Aswin Krishnan Ajit, Shahul Ameen

20. **Advances in Brain Stimulation Therapies**   212
    Nand Kumar, Saurabh Kumar

21. **Surgical Interventions for Neuropsychiatric Disorders**   224
    Bikash R Behera, Paresh K Doshi

Index   247

CHAPTER 1

The March of Advancing Frontiers: An Overview

PK Singh

INTRODUCTION

The border which faces all the onslaughts and still marches further forward is the frontier. We are referring here to the frontier of knowledge which makes excursions into the domain of the unknown and wins it over step by step through persistence and perseveration. This is what we call "advancement." The realm of the unknown is presumably much larger and undefined compared to what is known to us. The unknown contains within itself the precious "secrets" of all-powerful Nature in a variably encrypted and selectively accessible format which is revealed to us in unpredictably incremental fashion through the valor of committed and dedicated pursuit. It is the tenacious human curiosity, combined with creativity that leads to discovery of unknown treasures in the form of revelations of secrets and new laws of the Nature. Within our own lifetime, we have seen the march of science in several areas of life. Mass media has moved from big box-like radios to televisions to palm-sized smartphones which have evolved to become an obligate all-in-one constant companion; it has made redundant many technological marvels of the yesteryears in one stroke. It has become an indispensable, ever-ready, ever accessible supplement to our mental faculties. If we were to stretch the imagination a little farther on the same timescale, may be a time will come when we will have gadgets for revisiting the past or foreseeing the future. It might appear a bit quixotic today but given the fact that the rate of change currently, in the area of science, is multiplying in geometric proportions, it may not be surprising to find that a wild imagination of today becomes a reality of tomorrow. Who would have imagined about a century ago that nearly 4.6 billion passengers would have flown across the skies of the world in 2019 alone in a flawless and increasingly more comfortable manner. We have now entered into the 21st Century, also known as the information age. In this information age, the models and paradigms of intervention for mental maladies have also been multiplying very fast. But unfortunately, the mainstream psychiatry keeps confined itself to only a few easily accessible and easily dispensable modes of intervention, ruled predominantly by prescription of pills. Prescribing a pill is the easiest intervention to deliver; therefore, if prescribed judiciously it can be cater to a larger population in a cost-effective manner. From this point of view, the overshadowing of other modes of therapeutic interventions by greater reliance on drugs may appear justified. But drugs alone have great limitations. They are highly inadequate when compared to the complexity and multiplicity of multi-level factors involved in causation and correction of mental derangements, deviations, and disorders that we come across in real life. We have to think and explore "out of the box" to devise innovative strategies to match the enormousness of this difficult task. We as mental health professionals must inculcate an eclectic approach and bring to the doorsteps of each suffering individual all possible ways of healing methods in a convergent manner. With this goal in mind, it was decided to pool together the talent of Indian Psychiatric Fraternity to overview most of the possible therapeutic strategies which are currently being given shape at the cutting edge of advancing frontiers of psychiatric therapeutics. The advancements are always made at the frontiers which are multifaceted, multidimensional, and generally interconnected.

Healing the hurt, at all levels of life, be it personal or social, somatic or psychic, spiritual or mundane, is the first duty of all practitioners of science of health. Health delivery is the executive arm of all Health Sciences. The art of practice of health delivery is to deploy the power of knowledge, be it scientific or experiential, in a most befitting manner to cater to the uniqueness of the individual, his milieu, and the disorder he is suffering from. It has to be used in a most effective and innovative manner so as to minimize any harm while at the same time ensuring maximal recovery from the disorderliness to reduce distress and dysfunction. Healing professionals work at the interface of Science and Society. They have the never ending duty to heal. It is from this social endpoint that all academics and therapeutic research derive their meaningfulness. From this viewpoint, it is imperative that all health practitioners keep themselves updated about all the latest and cutting edge principles, concepts, and technologies so that they are maximally enabled and empowered to function as an effective healer. In fact, the healing hand may be viewed as the adaptive loop of human race to maximize its survival potential. This therapeutic loop, which is the corrective loop for constantly unleashing disorderliness, will determine not only the survival but also the quality of life of individual human beings.

It was with this outlook that the theme of this issue of "Different Strokes" was chosen as "Advancing Frontiers of Psychiatric Therapeutics." There are 20 additional chapters in this booklet, which cover a very wide range of intervention strategies. It ranges from Spirituality to Psychosurgery, from the most esoteric to the most mundane of all therapeutic strategies.

THE ANCIENT TIMES

Historically, there always has been need and also attempts at modifying the behavior of people who exhibit altered, abnormal, and/or dangerous behavior through various means called therapy. The nature of intervention depended on the understanding and convictions of that period about the cause of such alterations. Such convictions have gradually changed and/or evolved over period of time. The earliest has been the belief that mental disorders are caused by supernatural forces in the form of being possessed by devils or demons. The belief in demoniac possession as a cause of mental illness led to two different kinds of reactions with the aim to either protect the individual from being possessed or getting the individual freed from possession. The corrective measures ranged from exorcism or trephining of skull to relieve the person from possession by spirit in some societies, to the other extreme of maintaining such piety so that these devils cannot take hold of the individual. Maintenance of personal purity was done by the ancient Persians, who took to precautionary measures in the form of ensuring purity of mind and body to pre-empt and reduce the chances of being possessed and thus keep oneself protected from mental illness.

The evidences obtained from the remnants of trephined skulls from a period dating back to 5000 BC, point toward the antiquity of this practice. It appears very barbaric from the perspectives of modern times. But paradoxically and most surprisingly, even today we drill holes in human skull to put in place slender wires of metal for a modern intervention, called brain stimulation therapy, albeit in a very sophisticated manner, vindicating though the aphorism that life moves in a circle. We also have a chapter on "Brain Stimulation Therapies" in this book.

Bleeding, purging, and vomiting to undo the bodily humoral imbalance, malaria therapy, metrazol therapy, hydrotherapy, insulin coma therapy, and frontal lobotomies have had their own hey days of being on the high, to the extent that some of them also having been recognized with the award of prestigious and coveted Nobel prize. Some of the other irrational therapies of yesteryears include blistering, dousing patients with boiling or ice-cold water, using physical restraints such as straitjackets or simply using sedatives to keep the patients sedated for long periods of time. Use of religious rituals and use of amulets and talisman are still quite prevalent. In many of the private madhouses run by clergymen in the west of those days, certain religious practices that were used for such patients included attending Churches, going on pilgrimages, engaging in confessions of sins, and undertaking repentance.

Only electroconvulsive therapy of that period, used to induce controlled seizure for therapeutic purposes, has survived because of its proven and rapid efficacy in certain severe mental conditions with high margin of safety. Even though this method has also undergone substantial modification and further technological sophistication, in keeping with the times, it has increasingly been brought under societal and legislative controls in different parts of the world. This is only reflective of the highly enigmatic, multifactorial and multifaceted nature of the mental disorders and the different aspects of life it interfaces with.

Egyptians have been recorded to advise recreational activities to help recovery from symptoms of mental illness. This is indicative of a very enlightened view that they held at that time, even though it must have been quite inadequate for inducing recovery from the different states of mental disorders.

Hippocrates probably was the first to suggest in 3rd-5th century BC that mental illnesses are because of natural occurrences in the body and not because of supernatural forces, wrath or curse of divine bodies, or possession by evil spirits. He suggested that it was because of the imbalances between four humors of the body. The methods of correction of these imbalances, such as bloodletting, purging, and vomiting, suggested in those days would not be acceptable today. However, Hippocrates had also suggested change of occupation and/or environment as a method of remedy for mental patients, which is quite consistent with current views and understanding of mental illnesses.

Mental illnesses were also thought to be a consequence of immoral behavior or sin having been committed by the individual or their family members. Mentally sick people were treated as less than human entities, at times like animal. In fact, at different times, they were subjected to sterilization and other forms of genital restrictions. The conditions of asylums and madhouses have been described as pathetic throughout history. A major turning point in the history of care of mentally ill has been the refreshingly reformist "Humanitarian Movement" ushered in by Philippe Pinel and William Tuke in France. They thought and practiced that mentally ill patients would improve if they were treated with "kindness and care" and "respect and compassion." This was to take them out of the neglectful, abusive, demeaning, and filthy environment of the yesteryears. It did have a positive impact in the lives of the mentally ill inmates; it also had a positive impact in the functioning of the asylums throughout the world and also on the coming generations.

After this, came the hospital movement in the 18th century with the stated objective of "protecting society and individual from harm, to cure those amenable to treatment, to improve the lives of the incurable, and to fulfill the humanitarian duty of caring for the insane."

THE MODERN TIMES

At the turn of the century came Dr Sigmund Freud, the Father of Psychoanalysis. With his lucid and coherent formulations of the structure of mind and psychodynamic causes of psychopathologies, he changed the mindset of professionals of the whole world that led to the wide acceptance of a completely new paradigm of intervention. It also had a deep impact on the literature as well as the general mindset of people of that time. Psychodynamic psychotherapy spread far and wide as one of the mainstream modes of intervention for mental illnesses, especially for the nonpsychotic ones. However, because of its highly subjective, conjectural, and nonverifiable nature of theories along with a very prolonged format of patient-therapist interaction requiring a highly skilled and trained therapist who are now not only very few but are also dwindling in number. The psychoanalysis later found itself on a weaker footing in face of strongly emerging bold and confident psychopharmacology. However, cognitive behavior therapy, more popularly known as CBT, has emerged to acquire the center stage of psychotherapeutic interventions. It focuses on the relationship between thoughts and emotions at the conscious level, analyzes their distortions, and suggests methods of correction.

With the introduction of chlorpromazine in early 50s and antidepressants in late 50s, the fate of mentally sick people took a quantum leap for the better. The speed and magnitude of predictable symptomatic improvement in psychotic and depressed patients was phenomenal. These drugs brought a sea change in their lives. Never before had such a thing happened that mentally ill patients could return back to their previous level of life in a predictable manner, very much like patients suffering from other medical illnesses. Based on these observations of clinical improvements with certain psychotropic drugs, many possible theories about their etiology, especially at the neurobiological levels, emerged in a retrograde fashion based on the putative mechanisms of actions of these drugs. Such theories are still being explored further. This definitely was a step forward but it seems to have very quickly led to a plateau. It is not showing up or leading to any newer doorsteps to either recovery or newer theories. Apart from the issues of short-term and long-term side effects, the efficacy rate and profile of effectiveness of even newer psychotropics are not showing any advancement. Their advancing edge needs to be emboldened further.

Stuck with a block on the traditional path, newer options for therapy are being explored at all possible levels, the physical, the psychic, and the spiritual levels. We have tried to include representative areas from each of them in this book. With the advancement in technologies, many hitherto unimagined and unthought of options for interventions have emerged and are being explored and experimented upon.

Mankind has now been able to fully analyze its own genome. Armed with the power of this knowledge, its applied potentials are also being examined with reference to mental health needs. One possible application of this knowledge is in the domain of developing personalized medicine as applicable to psychiatry in the form of pharmacogenomics which will allow pharmacotherapy to be tailored to the needs, uniqueness, and idiosyncracies of the individual. Further advancements in genetic technologies have made possible the power to edit the genes. With increasing understanding of the relationship between genes, endophenotypes, and the phenotype-behavior, it is possible that in near future we may have gene therapy as one of the established modes of psychiatric therapeutics. Another area full of potentials is the use of pluripotent cells in refreshing and replenishing the old and the crooked cells and tissues by way of stem cell therapy. Gut has been described as the second brain and increasingly the communications between the two for maintenance of mental health and execution of mental operations are being deciphered. This knowledge is being used as Psychobiotic Therapy for mental health.

Human intelligence is proving to be inadequate to meet mankind's own dreamy and imaginative aspirations. Human intelligence is being assisted in all walks of life by the artificial intelligence, at times threatening to overtake it. It is getting supplemented, assisted, and augmented by gadgets of artificial intelligence which of course is man's own creation. Artificial intelligence has spread its wings in many areas of life, predominantly in hospitality, in commerce, transport, defense and also very substantially in the area of medical investigation and intervention. Its use in mental health cannot be left behind. Already we have online psychotherapies and Avatar therapy. The full potential and role of this augmented power in psychiatric therapeutics will continue to remain an active area of professional and scientific explorations.

Further advancements of scientific technologies have empowered and also emboldened scientific researchers and practicing professionals to foray into hitherto unchartered caves, crevices, land and islands of mental health therapeutics. Lately, the technology of functional brain scans has opened a completely new window to the understanding of the functions of brain. The functional magnetic resonance imaging (fMRI) of brain taken after activating it with specific mental tasks or with experience of specific emotional states, are presenting very interesting pictures. In fact, there are scientists who claim that they can decipher from the brain scans as to what emotional state the individual is experiencing or what number he is holding in his mind. These claims are very interesting and are at the verge of immeasurable possibilities of futuristic nature. But how far this tech-toy will take us in our quest of trying to understand the true nature of mind and mental disorders, remains an unanswered question. One is reminded here of the hope and hype that was generated at the time of discovery of X-rays or invention of electroencephalography (EEG). In their euphoria at the time of their discovery, people thought that it will now lead to uncovering of all the mysteries of medical science. With the passage of time, we have now fully realized the stark limitations of both these technologies as regards their potential in providing answers to the perpetual questions relating to the mental dimension.

The preferred place and physical setting for treatment of mental disorders as well as goals of such treatments, have also undergone fundamental changes. It has moved from lunatic asylums to mental hospitals to institutes of mental health to the community; similarly the goals of treatment have also evolved from the initial position of providing protection to the society from the mentally insane to providing cure with recovery and rehabilitation back in the community, to realizing one's own full potential. The mental health scenario of today is completely different from that of yesteryears and is likely to get transformed for the better in future.

CONCLUSION

The area of mental health is going to increasingly acquire more and more importance and significance. In the information age, the psychological sophistication of people is bound to increase. People are likely to focus and seek more and more help for promotion and maintenance of their mental health. Even otherwise mental health is a very important determinant of all other dimensions of health. It is quite natural that all different, multilateral, and innovative approaches be brought together in a convergent manner for the rescue, restoration, and rejuvenation of mental health of the masses. Given the current level of ignorance about the nature, affiliations and dimensions of mind, we will have to try all possible weapons and strategies in our store to eventually win the race to provide foolproof shield and immunity to everyone's mental health.

SUGGESTED READING

1. Hardy J (2015). A beautiful mind: the history of the treatment of mental illness. [online] Available from https://historycooperative.org/a-beautiful-mind-the-history-of-the-treatment-of-mental-illness/ [Last accessed December, 2019].
2. Oosterwijk S, Lindquist KA, Anderson E. States of mind: emotions, body feelings, and thoughts share distributed neural networks. Neuroimage. 2012;62(3):2110-28.
3. Jutras M. Historical perspectives on the theories, diagnosis, and treatment of mental illness. BCMJ. 2017;59(2):86-8.
4. Hussung T (2016). A History of Mental Illness Treatment: Obsolete Practices. [online] Available from https://online.csp.edu/blog/psychology/history-of-mental-illness-treatment [Last accessed December, 2019].
5. SA Mind (2017). Is Your Happy the Same as My Happy? [online] Available from https://www.scientificamerican.com/article/can-you-tell-someones-emotional-state-from-an-mri/ [Last accessed December, 2019].
6. Wikipedia. Treatment of Mental Disorders. [online] Available from https://en.wikipedia.org/wiki/Treatment_of_mental_disorders. [Last accessed December, 2019].
7. Wikipedia. History of Mental Disorders. [online] Available from https://en.wikipedia.org/wiki/History_of_mental_disorders [Last accessed December, 2019].

CHAPTER 2

Artificial Intelligence-based Therapies

Debasish Sanyal

INTRODUCTION

Tremendous advancement in the field of computer science and information technology over last few decades has touched every facet of human life. Computers, internet, and smartphones are everywhere and being its user includes academics, technologists, businessmen as well as common people. Medical science including the field of mental health and psychiatry has also been influenced by this revolution of technology. Computers cannot only do huge calculations, handle huge information accurately, but also they have intruded into areas which were assumed to be prerogative of human intelligence. Thus, computers can now defeat even Grandmasters in game of chess. People began to talk about computers becoming intelligent like human beings and possibly exceed human capacity. IBM's Watson supercomputer may be able to beat humans at game of jeopardy, but currently match the cognitive capacity of a human being.

Controversies exist about what exactly is human intelligence. Large number of academics from diverse areas has argued against machine being able to truly approximate functions of human mind. Philosophers like Searle[1] and physicists like Penrose[2] to name a few have strongly emphasized eminence of human intelligence over computer.

Many researchers have proposed following essential requirements of artificial intelligence (AI):[3-6]

- Reason
- Use strategy
- Make judgments
- Plan
- Learn
- Natural language communication capability
- Work toward common goal.

Humans can recognize patterns, learn new knowledge by applying insights and experience, create mental models of reality, think abstractly, and innovate.[7]

However, our thinking is extremely slow due to slow neural transactions.

Machine intelligence includes the ability to remember billions of facts precisely and recall them instantly. And, can share their knowledge at extremely high speed.

John McCarthy, the father of AI; coined the term "artificial intelligence" in 1956.

The modern definition of AI is "the study and design of intelligent agents" where an intelligent agent is a system that perceives its environment and takes action which maximizes its chances of success.

TYPES OF ARTIFICIAL INTELLIGENCE

There are three types of AI:
1. *Narrow AI:* Developed and trained for a particular task—weather forecast.
2. *Artificial general intelligence (AGI):* It is an AI system with generalized cognitive abilities which find solutions to the unfamiliar task it comes across, still not achieved.
3. *Artificial superintelligence (ASI):* It refers to the position where computer/machines will surpass humans and machines would be able to mimic human.

APPLICATIONS OF ARTIFICIAL INTELLIGENCE IN PSYCHIATRY

- AI in psychiatric diagnosis
- AI in psychiatric treatment.

AI in Psychiatric Diagnosis: How Machine Learning Algorithms are Used in Psychiatry

Limitations of current psychiatric diagnosis are that many conditions overlap. At least 50% of patients receive more than one psychiatric diagnosis. People visiting more than one provider may be diagnosed differently, leading to confusion, straining trust, and complicating recovery planning.

Approaching psychiatric diagnosis by using mathematical tools to search for consistent patterns inherent in clinical data, avoid error from human bias and the risk of holding onto familiar categories in favor of more accurate approaches. By using AI type approaches, researchers can leverage computation power to see consistencies in how symptoms cut across received diagnostic categories to develop "transdiagnostic" perspectives. Machine learning has already made its way into clinical research and analyzes the psychological traits of the patients using unsupervised techniques (unlabeled samples are to be divided into groups of related cases) and semi-supervised techniques (both labeled and unlabeled cases are present).[8,9] This method is used to broadly classify depressed individuals from the healthy ones.

Below I describe some areas where AI approach has been used in psychiatric diagnosis.

Psychosis Early Detection[10]

Artificial intelligence could be used to notice relevant symptoms and acts as an early detection mechanism, as demonstrated by two recent case studies.

Veterans are considered as a typical high-risk group for developing mental health difficulties. Cogito—a company funded by the Defense Advanced Research Projects Agency—teamed up with the US Department of Veterans Affairs to try an application named Companion, to monitor veteran subject's phone 24/7. The sound of the user's voice and their frequency of mobile phone usage, changes in inflection, energy of pitch may translate into mental health indicator using AI.

IBM's Computational Psychiatry and Neuroimaging group, alongside several universities, built an AI that used a method called natural language processing (NLP) analyzing patient's speech for different indicators, such as coherence of speech and ideas and achieved 83% retrospective accuracy of detection.

- Researchers from Harvard University and the University of Vermont used color analysis, metadata, and algorithmic face detection using AI to get 70% accuracy in detecting signs of depression from Instagram pictures. Depression patients were more likely to post bluer, grayer, and darker-colored photos. Using computer vision to diagnose attention-deficit hyperactivity disorder (ADHD) in children.

  Scientists at the University of Texas at Arlington and Yale University used computer vision and machine learning to assess children while they are performing exercises to test a child's attention, decision-making, and ability to manage emotions and were able to diagnose ADHD more accurately.

  Computer game Cyberball, which measures social rejection can be used to assess borderline personality disorder.

- Virtual reality offers method to study behavior under controlled conditions such as assessing interpersonal behaviors such as distance regulation, gaze direction, and posture.

Neuroimaging biomarkers: They have been studied for major depressive disorder (MDD), schizophrenia, obsessive-compulsive disorder (OCD), and chronic pain syndromes. Taking data from 200 patient samples, and looking at 10,000 neuroimaged connections and 140 brain lesions, and using sophisticated AI algorithms to select the 16 functional connections that are specific for and discriminate autism spectrum disorder (ASD) from normal (typically developed) brains, could not distinguish MDD patients from their controls, but showed some ability to discriminate between patients with schizophrenia and controls. By pinpointing the lack of emotional response in the brain, an artificially intelligent system can alert a doctor to psychotic symptoms, and calculate the probability of a patient developing schizophrenia by analyzing the functional magnetic resonance imaging (fMRI) and speech pattern data that the program has gathered. The sum of the information a computer gathers allows the system to develop a full mental profile of a patient, which can then be shared with a psychologist or psychiatrist for double-checking and administration of care. Patterns of disjointed speech may appear in very mild form years before a patient develops schizophrenia and the breaks may be so subtle that even a trained *professional* could miss them.

AI in Psychiatric Treatment

Improve Mental Health Access[10,11]

Less than *one psychiatrist for every 100,000 people* in more than 45% of world populations. AI enabled programs may be used to screen people for mental illness.

AI Provides Personalized Treatment

An online platform Ginger.io can tailor its suggestions to the needs of the user and provide access to a variety of treatments.

Stigma Avoidance

Stigma of mental illness makes people reluctant to seek help. As opposed to fellow humans, an AI does not necessarily form part of any wider social construct and may be perceived as *nonjudgmental, nonopinionated* and neutral.

Psychotherapy Uses

The main advantages offered by the use of information technology in psychotherapy are:
- Supplementary time for supervised treatment gained by the patient
- Decrease the time append in direct interaction with the practitioner
- Decrease the cost of the treatment
- Some help in taking treatment decisions.

The main applications of computer in psychology refer especially to psychotherapy:[12]
- Self-help internet sites
- Computer administered therapy
- Screening and assessment using web applications over the internet
- Adjunctive palmtop computer therapy
- Online consultation
- Advocacy
- Virtual reality therapy
- Interactive voice messaging systems
- Biofeedback via ambulatory physiological monitoring

- Virtual spaces for support groups (can be based on social network instruments or by a custom solution).

STRESS MANAGEMENT

Macquarie University in Sydney helps students develop better coping techniques, particularly in connection with examination stress using AI techniques.

Kavakli and colleagues proposed a virtual companion that can be readily available to provide support. The virtual counselor offers advice and support with stress management. AI can play in making people feel socially more connected. Example, being Melbourne, Australia, Moderated Online Social Therapy (MOST) project.

CHATBOTS AND VIRTUAL AI THERAPIST[10,13,14]

Online cognitive behavioral therapy (CBT) which is available 24/7, accessible easily and instantaneously is just as effective as human counselor-based CBT. The first randomized control trial with Woebot showed that after just 2 weeks, participants experienced a significant reduction in depression and anxiety. A virtual therapist named Ellie has also been launched and trialed by the University of Southern California's Institute for Creative Technologies (ICT). Initially, Ellie was designed to treat veterans experiencing depression and post-traumatic stress syndrome. What is so special about the technology is that Ellie can detect not only words but also nonverbal cues (e.g. facial expression, gestures, and posture), which are subtle and difficult to pick up.

FUTURE SCENARIO

Artificial intelligence in future may be used for finding the neurodevelopmental trajectory of humanity by doing dataset clustering and letting unsupervised machine learning and find the potential points where interventions can change trajectory of development, and thereby develop probable therapy for neurodevelopmental diseases and possible answer to aging.

Other possible ways in which AI may be used in future are as follows:
- Smartphone behaviorometrics
- Body sensor behavioriometrics
- Social media behaviorometrics
- Natural language processing monitoring
- Behavioral assessments from real-life behavioral observation
- Social media behavioral assessment
- Regular assessment of various biomarkers in a transdiagnostic way
- AI-based rehabilitation of neurodevelopmental and neurodegenerative disorders
- Whole brain simulation or mind transfer—immortal humans!!
- Robotic playmates and companions
- Social AI for social reintegration

- Enhancement by implants, merger of human and AI for augmented human intelligence
- Detailed microscopic level knowledge about organization of human brain and connectomes so that its interactions can be understood (Blue Brain Project, Human Connectome Project).

CONCLUSION

Amidst the technological revolution we are witnessing, it is hoped that proper and judicious use of artificial intelligence is going to help psychiatry and patients in near future. It is a powerful resource. The way we use it will decide whether it proves to be a bane or boon for us.

REFERENCES

1. Searle JR. Is the Brain a Digital Computer? Proceedings and Addresses of the American Philosophical Association. 1990;64(3):21-37.
2. Penrose R. Shadows of the Mind: A Search for the Missing Science of Consciousness. Oxford: Oxford University Press; 1994.
3. Russell S, Norvig P. Artificial Intelligence: A Modern Approach, 2nd edition. India: Pearson Education; 2003.
4. Luger GF, Stubblefield WA. Artificial Intelligence: Structures and Strategies for Complex Problem Solving. New York: Addison-Wesley; 2004.
5. Poole D, Mackworth AK, Goebel R. Computational Intelligence: A Logical Approach. New York: Oxford University Press; 1998.
6. Nilsson NJ. Artificial Intelligence: A New Synthesis. New York: Morgan Kaufmann Publishers Inc.; 1998.
7. Kurzweil R. The Singularity Is Near: When Humans Transcend Biology. New York: Viking Penguin; 2005.
8. Non-technical person's guide to entering the machine learning industry. [online] Available from https://www.analyticsindiamag.com/non-technical-persons-guide-to-entering-the-machine-learning-industry/ [Last accessed January, 2020].
9. Opinions using neural networks to forecast sun's sunspot time series (2019). [online] Available from https://www.analyticsindiamag.com/using-neural-networks-to-forecast-suns-sunspot-time-series/ [Last accessed January, 2020].
10. World Economic Forum. 3 ways AI could help our mental health. (2018) [online] Available from https://www.weforum.org/agenda/2018/03/3-ways-ai-could-could-be-used-in-mental-health/ [Last accessed January, 2020].
11. There's an App for That? Merging Technology and Mental Health. (2020) [online] Available from https://blog.ozobot.com/2018/01/18/theres-app-merging-technology-mental-health/ [Last accessed January, 2020].
12. Newman MG. Technology in psychotherapy: an introduction. J Clin Psychol. 2004; 60:141-5.
13. Rucker M, Fogoros RN. Using artificial intelligence for mental health (2019). [online] Available from https://www.verywellmind.com/using-artificial-intelligence-for-mental-health-4144239 [Last accessed January, 2020].
14. Bemelmans R, Gelderblom GJ, Jonker P, de Witte L. Socially assistive robots in elderly care: a systematic review into effects and effectiveness. J Am Med Dir Assoc. 2012;13:114-20.e1.

CHAPTER 3

Recent Advances in Biofeedback Therapy

Vijendra Nath Jha

INTRODUCTION

The term "biofeedback" has two components "bio" and "feedback" which literally translates into, giving back to the subject, information about some of the biological/physiological functions. This information about the biological/physiological functions is usually in the form of signals, with the goal that, in due course, the subject can manipulate these functions at will. There are certain functions which we carry out voluntarily or consciously, e.g. walking, running, and holding a glass. And there are other functions which seem to be outside our control or are involuntary, such as heart rate, respiration, pain perception, skin temperature, and gastrointestinal function. Biofeedback can help one to control the latter set of physiological functions that were thought to be autonomic or outside one's control. Although there is much to be researched as to how does biofeedback work, one thing is for certain that it provides relief in certain conditions related to stress by providing relaxation.[1] As with advances in other fields of medicine, the field of biofeedback also has seen advances (such as ability to modify brain waves) which we shall be discussing in this section.

WHAT IS KNOWN ABOUT BIOFEEDBACK THERAPY?

The concept of biofeedback was not new to Indian medicine. Indian Yogis used to practice this in the form of yoga and transcendental meditation.[2] However, the term biofeedback was coined in 1969 at a landmark conference in Santa Monica, in which mathematician Norbert Wiener explained that systems can be controlled by monitoring their results (*cybernetics theory*).[3] Biofeedback therapy was given a standard definition in the year 2008 as "a process that teaches a person how to alter his or her physiological activity for the purpose of improving health and physical performance."[4] Simplifying it further, it is a therapy which helps a person to modify his physiological functions. Depending upon various physiological functions, electrodes and other apparatus are used to monitor those functions, such as cardiac activity/heart rate, respiratory patterns, musculoskeletal activity, cutaneous temperature, and, of late, brain waves. The readings from those physiological functions are relayed to special equipment which then convert the readings into signals and feedback the information to the user in audio or visual form, in real time. Over the period of several sessions, the user observes changes in those signals with changes in thinking, emotions, and behavior, and through the principles of classical and operant conditioning learns to control those parameters without the equipment.

BIOFEEDBACK METHODS

There are several types of equipment which are used to measure a variety of bodily functions:
- *Electromyogram*: As the name implies, it measures electrical changes in various muscle groups which are then displayed over the monitor. The patient then hears or sees the signal which is proportional to the muscle activity.
- *Electrodermal activity*: Apart from the electrical activities in muscle groups, skin also shows electrical activities, which can be measured directly in the form of dermal conductance and dermal potential and also indirectly in the form of dermal resistance.
- *Electroencephalographic activity*: It measures the electrical activity from the brain through electrodes placed over the scalp.
- *Thermal biofeedback*: Feedback of skin temperature is another useful method and it helps patients to learn to control their blood flow.
- *Electrocardiogram*: This is a common investigation but biofeedback therapists measure the heart rate variability (HRV) to treat various illnesses such as asthma, chronic obstructive pulmonary disease (COPD), and anxiety.
- *Pneumograph*: This device is used to measure respiratory rate and chest wall expansion. This helps clinicians to detect and correct dysfunctional breathing pattern and behavior.

CLINICAL APPLICATIONS

Biofeedback has been the mainstay of nonpharmacological treatment of various common conditions such as:
- *Headache*: Frontalis muscle electromyographic feedback and thermal feedback are the main biofeedback techniques for relief of headaches.
- *Cardiovascular disorders*: Hypertension, arrhythmias, and Raynaud's are some disorders that are being successfully managed by this method.
- *Urinary and fecal incontinence*: Mowrer's bedwetting alarm for nocturnal incontinence and Kegel perineometer for urinary incontinence have been very helpful.
- *Anxiety and stress reduction*: Patients with anxiety and stress disorder benefit a lot when they become aware of the variation in physiological functions with changes in anxiety levels. They gradually learn to control these variations and manage their anxiety.

- *Chronic constipation*: Impairment in neuromuscular system resulting in symptoms of outlet obstruction can also benefit by these techniques.

RECENT ADVANCES IN BIOFEEDBACK

Neurofeedback

Neurofeedback or neurotherapy is a new advancement in the field of biofeedback by which one can learn to modulate one's brain waves. Just like other forms of biofeedback, the brain wave recordings and other physiological variables are modified using the software and fed back to the subject. The recordings of brain waves of the subject are registered, transformed, and enlarged into signals that can be presented to the subject in various forms, such as bonus points in a video game, picture quality/brightness of a video clip or sound pattern of a beautiful music. Subsequently, these signals help the patient in learning how to modify changes produced in his brain waves, through principles of classical and operant conditioning. The main objectives of neurofeedback are the same as with other feedback methods—controlling the system of physiological responses (in this case brain waves) with training, maintaining this control over physiological responses even without feedback, and generalizing the self-control achieved in due process.

There has been noticeable increase in the number of research papers focusing on neurofeedback and its applications to induce behavioral changes.[5]

If we trace back the origin of neurofeedback, we see that in early 1930s there were several studies which highlighted the fact that human electroencephalograph (EEG) was also susceptible to the principles of classical conditioning.[6,7] Few decades later, MB Sherman supported these findings when he was able to successfully demonstrate the changes in EEG with operant conditioning. He was able to produce the same EEG changes in a cat as in wakefulness [(also called sensorimotor rhythm (SMR)]. This helped increase in sleep spindles during sleep thereby improving sleep quality.[8] Around the same time, Dr Kamiya also found that given the correct feedback, the amplitude and frequency characteristics of EEG can be controlled by his subjects.[9] In 1976, Lubar described sensorimotor rhythm NF in hyperkinetic child and observed clinical benefits.

Neurofeedback have been used in combination with several brain imaging techniques such as quantitative electroencephalography (QEEG), functional magnetic resonance imaging (fMRI),[10] near-infrared spectrography (NIRS), positron emission tomography (PET),[11] and single-photon emission computed tomography (SPECT). However, only fMRI-NF (fMRI–neurofeedback) and EEG-NF (electroencephalography–neurofeedback) have acceptable applications in clinical studies and NIRS studies are ongoing.

Electroencephalograph Neurofeedback

In a typical EEG-NF system, EEG electrodes are placed over scalp to record brain waves. These waves are then fed into software which converts them into signals for display to the subject. These waves are usually grouped into three bands based on the wave frequency; delta (2-4 Hz) and theta (4-8 Hz) waves as slow frequency band, alpha waves (8-12 Hz) as medium or intermediary band, and beta (12-38 Hz) and gamma (38-42 Hz) waves as fast frequency band. Higher the frequency, higher is the level of arousal. Extreme arousal is seen in frequencies beyond 21 Hz in the form of anxiety and/or anger. Most people would benefit from frequencies that are in the range of 12-21 Hz and are associated with a calm and relaxed state. Thus, during a hypothetical therapeutic session, the subject might be asked to play an electronic game where the movement of the virtual player depends or is proportionate to the user keeping his brain waves in the midrange frequency. Session by session, the ease of maintaining the brain waves in the midrange frequency increases and corresponding improvement in scores on psychometric testing is also evident.

Electroencephalograph neurofeedback has several advantages such as being widely available and accessible in mobile settings. However, it has some disadvantages such as low spatial resolution, signal attenuation from the source to the scalp, and considerable inter-individual variability.[12]

Functional Magnetic Resonance Imaging Neurofeedback

Functional magnetic resonance imaging in real time, also known as rtfMRI, is a recent and welcome development in the field of neurofeedback. This method uses blood oxygen level dependent (BOLD) signal to present appropriate feedback to the subject and to enable modulation of brain activity. Depending upon the computational software available, the analysis is performed almost instantly or with a delay of few seconds.[13]

The field of rtfMRI has seen several advances which have been reviewed in detail.[14] Some of these technical advances are—use of implicit protocols, the development of multivariate analysis technique, use of external rewards, and connectivity-based neurofeedback.

Implicit neurofeedback: Contrary to conventional neurofeedback methods, in implicit neurofeedback, subjects are not told what behaviors are being targeted or even that they are being trained at all. They are simply presented with a stimulus and asked to follow certain commands and the resultant changes in brain activities are being interpreted by the experimenter without the knowledge of the subject. The advantage of this implicit neurofeedback is that it reduces the "experimenter effect". It is seen that the subjects may knowingly or unknowingly learn to exhibit results in order to match the expectations of the experimenter. It can be very useful in cases like post-traumatic stress disorder (PTSD), where repeated presentation of aversive stimuli (to extinguish fear) can lead to extreme levels of anxiety and high dropout rates. Similarly this method is helpful in patients with impaired cognitive ability who might not understand complex training instructions.

Multivariate methods: Conventional fMRI-NF methods are unidimensional, i.e. they may change the fMRI signals averaged across a region of interest (ROI) in the brain in one dimension only. However, with the use of multivariate analysis, neurofeedback gets multidimensional. It displays what is known as "voxel patterns" or three-dimensional patterns of fMRI signals in the ROI. This multidimensional activation pattern is considered more specific and spatially sensitive.

Role of external reward: Although feedback scores provided to subjects during feedback sessions are good reinforcement signals, it is seen that, in addition, if external reward (such as money) is also provided, it leads to greater enhancement of feedback scores than either given alone.

Connectivity-based Neurofeedback

Brain functions are formed not only by activation of specific ROIs, but also by network of brain regions which are highly interacting and correlated with each other. This new feature of neurofeedback based on connectivity has enabled the modification of connectivity of a targeted brain network via two main methods. First is dynamic causal modeling (DCM); in this method causal relationship and mutual influences between different brain regions in a network are tested. One model/network is selected as the target model and two or more alternate models are also selected. Next, the participant is asked to increase the feedback scores to match the targeted model. A positive feedback is given when it matches the targeted model and negative feedback if it matches one of the alternate models. The model with the largest degree of fitness is selected as the right model. Second method is correlation-based which uses Pearson's correlation coefficients of activity time courses between two ROIs to assess correlation between them.

The above-mentioned four techniques in fMRI neurofeedback have made more advancements in the field of neurofeedback. These are *decoded neurofeedback* or *DecNef* and *functional connectivity-based neurofeedback* or *FCNef*. DecNef involves studying specific brain regions, whereas FCNef studies the connectivity between different brain regions. These newer techniques have been proposed to help neuroscientists in establishing a causal relationship between neural activity and specific behavior. The goal of DecNef is for participants to learn to induce a specific activity pattern within a target brain region. Hence, in DecNef implicitness, reinforcement schedule with external reward, and multivariate analyses have been included. The goal of FCNef is to change specific functional connectivity between two brain regions for which FCNef integrates aspects such as implicitness, reinforcement schedule with external reward, and connectivity analyses.

With a high spatial resolution, rtfMRI allows for a refined delineation of cortical and subcortical targets.[15] Better access to deep subcortical structures, noninvasiveness, and accuracy are some of the advantages of rtfMRI neurofeedback. It has some limitations as well; foremost being that it is not "real-time" in true sense. The fMRI signal is created by the hemodynamic delay of up to 5 seconds between the actual neural activity and the vascular response; whereas the delay in EEG signaling is only few milliseconds.[16] Another disadvantage is the fact that the subject has to remain in a magnetic resonance system throughout the period of task.

Near-infrared Spectrography

This is another recent advancement in neurofeedback which employs the use of near infrared spectroscopy. NIRS is a method of spectroscopy that uses near infrared region of the electromagnetic spectrum (from 780 nm to 2,500 nm), the advantage being, that NIRS can penetrate much further into a tissue than any other radiation. Regular blood hemoglobin monitoring and determining optical absorption coefficients by NIRS can help in locating a specific brain region and the activity of that region. Being noninvasive, it can help in the assessment of brain function/neural activity by detecting changes in blood hemoglobin concentrations.[17] This particular method has also been called hemoencephalography (HEG).

Use of Neurofeedback in Various Disorders

Attention deficit hyperactivity disorder (ADHD): With regards to the brain waves, the major findings in ADHD children (inattentive type) are an excess of low frequency waves (theta, 4–7 Hz) and a deficit of high frequency waves (beta, 13–21 Hz) in midline and frontal cortices.[18] It is also called as high theta to beta ratio. Thus the neurofeedback protocol used is decreasing theta to beta ratio meaning thereby, increasing beta waves and decreasing theta waves.[19]

Depression: There are basically two commonly used protocols for NF in depression. The first is based on asymmetry of alpha activity in prefrontal cortex such that there is high alpha activity in left prefrontal area and low in corresponding right hemisphere. Hence, the subject is trained to decrease alpha activity on the left side and increase it on the right prefrontal area.[20] The second protocol focuses on the increased theta to beta ratio in left prefrontal area. Theta activity is associated with lowered brain activity and it is increased in depression, whereas beta activity which is associated with motivational and executive functions is lowered in depression, hence increased theta to beta ratio.[21] Subjects are trained to lower theta activity and enhance beta activity to 13–20 Hz range as increasing beta activity beyond that range can precipitate or worsen pre-existing anxiety state in a depressed subject.

Stroke rehabilitation: Real-time fMRI neurofeedback has proved to be helpful in stroke patients as is evident by systematic review studies. It has been seen that neuronal connectivity and activity between impaired brain regions can be modulated by stroke patients using real-time feedback. It has also been evident in these studies that cognitive and motor functions are also significantly improved by neurofeedback. However, it was also reported that the effectiveness varies across different target areas.[22]

Neurofeedback as a treatment modality differs from other techniques (like electroconvulsive therapy, transcranial magnetic stimulation) in the fact that it does not force the brain waves to change. It only provides a signal to the subject so that the subject is the only one who can voluntarily learn, recognize, and produce their optimum brain state. Hence the brain resets itself to a new steady state and this is felt by the subject as a real reward and during every session, the neural network is strengthened.

LIMITATIONS AND FUTURE TRENDS

Limitations

Though biofeedback does not have any side effects of its own unlike pharmacotherapy, it does have certain limitations. The various mechanical devices and electrodes used can cause apprehension in some patients causing irregularity in readings. As is the case with other devices, unwanted "noise" can come from poor placement of electrodes. Patients with cognitive impairment can find it difficult to understand and execute the instructions and the necessary steps. As it is a time-consuming procedure and with the cost involved, it can be difficult to employ this in setups with large patient population and insufficient manpower.

It may be difficult to use biofeedback in disorders in which there is low physiological reactivity. Similarly its use is limited in disorders such as personality disorders in which physiological mechanisms cannot be implicated to be directly involved.

Future Trends

Several reviews have highlighted the lack of standardization amongst feedback studies. A consensus is to be made regarding what functions are to be targeted and what should be the outcome measures, as well as the optimal number and timing of sessions. Keeping these in mind, large scale double blind randomized controlled studies should be planned to properly assess the efficacy and effectiveness of biofeedback methods. More systematized neurofeedback studies may, in future, help us localize regional neural activity and interconnectivity with specific behaviors.

CONCLUSION

Biofeedback methods have been evolving and advancing with time and have provided a good alternative to medications, especially in chronic, treatment-resistant cases and patients with intolerable side-effects to medications. Although the beneficial effects may take time to appear, they are long-lasting and without side effects. Neurofeedback, a welcome advancement in this field, has shown promising results, however, more standardized studies are warranted before it can be accepted as an accessible and valid therapeutic modality.

REFERENCES

1. Schoenberg PL, David AS. Biofeedback for psychiatric disorders: a systematic review. Appl Psychophysiol Biofeedback. 2014;39(2):109-35.
2. Blumenthal JA. Relaxation therapies and biofeedback: applications in medical practice. In: Jesse OC Jr. (Ed). Consultation Liasion Psychiatry and Behavioural Medicine. Philadelphia: WB Saunders; 1988. pp. 272-83.
3. Wiener N. Cybernetics or Control and Communication in the Animal and the Machine, 2nd edition. Cambridge: MIT Press; 1969.
4. Schwartz MS, Andrasik F (Eds). Biofeedback: A Practitioner's Guide, 4th edition. New York: Guildford Press; 2016.
5. Sulzer J, Haller S, Scharnowski F, et al. Real-time fMRI neurofeedback: progress and challenges. NeuroImage. 2013;76:386-99.
6. Loomis AL, Harvey EN, Hobart G. Electrical potentials of the human brain. J Exp Psychol. 1936;19(3):249.
7. Jasper H, Shagass C. Conditioning of the occipital alpha rhythm in man. J Exp Psychol. 1941;28(5):373.
8. Sterman M, Wyrwicka W, Roth S. Electrophysiological correlates and neural substrates of alimentary behavior in the CAT. Ann N Y Acad Sci. 1969;157(2):723-39.
9. Nowlis DP, Kamiya J. The control of electroencephalographic alpha rhythms through auditory feedback and the associated mental activity. Psychophysiology. 1970;6(4):476-84.
10. Beauregard M, Levesque J. Functional magnetic resonance imaging investigation of the effects of neurofeedback training on the neural bases of selective attention and response inhibition in children with attention deficit/ hyperactivity disorder. Appl Psychophysiol Biofeedback. 2006;31(1):3-20.
11. Lou HC, Henriksen L, Bruhn P. Focal cerebral hypoperfusion in children with dysphasia and/or attention deficit disorder. Arch Neurol. 1984;41(8):825-9.
12. Bledowski C, Linden DE, Wibral M. Combining electrophysiology and functional imaging–different methods for different questions. Trends Cogn Sci. 2007;11(12):500-2.
13. Scharnowski F, Veit R, Zopf R, et al. Manipulating motor performance and memory through real-time fMRI neurofeedback. Biol Psychol. 2015;108:85-97.
14. Watanabe T, Sasaki Y, Shibata K, et al. Advances in fMRI real-time neurofeedback. Trends Cogn Sci. 2017;21(12):997-1010.

15. Ruiz S, Buyukturkoglu K, Rana M, et al. Real-time fMRI brain computer interfaces: Self-regulation of single brain regions to networks. Biol Psychol. 2014;95(1):4-20.
16. Weiskopf N, Mathiak K, Bock SW, et al. Principles of a brain-computer interface (BCI) based on real-time functional magnetic resonance imaging (fMRI). IEEE Trans Biomed Eng. 2004;51(6):966-70.
17. Kober SE, Wood G, Kurzmann J, et al. Near-infrared spectroscopy based neurofeedback training increases specific motor imagery related cortical activation compared to sham feedback. Biol Psychol. 2014;95:21-30.
18. Matousek M, Rasmussen P, Gillberg C. EEG frequency analysis in children with so-called minimal brain dysfunction and related disorders. Adv Biol Psychiatry. 1984;15:102-8.
19. Gevensleben H, Holl B, Albrecht B, et al. Neurofeedback training in children with ADHD: 6-month follow-up of a randomised controlled trial. Eur Child Adolesc Psychiatry. 2010;19(9):715-24.
20. Hammond DC. Neurofeedback treatment of depression and anxiety. J Adult Dev. 2005;12(2-3):131-7.
21. Linden DE. Neurofeedback and networks of depression. Dialogues Clin Neurosci. 2014;16(1):103-12.
22. Wang T, Mantini D, Gillebert CR. The potential of real-time fMRI neurofeedback for stroke rehabilitation: a systematic review. Cortex. 2018;107:148-65.

CHAPTER 4

Current Status of Yoga and Other Spiritual Therapies in Psychiatry

Hemant Bhargav, Jitender Jakhar, Nishitha Jasti, Rashmi Arsappa, Shivarama Varambally, BN Gangadhar

INTRODUCTION

Yoga holds a place of pride among all the alternative system of therapies which are required to supplement the mainstream therapies. Yogic philosophy and practices extend across the physical, the psychic, and also the spiritual dimensions of man. Therefore, a brief discussion of other spiritual therapies along with role of yoga in therapy, is quite consistent with the theme of the book. Having originated in India, Yoga has now received acceptance from all parts of the world. The crowning glory has been the declaration of 21st June as "International Yoga Day" by the United Nations in 2014.

YOGA

Yoga, an ancient Indian system of holistic living, was originally designed for enhancing spiritual progress, but it is gaining popularity among the clinicians and researchers for its therapeutic applications now.[1] Currently available treatments for psychiatric disorders, drugs in particular, offer some benefits, but at the cost of unwanted side effects. In many situations, the drugs merely address symptoms because the cause of illness is unclear. It is due to this reason that surveys show substantial number of patients and families frequently seek traditional treatment approaches.[2] Studies have shown that yoga has the potential to influence several brain processes, from attention to plasticity, and hence it is a therapeutic intervention in the area of mental health that deserves further exploration.[3] Numerous studies have demonstrated the proficiency of yoga-based interventions in treating various psychiatric disorders over the past two decades.[4] Major psychiatric disorders where yoga-based lifestyle interventions have been found useful as an adjuvant are: (1) depression, (2) schizophrenia, (3) anxiety-related disorders, (4) cognitive disorders, (5) substance use disorders, and (6) somatoform disorders. More recent researches also point to significant neurobiological effects of yoga.[5,6]

OTHER SPIRITUAL THERAPIES

Sullivan defined spirituality as a distinct element that relates the self to others and the universe, and may or may not encompass belief in god.[7] Puchalski

(2012) construed spirituality as an approach to find purpose of the life while connecting self with the sacred.[8]

Literature survey shows that there are two main lines of approaches under spiritual therapies: (1) Religious and (2) spiritual. Spiritual approaches include themes such as virtuous values, prayers, resilience, transcendence, and meditation. Religious outlook explores the beliefs and explicit customs of religion such as Hinduism, Catholics, Jews, Muslims, etc. Regarding the role of spiritual therapies in mental health, there are mixed results. A few studies have exhibited a strong relationship between spirituality/religiosity and psychological well-being in terms of satisfaction, happiness, and moral values.[9,10] Similarly, another review article found a strong correlation of spirituality with purpose and meaning of life, social support, well-being, optimism, and hope.[11] However, there are also reports mentioning the adverse effects of religiosity. A significant association with thoughts of remorse, abandonment or penance translated into higher prevalence of depression, anxiety, and mortality in this population was observed.[11,12] Although there is substantial growth in this area, the approaches are quite varying and lack standardization.

ROLE OF YOGA IN MAJOR PSYCHIATRIC DISORDERS: CURRENT EVIDENCE

Yoga in Depression

A recent systematic review assessed efficacy of yoga in depression.[13] The review found a total of 23 trials between 2011 and May 2016. These trials used three kinds of study designs: randomized control trials (RCTs), pre-test/post-test and quasi-experimental, with most of them being RCTs. Techniques from different yoga schools were taken as interventions, with the most common being *Hatha Yoga*. The subjects recruited in these studies ranged from 14 to 136, suggesting a small sample size in majority of the studies. Also, the studies used interventions with varied duration, average duration of intervention being 9 weeks which indicates that only short-term effects of yoga were assessed. Despite the limitations, efficacy of yoga interventions in reducing depression is accepted to be remarkable.[13]

A recent RCT examined the potential of 8-week Hatha Yoga as monotherapy for mild-to-moderate major depression with blinding outcome assessors.[14] 38 adults with major depression of mild-to-moderate severity scoring 14–28 on Beck Depression Inventory-II (BDI-II) were randomized into Hatha Yoga and attention control groups. 20 subjects were recruited in the earlier and 18 subjects into the latter group, respectively. Both the interventions were for a duration of 90 minutes and continued for 8 weeks. A significantly greater reduction in BDI scores was observed in the yoga group than the controls after 8 weeks ($p = 0.034$). Subanalyses showed that subjects in the yoga group were much likely to attain remission among the subjects completing the 8-week intervention, i.e. BDI score ≤9. Further, the effect size was observed to be large in reducing BDI scores with yoga as intervention with Cohen's d = – 0.96.

Another recent study assessing the effect of 12-week yoga and meditation-based lifestyle intervention (YMLI) on depression severity and systemic neuroplasticity biomarkers in adults with major depressive disorder (MDD) receiving routine drug treatment. 58 patients with MDD were randomized and recruited into yoga or control group. BDI-II scale was applied to assess the severity of depression. A significant increase in BDNF and a significant decrease in BDI-II scores after YMLI was noted, compared to control group. Sirtuin 1, dehydroepiandrosterone sulfate (DHEAS), and telomerase activity levels also showed significant increase with YMLI. Further, decreased IL-6 and cortisol levels, in addition to decreasing DNA damage and balance in oxidative stress, were noted in this population. Multiple regression analyses suggest that yoga group displayed higher BDNF colinearly with less BDI-II scores in comparison to the controls. Decreased cortisol and rise in sirtuin 1 and telomerase activity significantly verify this association (all $p < 0.05$). Authors opined that the improvement in systemic neuroplasticity biomarkers significantly resulted in reduction in depression severity after YMLI and concluded that YMLI can be considered as a therapeutic intervention in management of MDD.[15]

Yoga in Psychosis

Psychosis, especially the chronic forms such as schizophrenia, is one among the severe mental disorders. Psychosis carries stigma and causes significant morbidity as well as disability. Treatment options for psychosis increased significantly in the last two decades but appear to have reached a deadlock in recent years. Effective medications are unavailable for negative and cognitive symptoms and they cause a variety of adverse effects, ranging from extrapyramidal side effects of the older antipsychotics to metabolic, cardiac, and hormonal effects of the second-generation drugs. Hence, complementary treatment options have emerged as a critical area of research, yoga being one of them.

Initial Randomized Controlled Studies in Inpatients of Schizophrenia

Duraiswamy et al.[16] investigated the effectiveness of yoga therapy (YT) in addition to the ongoing antipsychotic treatment in 61 moderately ill schizophrenia inpatients. Subjects were randomly assigned and recruited into YT ($n = 31$) and physical exercise therapy (PT; $n = 30$). The respective interventions were given for 4 months. A rater who was blind to the group status of the subjects had assessed them at the baseline and after 4 months of intervention. At the end of 4 months, subjects in the YT group displayed significantly less psychopathology than the PT group. They also showed significantly greater quality of life and socio-occupational functioning. The authors concluded that the reduction in symptoms was seen with both nonpharmacological interventions with YT having better efficacy.

Facial emotion recognition deficits (FERDs) have been persistently being observed in patients with schizophrenia, resulting in the impairment of their socio-occupational functioning. Therapeutic options to improve these deficits have not been explored well in antipsychotic-stabilized patients. A study aimed at evaluating the efficacy of yoga therapy on symptoms, functioning, and facial emotion recognition deficits in patients with schizophrenia.[17] The subjects were antipsychotic-stabilized patients, randomized into yoga ($n = 27$), exercise ($n = 17$) or waitlist group ($n = 22$). The raters who were blind to the group status had assessed the subjects at baseline, 2nd month, and 4th month of follow-up. Positive and Negative Syndrome Scale (PANSS), Socio-Occupational Functioning Scale (SOFS), and Tool for Recognition of Emotions in Neuropsychiatric Disorders (TRENDS) were used to assess the subjects at timepoints mentioned above. Yoga module used in this study was devoid of meditation and included practices like jogging, twisting, hand stretch breathing, forward–backward bending, tiger breathing, Trikonasana, Shashankasana breathing, Surya Namaskar, Vakrasana, Ushtrasana, Makarasana, Bhujangasana, Shalabhasana, Dhanurasana, Viparita Karani, Matsyasana, Bhastrika Pranayama, Nadi Shuddhi Pranayama, and Nadanusandhana. A significant positive correlation was noted between FERD and socio-occupational functioning ($r = 0.3$, $p = 0.01$) at the baseline. A significant improvement in positive and negative symptoms, socio-occupational functioning, and performance on TRENDS ($p < 0.05$) in the yoga group was observed and not in the other two groups. The maximum improvement was found at the end of 2 months. Of which, the improvement in negative and positive symptoms persisted even at the end of 4 months. Worsening of positive symptoms with yoga therapy was reported by none.

Barriers to yoga therapy: To evaluate the effectiveness of yoga as an adjunct therapeutic option for persons with schizophrenia, a single blind randomized controlled study at tertiary mental healthcare hospital was conducted in India. It was observed that many patients were not able to avail the yoga training, even though detailed and well-instructed yoga sessions were offered free of cost with provision of monetary assistance for travel. It is very important to understand the potential barriers to yoga therapy for patients with schizophrenia to improve its availability and acceptability in the patient population. Baspure et al. made an attempt in this direction in 2012.[18] They identified primary reasons for decline in the attendance of the schizophrenia patients in larger randomized controlled yoga study as: (1) radius from the center ($n = 83$; 37.2%); (2) unavailability of a person to escort and assist

(n = 25; 11.2%); (3) extra-occupied work schedule (n = 21, 9.4%); (4) reluctance to attend more than a month (n = 11; 4.9%), (5) resistance toward yoga therapy (n = 9, 4.0%); (6) personal reasons (n = 3, 1.3%); and (7) religious reasons (n = 1, 0.4%). No reasons were imputed by 70 patients (31.6%). None of the patients refused citing research characteristic of the intervention as a reason. Authors noted that majority of the patients suitable for practicing yoga did not consent to the study. The need for continual day-to-day training and practice under supervision for long periods of time in specialized centers is one of the most challenging barriers for the patients with schizophrenia to avail yoga therapeutic services. Furthermore, there is a need for exploring the alternative models/schedules that are patient-centered to deliver the proper efficacy of yoga to patients with schizophrenia.

As discussed above, practicing yoga in yoga center on a daily basis, though effective, was not observed to be feasible for most of the patients for various reasons. Hence, Govindaraj et al. (2015) determined the willingness of patients with schizophrenia to participate in yoga therapy programs on outpatient basis.[19] They observed that nearly 90% of the patients with schizophrenia reported that they can participate in add-on yoga therapy programs, when they were given the options of choosing outpatient-based yoga therapy sessions weekly, fortnightly or monthly as per their convenience. Logistic reasons such as long distance travel and financial problems which were found to be the main barriers for participating in daily yoga therapy programs according to a previous study in the same setting did not become significant factors in this study as patients were given convenient options such as weekly, fortnightly, and monthly sessions instead of a fixed daily basis regimen.

Randomized Controlled Study in Outpatients of Schizophrenia

Thus, considering the need for more pragmatic approach, another RCT was conducted to test the efficiency of yoga therapy as an additional therapy in outpatients with schizophrenia by Varambally et al. (2012).[20] This study was done at NIMHANS (Bengaluru) with involvement of active control and waitlist groups, using a single-blind randomized controlled design. The patients with schizophrenia were randomized into yoga, exercise, or waitlist group after obtaining their consent. Their pharmacological therapy was kept unchanged during the entire duration of the study. Supervised yoga or exercise sessions were imparted for 1 month for the respective groups. The rater, who was blind to the group allotment of the subjects, assessed the participants at the start of the intervention and at the end of 4 months. Significantly greater number of patients in the yoga group improved on PANSS negative and total PANSS scores along with social functioning scores as compared to the exercise and waitlist group. The likeliness of improvement in yoga group, especially the negative symptoms, appears to be five times greater than either of the groups from the odds ratio analysis. The authors concluded that a month's yoga training succeeded by 3 months home-practice of yoga in addition to their conventional treatment, displayed a significant advantage over the other two groups in patients with chronic schizophrenia with stabilized pharmacological therapy.

Yoga for Antipsychotic-induced Side Effects

The management of schizophrenia is majorly based on antipsychotic medications (APMs). First-generation or traditional antipsychotics have been very effective in the treatment of the positive symptoms of psychosis such as delusions and hallucinations. However, they commonly result in extrapyramidal side effects (EPS) such as dystonia, akathisia, and drug-induced parkinsonism at clinically effective dosages. This results in major distress, disabling a patient significantly to carry on his routine. The second-generation antipsychotics result in weight gain, dyslipidemia, and insulin resistance (metabolic syndrome), even though they cause less EPS. Thereby, anticholinergics (e.g. trihexyphenidyl) are commonly added to APMs to manage EPS. But again, these medications have their own side effects such as constipation, xerostomia, and indigestion. Evidence also suggests that memory impairment typically observed in patients with schizophrenia might be attributed to the usage of anticholinergic medications. Hence, considering the need for further exploration on the effective methods to manage and alleviate antipsychotic-induced side effects in patients with chronic psychoses, the efficacy of 5-month yoga therapy on antipsychotic-induced side effects was performed by Verma et al. (2017) on chronic schizophrenia patients residing in a Schizophrenia Rehabilitation center in Bengaluru.[21] The recruited subjects were 21 (12 females) in the ages 52.87 + 9.5 years and suffering from 24.0 ± 3.05 years. All subjects were receiving antipsychotic medications and had been stabilized for more than a month. Antipsychotic-induced side effects were assessed by Simpson Angus Scale (SAS) and Udvalg for Kliniske Undersogelser (UKU) side effect rating scale at three points of time: (1) baseline, (2) after 1 month of treatment as usual (pre), and (3) after 5 months of validated integrated yoga (IY) intervention (post). In addition, secondary variables such as cognitive functions (using Trail making Test A and B), clinical symptoms, and anthropometry were assessed. The intervention was the practice of a validated 1-hour yoga module (consisting of asanas, pranayama, relaxation techniques, and chanting) which was practiced for 5 months with the frequency of five sessions per week. A significant reduction in 38 items of UKU scale and drug-induced parkinsonian symptoms (SAS score; $p = 0.001$) was observed along with significant improvement in their executive functions, processing speed, and negative symptoms of schizophrenia patients after 5-month intervention. There was no report of any side effects of the intervention. The effectiveness of yoga intervention in managing antipsychotic-induced side effects was demonstrated and could be considered a preliminary evidence to explore much in this direction.

Yoga for Caregivers of Patients with Schizophrenia

Schizophrenia not only affects the patient, it also puts strain on financial and human resources, leading to social and psychological agony for their families also. It was observed that higher levels of stress and depression were found in the caregivers of the patients with any illness than the non-caregivers. The caregivers also reported lower levels of physical health, subjective well-being, and self-efficacy than non-caregivers. The caregivers of patients with schizophrenia reported greater burden than the caregivers of patients with any other chronic medical illness, both subjectively and objectively. This was particularly observed in the families with poor social support. This led to the systematic development and feasibility testing of yoga program to cater the needs of the caregiver of patients with schizophrenia by Jagannathan et al. (2012).[22] In 2013, this module was further investigated in a randomized controlled pilot trial by Varambally et al.[23] In this study, the caregivers of outpatients with functional psychosis who consented to participate in the study ($n = 29$) were recruited. They were randomized into yoga ($n = 15$) or waitlist group ($n = 14$) and the subjects in the yoga group were offered supervised yoga session with a frequency of thrice a week for 4 weeks. They were also instructed to practice the same practices at home for the next 2 months. The assessments were done at the baseline and after 3 months of the intervention. At the end of 3 months, yoga group showed a significant reduction in burden scores and improvement in the scores of quality of life as compared to the waitlist group.

Yoga for Inpatients Acutely Treated for Psychosis

All the abovementioned yoga studies were conducted in stabilized patients of schizophrenia. But it is observed that in acute functional psychotic state too, despite the extensive role played by first and second generation antipsychotics (FGA and SGA) in reducing symptoms and disability, a significant number of patients still remain quite symptomatic signaling the inputs of other therapeutics options. Thus, an attempt was made by Manjunath et al. (2013) using single blind randomized controlled design to test the efficacy of yoga therapy as an add-on to medication in inpatients with functional psychotic disorder.[24] The subjects receiving antipsychotic and antiparkinsonian drugs (as needed), who gave consent to participate ($n = 88$) in the study were equally randomized to yoga or exercise therapy sessions within 3-4 days of their admission. The recruited subjects were given respective interventions in their wards daily for a period of 2 weeks so that at least 10 sessions of intervention are delivered. Each session lasted for an hour. For the subsequent 4 weeks, the patients were advised to continue the same practices at home. Their caregivers who observed the sessions during their stay at the center were requested to monitor their performance at home. The management of drug doses was done by their psychiatrist, who was external to this trial. The two groups did not vary on clinical syndrome scores at the end of 2 weeks. However, subjects in the yoga group had lesser mean scores on Clinical Global Impression Severity (CGIS), PANSS, and Hamilton Depression Rating Scale (HDRS) at the end of 6 weeks ($p < 0.05$). Yoga intervention was detected to be advantageous over exercise in curtailing the clinical CGIS and HDRS scores on repeated measure analysis of variance. This led to a conclusion that yoga intervention as an add-on to conventional treatment is feasible and beneficial in the early and acute stage of psychosis also.

Yoga in Anxiety-related Disorders

The effect of Hatha Yoga on anxiety disorder was examined through a meta-analysis. A total of 501 participants from 17 studies (11 waitlist-controlled trials) were identified. The studies in which subjects received Hatha yoga and reported their anxiety levels before and after the intervention were included. The Hedges' g for pre-post within group and controlled effect sizes were, Hedges' $g = 0.44$ and Hedges' $g = 0.61$, respectively. The authors observed that efficacy of the intervention was positively associated with duration of the practice. Also, it was noted that subjects with elevated levels of anxiety benefitted the most, concluding Hatha yoga might be a promising method for alleviating anxiety.[25]

A recent systematic review and meta-analysis by Cramer et al. (2018)[26] examined the effectiveness and safety of yoga for anxiety.[26] They had searched the databases for yoga-related RCTs for individuals with anxiety disorders till October, 2016. Anxiety scores and remission rates were fixed as the primary outcomes. Quality of life, depression, and safety of the intervention were the secondary outcomes. Meta-analyses demonstrated large effects of yoga compared to active controls and small short-term effects of yoga on anxiety in comparison to no treatment. Effects were sturdy even on the grounds of no methodological bias. Intervention-related safety data was only reported in three RCTs. The reports have revealed that yoga was not associated with any increase in trauma and injuries, concluding that yoga might be a safe as well as an effective therapeutic option for individuals with elevated levels of anxiety, but evidence still stands inconclusive for those with DSM-based diagnosis of anxiety disorders.

Yoga for Cognitive Disorders

Many studies have exhibited the effectiveness of yoga on cognitive variables in healthy individuals, especially in the elderly,[27] and in subjects with primary psychiatric disorders such as depression[28] and psychosis.[29] Preliminary studies investigating the effect of a meditation program on patients suffering from mild cognitive impairment have also shown positive effects. Adults residing in community homes with a diagnosis of mild cognitive impairment (MCI) or early-stage Alzheimer's disease were enrolled in the pilot study along with their live-in caregivers. A short comprehensive yoga training was given after which, they were instructed to meditate for 11 minutes, twice a day for 8 weeks. This exploratory trial has indicated that the 8-week meditation program was acceptable and effective in improving mood, sleep quality, and memory along with reduction in perceived stress in subjects with cognitive impairment and their caregivers.[30] Thus, yoga therapy may be potentially useful in cognitive disorders and this area needs further exploration by clinical trials with systematic methodology.

Yoga in Substance Use Disorders

Substance use disorders (SUDs) are another area where preliminary studies point toward potential clinical utility of yoga therapy as an adjuvant to conventional line of treatment. Different types of yoga programs have been explored as an interventional strategy in patients with substance abuse. Shaffer et al. found that Hatha yoga therapy was comparable to conventional methadone treatment with traditional group psychotherapy in 61 randomly assigned IV drug users on various measures of sociological, psychological, and biological aspects.[31] Another study demonstrated that practice of Sudarshan Kriya (SK) and Pranayama (P) in cancer patients with nicotine addiction who had completed their conventional therapy, reduced tobacco habit in 21% of individuals after the 6 months follow-up of the practice.[32] Further, in a pilot study conducted in India, it was observed that a 90-day comprehensive yoga-based lifestyle residential program improved various psychological self-reported measures which include the Quality of Recovery Index and Behavior and Symptom Identification Scales.[33] Shahab et al. showed that a 10-minute yogic breathing exercises in abstaining smokers had an acute effect of reduction in craving compared to a control group who watched videos.[34] Similarly, another feasibility study tested the feasibility of a 10-week yoga program on 18 subjects with alcohol dependence and found the program to be feasible and well accepted adjunct for treatment of alcohol dependence and concluded that studies with larger sample size and longer duration are required in future.[35] The usefulness of yoga and mindfulness in substance use disorders has been elusively summarized in a recent narrative review suggesting the rise in the support toward inclusion of yoga and mindfulness as promising complementary interventions for managing and preventing addictive behaviors.[36]

Yoga for Somatoform Disorders

There is sufficient evidence for usefulness of yoga for short- and long-term reductions of pain.[37] A randomized controlled trial (RCT) on 150 female patients with menstrual disorders and somatoform symptoms tested efficacy of 6 months of yoga nidra practice in comparison to the control and observed significant improvement in several somatoform symptoms.[38] Another recent open label trial was conducted on 64 patients with diagnosis of somatoform pain disorder. The study used a generic yoga program and found significant reduction in pain scores and improvement in quality of life, anxiety, and sleep in the subjects toward the end of 12-week intervention period.[39] Though preliminary results are encouraging, systematic and long-term follow-up studies are needed to confirm the efficacy of yoga in somatoform pain disorders.

BIOLOGICAL MECHANISMS FOR ROLE OF YOGA IN PSYCHIATRY

Studies have started to explore the biological underpinnings for the effects of yoga in mental disorders and evidence generated so far reveals that yoga may act through multiple mechanisms. These mechanisms involve: (1) downregulation of hypothalamic-pituitary-adrenal (HPA) axis, thereby reducing cortisol levels,[40] (2) modulating the autonomic nervous system toward homeostasis,[41] (3) affecting brain hemodynamics,[42] (4) affecting neurotransmitter levels,[43,44] (5) enhancing brain volume[45] and the mediators of neuroplasticity,[46,47] (6) reducing the markers of inflammation and enhancing endorphins,[48] (7) affecting genetic and epigenetic expressions,[49] and (8) through improvement in cognition.[50]

In a study conducted by Jayaram et al., it was found that 4 weeks of yoga postures, breathing techniques, and meditation increased the socio-occupational functioning, plasma oxytocin levels, and facial emotion recognition in patients suffering from schizophrenia in the yoga group compared to the waitlist.[43] Streeter et al. in 2010 conducted an RCT to examine the impact of yoga intervention on gamma aminobutyric acid (GABA) levels. The two arms chosen were yoga and exercise in the form of walking. Three yoga sessions a week for 12 weeks have shown a positive correlation between improvements in scores of anxiety and mood, and acute rise in thalamic GABA levels in the yoga group compared to the controls.[44] Similarly, number of studies have demonstrated the biological basis for the action of yoga in health and disease.[51]

DIFFERENTIATING PSYCHOPATHOLOGY FROM STATES OF SPIRITUAL ADVANCEMENTS

It has been observed that numerous features of spiritually awakening experiences are analogous in terms of content and form with the symptoms of psychosis. These similarities suggest a confusing overlap between the spiritually advanced and schizophrenia patients which has been noticed in many documented case studies. Also, there are no apparent clinical practice guidelines to distinguish them. Bhargav et al. (2015) used the literature survey and qualitative case analysis to deduce clinically relevant features distinguishing spiritually advanced persons from patients with schizophrenia. A case report with four major complaints from a 34-year-old unmarried male, repetitive thoughts questioning his existence, lack of sense of self since childhood, inability to hold on to any occupation, and social withdrawal, was elaborated by the author. The above symptoms appear to be identical to that of spiritually advanced personalities described in the ancient texts. Therefore, an elusive qualitative case analysis was done discussing the descriptions from modern psychology and ancient texts. This has provided a clear diagnosis of schizophrenia rather than spiritual advancement for the above case. A conclusion was drawn that the sense of "self" was found disorganized in spiritually advanced people as well as patients suffering from psychopathology. Further, the authors have elaborated that the psychotic experiences arise from their personality derangement. On the other hand, spiritual experiences lead to gradual and orderly diminishment of the selfish ego, enabling the individual consciousness to unite with the universal consciousness.[52]

CONCLUSION

Yoga therapy has been found useful as adjunct in management of high burden psychiatric illnesses such as schizophrenia and depression. There is a preliminary evidence toward the effectiveness of add-on yoga therapy in treating cognitive disorders, anxiety disorders, somatoform pain disorders, and substance use disorders. Systematic trials with long-term follow-up are needed to further concretize the role of yoga and other spiritual therapies in clinical psychiatric settings.

ACKNOWLEDGMENTS

Authors acknowledge Central Council for Research in Yoga and Naturopathy (CCRYN), an autonomous body, Under Ministry of AYUSH, Government of India, New Delhi for funding a Collaborative Research Centre at the NIMHANS Integrated Centre for Yoga, Bengaluru.

REFERENCES

1. Rao NP, Varambally S, Gangadhar BN. Yoga school of thought and psychiatry: Therapeutic potential. Indian J Psychiatry. 2013;55(Suppl 2):S145.

2. Cabral P, Meyer HB, Ames D. Effectiveness of yoga therapy as a complementary treatment for major psychiatric disorders: a meta-analysis. Prim Care Companion CNS Disord. 2011;13(4).
3. Gothe NP, McAuley E. Yoga and cognition: a meta-analysis of chronic and acute effects. Psychosom Med. 2015;77(7):784-97.
4. Balasubramaniam M, Telles S, Doraiswamy PM. Yoga on our minds: a systematic review of yoga for neuropsychiatric disorders. Front Psychiatry. 2013;3:117.
5. Streeter CC, Jensen JE, Perlmutter RM, et al. Yoga Asana sessions increase brain GABA levels: a pilot study. J Altern Complement Med. 2007;13(4):419-26.
6. Kalyani BG, Venkatasubramanian G, Arasappa R, et al. Neurohemodynamic correlates of 'OM' chanting: a pilot functional magnetic resonance imaging study. Int J Yoga. 2011;4(1):3-6.
7. Sullivan WP. "It helps me to be a whole person": The role of spirituality among the mentally challenged. Psychiatr Rehabil J. 1993;16(3):125-34.
8. Puchalski CM. Spirituality in the cancer trajectory. Ann Oncol. 2012;23(suppl_3):49-55.
9. Bonelli R, Dew RE, Koenig HG, et al. Religious and spiritual factors in depression: review and integration of the research. Depress Res and Treat. 2012;2012:962860.
10. Moreira-Almeida A, Koenig HG, Lucchetti G. Clinical implications of spirituality to mental health: review of evidence and practical guidelines. Revista Brasileira de Psiquiatria. 2014;36(2):176-82.
11. Koenig HG. Religion, spirituality, and health: the research and clinical implications. ISRN Psychiatry. 2012;2012:278730.
12. Hackney CH, Sanders GS. Religiosity and mental health: a meta–analysis of recent studies. JSSR. 2003;42(1):43-55.
13. Bridges L, Sharma M. The efficacy of yoga as a form of treatment for depression. J Evid Based Complementary Altern Med. 2017;22(4):1017-28.
14. Prathikanti S, Rivera R, Cochran A, et al. Treating major depression with yoga: a prospective, randomized, controlled pilot trial. PloS one. 2017;12(3):e0173869.
15. Tolahunase MR, Sagar R, Faiq M, et al. Yoga- and meditation-based lifestyle intervention increases neuroplasticity and reduces severity of major depressive disorder: A randomized controlled trial. Restor Neurol Neurosci. 2018;36(3):423-42.
16. Duraiswamy G, Thirthalli J, Nagendra HR, et al. Yoga therapy as an add-on treatment in the management of patients with schizophrenia: a randomized controlled trial. Acta Psychiatr Scand. 2007;116(3):226-32.
17. Behere RV, Arasappa R, Jagannathan A, et al. Effect of yoga therapy on facial emotion recognition deficits, symptoms and functioning in patients with schizophrenia. Acta Psychiatr Scand. 2011;123(2):147-53.
18. Baspure S, Jagannathan A, Kumar S, et al. Barriers to yoga therapy as an add-on treatment for schizophrenia in India. Int J Yoga. 2012;5(1):70.
19. Govindaraj R, Varambally S, Gangadhar BN. Yoga for schizophrenia: Patients' perspective. Int J Yoga. 2015;8(2):139-41.
20. Varambally S, Gangadhar BN, Thirthalli J, et al. Therapeutic efficacy of add-on yogasana intervention in stabilized outpatient schizophrenia: Randomized controlled comparison with exercise and waitlist. Indian J Psychiatry. 2012;54(3):227-32.

21. Verma M, Bhargav H, Varambally S, et al. Effect of integrated yoga on antipsychotic induced side effects and cognitive functions in patients suffering from schizophrenia. J Complement Integr Med. 2018;16(1).
22. Jagannathan A, Hamza A, Thirthalli J, et al. Development and feasibility of need-based yoga program for family caregivers of in-patients with schizophrenia in India. Int J Yoga. 2012;5(1):42-7.
23. Varambally S, Vidyendaran S, Sajjanar M, et al. Yoga-based intervention for caregivers of outpatients with psychosis: a randomized controlled pilot study. Asian J Psychiatr. 2013;6(2):141-5.
24. Manjunath RB, Varambally S, Thirthalli J, et al. Efficacy of yoga as an add-on treatment for in-patients with functional psychotic disorder. Indian J Psychiatry. 2013;55(Suppl 3):S374-8.
25. Hofmann SG, Andreoli G, Carpenter JK, et al. Effect of Hatha yoga on anxiety: a meta-analysis. J Evid Based Med. 2016;9(3):116-24.
26. Cramer H, Lauche R, Anheyer D, et al. Yoga for anxiety: a systematic review and meta-analysis of randomized controlled trials. Depress Anxiety. 2018;35(9):830-43.
27. Hariprasad VR, Koparde V, Sivakumar PT, et al. Randomized clinical trial of yoga-based intervention in residents from elderly homes: Effects on cognitive function. Indian J Psychiatry. 2013;55(Suppl 3):S357-63
28. Sharma VK, Das S, Mondal S, et al. Effect of Sahaj Yoga on neuro-cognitive functions in patients suffering from major depression. Indian J Physiol Pharmacol. 2006;50(4):375-83.
29. Bhatia T, Agarwal A, Shah G, et al. Adjunctive cognitive remediation for schizophrenia using yoga: an open, non-randomised trial. Acta neuropsychiatrica. 2012;24(2):91-100.
30. Innes KE, Selfe TK, Brown CJ, et al. The effects of meditation on perceived stress and related indices of psychological status and sympathetic activation in persons with Alzheimer's disease and their caregivers: a pilot study. Evid Based Complement Alternat Med. 2012;2012:927509.
31. Shaffer HJ, LaSalvia TA, Stein J. Comparing Hatha yoga with dynamic group psychotherapy for enhancing methadone maintenance treatment: a randomized clinical trial. Altern Ther Health Med. 1997;3(4):57-67.
32. Kochupillai V, Kumar P, Singh D, et al. Effect of rhythmic breathing (Sudarshan Kriya and Pranayam) on immune functions and tobacco addiction. Ann N Y Acad Sci. 2005;1056(1):242-52.
33. Khalsa SB, Khalsa GS, Khalsa HK, et al. Evaluation of a residential Kundalini yoga lifestyle pilot program for addiction in India. J Ethn Subst Abuse. 2008;7(1):67-79.
34. Shahab L, Sarkar BK, West R. The acute effects of yogic breathing exercises on craving and withdrawal symptoms in abstaining smokers. Psychopharmacology. 2013;225(4):875-82.
35. Hallgren M, Romberg K, Bakshi AS, et al. Yoga as an adjunct treatment for alcohol dependence: a pilot study. Complement Ther Med. 2014;22(3):441-5.
36. Khanna S, Greeson JM. A narrative review of yoga and mindfulness as complementary therapies for addiction. Complement Ther Med. 2013;21(3):244-52.

37. Büssing A, Ostermann T, Lüdtke R, et al. Effects of yoga interventions on pain and pain associated disability: a meta-analysis. J Pain. 2012;13(1):1-9.
38. Rani K, Tiwari SC, Singh U, et al. Six-month trial of Yoga Nidra in menstrual disorder patients: effects on somatoform symptoms. Ind Psychiatry J. 2011;20(2):97-102
39. Sutar R, Desai G, Varambally S, et al. Yoga-based intervention in patients with somatoform disorders: an open label trial. Int Rev Psychiatry. 2016;28(3):309-15.
40. Thirthalli J, Naveen GH, Rao MG, et al. Cortisol and antidepressant effects of yoga. Indian J Psychiatry. 2013;55(Suppl 3):S405-8.
41. Jerath R, Edry JW, Barnes VA, et al. Physiology of long pranayamic breathing: neural respiratory elements may provide a mechanism that explains how slow deep breathing shifts the autonomic nervous system. Med Hypotheses. 2006;67(3):566-71.
42. Bhargav H, Raghuram N, HR N. Frontal hemodynamic responses to high frequency yoga breathing in schizophrenia: a functional near-infrared spectroscopy study. Front Psychiatry. 2014;5:29.
43. Jayaram N, Varambally S, Behere RV, et al. Effect of yoga therapy on plasma oxytocin and facial emotion recognition deficits in patients of schizophrenia. Indian J Psychiatry. 2013;55(Suppl 3):S409-13.
44. Streeter CC, Whitfield TH, Owen L, et al. Effects of yoga versus walking on mood, anxiety, and brain GABA levels: a randomized controlled MRS study. J Altern Complement Med. 2010;16(11):1145-52.
45. Lazar SW, Kerr CE, Wasserman RH, et al. Meditation experience is associated with increased cortical thickness. Neuroreport. 2005;16(17):1893-7.
46. Naveen GH, Varambally S, Thirthalli J, et al. Serum cortisol and BDNF in patients with major depression—effect of yoga. Int Rev Psychiatry. 2016;28(3):273-8.
47. Froeliger B, Garland EL, McClernon FJ. Yoga meditation practitioners exhibit greater gray matter volume and fewer reported cognitive failures: results of a preliminary voxel-based morphometric analysis. Evid Based Complement Alternat Med. 2012;2012:821307.
48. Yadav RK, Magan D, Mehta N, et al. Efficacy of a short-term yoga-based lifestyle intervention in reducing stress and inflammation: preliminary results. J Altern Complement Med. 2012;18(7):662-7.
49. Kumar SB, Yadav R, Yadav RK, et al. Telomerase activity and cellular aging might be positively modified by a yoga-based lifestyle intervention. J Altern Complement Med. 2015;21(6):370-2.
50. Zeidan F, Johnson SK, Diamond BJ, et al. Mindfulness meditation improves cognition: Evidence of brief mental training. Conscious Cogn. 2010;19(2):597-605.
51. Gard T, Noggle JJ, Park CL, et al. Potential self-regulatory mechanisms of yoga for psychological health. Front Hum Neurosci. 2014;8:770.
52. Bhargav H, Jagannathan A, Raghuram N, et al. Schizophrenia patient or spiritually advanced personality? A qualitative case analysis. J Relig Health. 2015;54(5):1901-18.

CHAPTER 5

The Interface of Psychopharmacology and Psychotherapy

Rakesh K Chadda, Rishi Gupta

INTRODUCTION

The medical model of mental illnesses assumes that the processes underlying the etiogenesis are of a biological nature, and thus attempts to alter these pathological processes using pharmacological and biological therapies to achieve a change in the disease processes.[1] On the other hand, the proponents of the psychological model of illnesses, as given by the school of thought supporting psychotherapy, suggest psychotherapeutic interventions based on a therapeutic bond formed between the patient and the therapist. It is now well known that mental disorders have a multifactorial etiology spanning across biological, familial, psychological, and sociocultural factors,[2] and hence their management needs to be targeting at these etiological factors, thus including a multidisciplinary management encompassing biological, psychological, and social interventions.

In many treatment settings, especially in the low- and middle-income (LAMI) countries, because of a lack of resources, trained professionals, time, and financial constraints, pharmacotherapy is used as the mainstay of treatment and psychotherapeutic interventions are not frequently opted as a treatment option. Additionally, in the complex family structures in collectivistic societies such as India, one needs to make suitable modifications while administering psychotherapies which are classically developed in the western world.[2] For many years, the pharmacological and psychotherapeutic interventions have been viewed in competition to each other, with advocates of each group claiming theirs to be superior to the other.[3] But lately, the advantage of collaboration over competition has been recognized and the importance of combining these two modes of treatment rather than choosing one over the other has been investigated with active interest by researchers worldwide.[4] With the advent of neurobiological research, the proponents of "biological" theories of mental illness advocated psychotropic drugs as the mainstay of treatment of mental illness based on the postulate that all mental illnesses are a culmination of aberrant levels and functioning of neurotransmitters in the neural circuits of the brain and can hence be treated by pharmacological agents designed to alter their physiology and chemistry. The biomedical research in this area has led to the development of many psychotropic drugs acting on various receptors and through varying mechanisms, but pharmacological management has yet not been able to cater to the entirety of managing mental illness. In addition, there have not been any remarkable developments in the last few decades in biological treatments with criticism of many psychotropic agents belonging to "me too" category, and also producing only a partial improvement, lacking especially in psychosocial dimensions. Visualizing mental illness from a biopsychosocial perspective, there are often a host of patient-specific psychological, cognitive, and social factors pertaining to the patient's macro- and microenvironments which also need to be taken care of. The role of psychotherapeutic interventions is increasingly being recognized in catering to these factors which are beyond the purview of pharmacological treatment alone. This chapter will look into the need and scope of integrating psychopharmacology and psychotherapy for the management of mental disorders and improving treatment outcomes.

WHY DO WE NEED AN INTEGRATED APPROACH?

Most psychiatric disorders are associated with abnormalities in the complex interplay of various neurotransmitters and neural circuitry. Despite burgeoning research, there is no unifying hypothesis that can explain the exact biological mechanisms underlying the psychopathology.

Many of the initial psychopharmacological agents such as chlorpromazine and imipramine were serendipitously recognized to have therapeutic effect in psychiatric illnesses such as psychosis and depression, respectively. But in the later period, in spite of proliferating research, the mechanism of action of the earlier as well as the newer and even the designer drugs is not yet fully understood.[5] In addition, many psychopharmacological agents are rather recognized as "dirty drugs" meaning that they bind to more than one molecular target or receptor in the body, and so tend to have a wide range of effects, some of which are not desirable.

There is a wide variation in response to pharmacological agents across patients with mental disorders of even similar nature. Patient with similar illness may respond differently to a drug belonging to the same class, and sometimes the same patient may show a different response to the same drug at different points of time in his/her illness. Although this variability is being addressed by different approaches including pharmacogenomics and stratified/personalized medicine, these sciences are still in their infancy and suffer from a lack of concrete biomarkers.

Psychopharmacological agents have also been demonstrated to have a high placebo effect.[6] In most of the major mental disorders such as schizophrenia and depression, only up to 30–40% of the patients have been found to respond satisfactorily to the medications, and about 20–30%

patients are unable to achieve remission and have treatment refractory symptoms.[7] Since most mental disorders tend to follow a chronic relapsing course requiring long-term treatment with drugs, side effects may accrue overtime leading to impairment of functioning, deterioration of quality of life, and poor adherence to treatment regimen, further increasing the risk of incomplete improvement, relapse, or recurrence.

To address these issues, an integrative approach is now being advised. For certain mental disorders such as depression and obsessive–compulsive disorder, a combination of psychopharmacological and psychotherapeutic interventions has been shown to have better treatment outcomes. Even in severe mental disorders such as schizophrenia, psychotherapeutic interventions such as psychoeducation, cognitive behavior therapy, and psychosocial rehabilitation are able to bring better improvement by ensuring treatment adherence, and also reduce the frequency of hospitalization, even though these therapies do not directly affect the course of the disease.[8]

NEED FOR RECOVERY-ORIENTED TREATMENT

In the last few decades, there has been a paradigm shift in the principle of treating mental illness from a unidimensional medical approach to a recovery-oriented practice.[9] Instead of focusing merely on rapid stabilization and symptom relief as a clinical outcome, recovery-oriented practice aims to enable the patients to gain a meaningful life, social inclusion, and community integration.[10] The aim of psychiatric treatment has broadened to include resolution of symptoms and a state of remission, reducing the probability of relapse/recurrence, ameliorating stress on the family, medication adherence, strengthening the psychosocial skills that were lost (or never learned) due to the psychopathology, teaching the patient and the family methods to cope with residual symptoms, and improving occupational, social and interpersonal functioning.[11] Thereupon, it becomes imperative to integrate psychotherapeutic interventions with psychopharmacological management in order to realize these goals of treatment and achieve a good functional outcome for the patient.

BIOLOGICAL UNDERPINNINGS OF PSYCHOTHERAPY

In the earlier period, psychopharmacology and psychotherapy were often viewed to belong to completely different theoretical paradigms without any connecting mechanism, with a view that psychotherapy is a treatment for "psychologically-based" disorders, while medication is for "biologically-based" disorders. However, advances in the psychobiological research and structural and functional neuroimaging have demonstrated evidence of the potential role of psychotherapy interventions in "rewiring" or altering functional connectivity of brain neural circuits. The techniques such as single-photon emission computed tomography (SPECT), positron emission tomography (PET), and functional magnetic resonance imaging (fMRI) have made it possible to study changes at the brain systems level (by measuring changes in the brain blood flow or metabolism), associated with various psychotherapy interventions, e.g. cognitive behavior therapy (CBT). Several published studies are consistent in demonstrating changes in brain activity following psychotherapy in patients with anxiety and depressive disorders when compared with healthy comparison subjects.[12] Two studies which compared interpersonal psychotherapy with paroxetine and venlafaxine, respectively in the treatment of depression found psychotherapy as effective in reversing the pretreatment abnormalities, similar to the effects of pharmacotherapy.[13,14] Amongst anxiety disorders, e.g. post-traumatic stress disorder (PTSD) and social anxiety disorder, fMRI studies have shown increased activity in the amygdala and insular regions.[15] In PTSD, hypoactivation has been observed in the anterior cingulate cortex and ventromedial prefrontal cortex which may be associated with aberrations in vigilance and emotional-contextual processing. CBT has been shown to reverse these changes in PTSD, leading to the view that CBT possibly reduces phobic avoidance mediated via neurobiological alterations.[16] These findings suggest that the theoretical schism between psychopharmacology and psychotherapy is gradually narrowing and the potential for both working synergistically even at a biological level is an area worth exploring and utilizing for developing effective treatment strategies.

In recent times, psychotherapy is being reconceptualized as a neurobiological probe capable of inducing epigenetic changes in brain circuits, and activating epigenetic mechanisms in brain circuits to reduce psychiatric symptoms by improving the efficiency of information processing in these circuits, similar to pharmacotherapy. Given the limits of psychotropic drugs alone, one of the most promising therapeutic advances will be to combine drugs with psychotherapy.

INTEGRATING PSYCHOPHARMACOLOGY AND PSYCHOTHERAPY

Integrating psychopharmacology and psychotherapy in a clinical setting would need some practical consideration like a multidisciplinary approach. One-person treatment model involves a psychiatrist who conducts the psychotherapy as well as prescribes medication for the same patient, which may not be feasible in contemporary clinical situation. Two-person treatment model involves a psychiatrist as a prescriber and another clinician as the psychotherapist.[1] In most clinical scenarios, two-person treatment model may be the standard. One-person treatment model demands that the psychiatrist approach the patient's illness from the perspective of brain dysfunction and the psychological distress of a human being. This dual role has been termed as "bimodal relatedness", based on the biopsychosocial model.[17] However, in recent periods, evidence-based psychotherapy methods have expanded to include a broad range of individual-based, group-based and family-based therapies with a variety of treatment goals. It is thus worthwhile to practice an integrated treatment approach and be familiar with the available therapeutic options, and develop a close collaboration with clinical psychologist in order to facilitate a multimodal and multidisciplinary therapeutic effort.

Clinical Considerations for Integration of Treatment

The process of integration needs to be patient-centric and should be decided on a case-to-case basis, i.e. before integration of psychotherapy with psychopharmacological treatment, it is of utmost importance to choose the psychotherapeutic intervention feasible and suitable to the mental disorder in question. Before adopting an integrated approach, it is important to be clear about the patient in whom it will yield positive results so that available treatment options are used judiciously with due regards to time- and resource-related issues. Not all the patients may require an integrative model of treatment. Mild depression has been shown to respond adequately to psychotherapy alone and additional pharmacotherapy may not provide any additional benefit.

It is also essential that the pharmacotherapy and psychotherapy interventions work synergistically. For example, it has been shown that the combination of CBT and antidepressant improves the outcome of panic disorder better than either modality alone but combining CBT with a benzodiazepine confers no advantage.[18] Similarly, benzodiazepines have been shown to interfere with effectiveness of exposure and response prevention in anxiety- and trauma-related disorders.[19]

Evidence Base for an Integrated Approach

An integrated approach of pharmacological and psychotherapeutic interventions can be followed in a range of mental disorders, principles of some of which are discussed as follows:

Schizophrenia

Schizophrenia is a severe mental disorder with often following chronic course, and is associated with substantial psychosocial impairment. Although, long-term maintenance on antipsychotic medications is considered to be one of the most important strategies in preventing rehospitalization in patients of schizophrenia,[20] psychotherapeutic interventions have been shown to improve functional outcome and recovery of patients. However, before integration, it is essential to choose the appropriate intervention for patients.

Certain psychotherapeutic interventions have been recommended to be avoided in schizophrenia. The Patient Outcomes Research Team (PORT) guidelines recommend that individual and group psychotherapies based on a psychodynamic model (defined as therapies that use interpretation of unconscious material and focus on transference and regression) should not be used in persons with schizophrenia since regression and psychotic transference may have harmful consequences in schizophrenia.[21] The PORT recommendations mention that "individual and group therapies employing well-specified combinations of support, education, and behavioral and cognitive skills training approaches designed to address the specific deficits of persons with schizophrenia can be utilized along with pharmacotherapy to improve functioning, and other targeted problems, such as medication adherence issues.[22]" A meta-analysis conducted in 1998 reported that psychosocial and psychotherapeutic treatments in patients with schizophrenia when combined with routine antipsychotic medication management produce better clinical outcome.[23] A randomized controlled trial (RCT) examining the efficacy of an integrated intervention model, Program for Relapse Prevention (PRP), which integrated pharmacological treatment with psychotherapeutic interventions such as psychoeducation and weekly group therapy for patients, and multifamily groups for schizophrenia patients, vis-à-vis pharmacological management found that the integrated treatment group had an early detection of relapse.[24] This has been further validated by subsequent studies which show that a combination of psychoeducational family therapy and antipsychotic medication produces dramatic improvements in the relapse rate compared to either modality alone.[25,26] CBT-based approaches delivered along with pharmacological management have also been shown to improve medication adherence in persons with schizophrenia.[27]

Depression

Integration of psychotherapeutic and pharmacological approaches in depression has been tested since early 1980s. In one of the earliest studies, Rounsaville et al. had reported that a combination of psychotherapy and pharmacotherapy gave better results in depression than the either treatment being used alone. The STAR*D (Sequenced Treatment Alternatives to Relieve Depression) trial suggests that psychotherapy used as augmentation of pharmacotherapy (psychotherapy added sequentially after incomplete antidepressant response) has a better impact on clinical symptoms of depression than medication alone.[28] Regarding data in adolescents, the Treatment for Adolescents with Depression Study (TADS) observed that response rates to a combination of CBT and fluoxetine were higher than with CBT or pharmacotherapy being used alone.[29] A 1997 "mega-analysis" by

Thase compared nonbipolar depressed patients treated with psychotherapy alone to those receiving combined treatment, and found that the advantage of the combination was particularly striking in patients with more severe and recurrent depression, though this difference was not observed in milder cases.[30] CBT and interpersonal therapy are the two most widely studied as psychotherapy intervention models integrated with pharmacological management in patients suffering from major depression.

The use of sequential integration of treatment has been found to be particularly effective in depression, where pharmacotherapy has been seen to provide initial rapid relief from acute distress, and psychotherapy has been demonstrated to help in bringing enduring changes in behavior and outlook thereafter, in combination with medications. In a preliminary meta-analysis of eight RCTs,[31] the sequential integration of psychotherapy and pharmacotherapy was found to be a viable strategy for preventing relapse and recurrence in major depressive disorder. A more recent meta-analysis of 13 RCTs examining the efficacy of the sequential integration of psychotherapy with pharmacotherapy after a positive response to acute-phase treatment with antidepressants in subjects with major depressive disorder has reported a significant reduction in risk of relapse with integrated treatment.[32]

Bipolar Disorder

Psychotherapeutic approaches which can be integrated with pharmacotherapy for bipolar disorder include psychoeducation, CBT, marital and family interventions, individual interpersonal therapy, and adjunctive therapies such as those for substance use.[33] A study examining integration of 6-week CBT with standard medication in patients of bipolar disorder reported a significantly enhanced compliance at 6-month follow-up evaluation in those who received a combined therapy.[34] Another study looking at the relative benefit of adding a structured psychoeducational intervention for married patients with bipolar disorder and their spouses to standard pharmacological treatment reported improved medication adherence, and significant incremental gains in overall patient functioning were noted with combined treatment.[35]

Interpersonal and Social Rhythm Therapy (IPSRT) is one of the most studied psychotherapeutic options for bipolar disorder, used in combination with medications. IPSRT addresses medication adherence, interpersonal stressors, and establishment of daily routines. The therapy aims at regulating circadian rhythms and improves regulation of sleep, energy, and mood, thereby having both therapeutic as well as prophylactic value.[36] A recent RCT testing the effectiveness of IPSRT combined with pharmacotherapy in patients with bipolar disorder II found a significant symptomatic improvement in the treatment group.[37]

Anxiety Disorders

Exposure-based techniques are some of the most commonly used behavior therapies used in treating anxiety disorders. Evidence supporting the integration of pharmacotherapy with psychotherapy is mixed for anxiety disorders, even though the practice is widespread. Foa et al. conducted an extensive review of the literature examining the combination of pharmacotherapy and CBT for all anxiety disorders and concluded that combination therapy for panic disorder seemed to provide an advantage over monotherapy but had a limitation of relapses after treatment ended. Combining medication and CBT is particularly helpful for patients with severe agoraphobia or for those who have an inadequate response to either treatment alone.[38] For obsessive compulsive disorder, the combination of exposure and response prevention with pharmacotherapy has been found to have better clinical outcomes than either treatment modality being used alone.[39]

Substance Use Disorders

Substance use disorders are also characterized by substantial psychosocial impairment and frequent relapses. While pharmacological management options are available for tobacco, alcohol, and opioid dependence, psychosocial management is an essential component of management plan. Psychosocial interventions help in overcoming issues such as poor motivation, noncompliance and expressed emotions in patients suffering from substance use disorders.[40] The COMBINE (combining pharmacotherapy and psychosocial interventions) study which evaluated the efficacy of specific pharmacotherapies, behavioral or psychosocial interventions, and their combinations for the treatment of alcohol dependence reported that the patient groups who demonstrated the best (statistical) drinking outcomes after 16 weeks of outpatient treatment had received naltrexone in combination with manual-guided counseling.[41]

CONCLUSION

The age-old stance of "psychopharmacology versus psychotherapy" is now giving way to the more modern "psychopharmacology with psychotherapy". Although significant advances have been made in this direction, true integration of the two is still in its infancy, with a lot remaining to be learnt regarding the best and most efficacious combinations, as well as the mechanisms underlying the combined efficacy of the two therapies. With a better understanding of the way in which these two therapies can be combined, psychiatrists will be able to benefit from the strengths of both, while at the same time ameliorating the shortcoming of each.

REFERENCES

1. Gabbard GO, Kay J. The fate of integrated treatment: whatever happened to the biopsychosocial psychiatrist? Am J Psychiatry. 2001;158(12):1956-63.
2. Chadda R, Deb K. Indian family systems, collectivistic society and psychotherapy. Indian J Psychiatry. 2013;55 (Suppl 2):S299-309.
3. Singh A, Singh S. Resolution of the polarisation of ideologies and approaches in psychiatry. Mens Sana Monogr. 2004;2(2):5-32.
4. Parikh SV, Hawke LD, Velyvis V, et al. Combined treatment: impact of optimal psychotherapy and medication in bipolar disorder. Bipolar Disord. 2015;17(1):86-96.
5. Hyman SE. Revitalizing psychiatric therapeutics. Neuropsychopharmacology. 2014;39(1):220-9.
6. Khan A, Brown WA. Antidepressants versus placebo in major depression: an overview. World Psychiatry. 2015;14(3):294-300.
7. Schwartz T. Psychopharmacology today: where are we and where do we go from here? Mens Sana Monogr. 2010;8(1):6-16.
8. Rector NA. Cognitive behavioural therapy reduces short term rehospitalisation compared with psychoeducation in inpatients with schizophrenia: commentary. Br Med J. 2005;8(1):8.
9. Waldemar AK, Arnfred SM, Petersen L, et al. Recovery-oriented practice in mental health inpatient settings: a literature review. Psychiatr Serv. 2016;67(6):596-602.
10. Farkas M. The vision of recovery today: what it is and what it means for services. World Psychiatry. 2007;6(2):68-74.
11. Glick ID. Adding psychotherapy to pharmacotherapy: data, benefits, and guidelines for integration. Am J Psychother. 2004;58(2):186-208.
12. Etkin A, Pittenger C, Polan HJ, et al. Toward a neurobiology of psychotherapy: basic science and clinical applications. J Neuropsychiatry Clin Neurosci. 2005;17(2):145-58.
13. Brody AL, Saxena S, Stoessel P, et al. Regional brain metabolic changes in patients with major depression treated with either paroxetine or interpersonal therapy: Preliminary findings. Arch Gen Psychiatry. 2001;58(7):631-40.
14. Martin SD, Martin E, Rai SS, et al. Brain blood flow changes in depressed patients treated with interpersonal psychotherapy or venlafaxine hydrochloride: Preliminary findings. Arch Gen Psychiatry. 2001;58(7):641-8.
15. Etkin A, Wager TD. Functional neuroimaging of anxiety: A meta-analysis of emotional processing in PTSD, social anxiety disorder, and specific phobia. Am J Psychiatry. 2007;164(10):1476-88.
16. Paquette V, Lévesque J, Mensour B, et al. "Change the mind and you change the brain": Effects of cognitive-behavioral therapy on the neural correlates of spider phobia. Neuroimage. 2003;18(2):401-9.
17. Docherty JP, Marder SR, Van Kammen DP, et al. Psychotherapy and pharmacotherapy: conceptual issues. Am J Psychiatry. 1977;134(5):529-33.
18. Mavissakalian M, Oldham J, Riba M, et al. Combined behavior and pharmacological treatment of anxiety disorders, volume 12. Washington, DC: American Psychiatric Press; 1993. pp. 565-84.

19. Singewald N, Schmuckermair C, Whittle N, et al. Pharmacology of cognitive enhancers for exposure-based therapy of fear, anxiety and trauma-related disorders. Pharmacol Ther. 2015;149:150-90.
20. Schooler NR, Keith SJ, Severe JB, et al. Relapse and rehospitalization during maintenance treatment of schizophrenia: the effects of dose reduction and family treatment. Arch Gen Psychiatry. 1997;54(5):453-63.
21. Lehman AF, Steinwachs DM. Translating research into practice: The Schizophrenia Patient Outcomes Research Team (PORT) treatment recommendations. Schizophr Bull. 1998;24(1):1 10.
22. Lehman AF, Kreyenbuhl J, Buchanan RW, et al. The Schizophrenia Patient Outcomes Research Team (PORT): updated treatment recommendations 2003. Schizophr Bull. 2004;30(2):193-217.
23. Mojtabai R, Nicholson RA, Carpenter BN. Role of psychosocial treatments in management of schizophrenia: a meta-analytic review of controlled outcome studies. Schizophr Bull. 1998;24(4):569-87.
24. Herz MI, Lamberti JS, Mintz J, et al. A program for relapse prevention in schizophrenia: a controlled study. Arch Gen Psychiatry. 2000;57(3):277-83.
25. Hogarty GE, Anderson CM, Reiss DJ, et al. Family psychoeducation, social skills training, and maintenance chemotherapy in the aftercare treatment of schizophrenia: II. Two-year effects of a controlled study on relapse and adjustment. Environmental-Personal Indicators in the Course of Schizophrenia (EPICS) Research Group. Arch Gen Psychiatry. 1991;48(4):340-7.
26. Zhang M, Wang M, Li J, et al. Randomised-control trial of family intervention for 78 first- episode male schizophrenic patients. An 18-month study in Suzhou, Jiangsu. Br J Psychiatry. 1994;(24):96-102.
27. Lecompte D, Pelc I. A cognitive-behavioral program to improve compliance with medication in patients with schizophrenia. Int J Ment Health. 1996;25(1):51-6.
28. Thase ME, Friedman ES, Biggs MM, et al. Cognitive therapy versus medication in augmentation and switch strategies as second-step treatments: A STAR*D report. Am J Psychiatry. 2007;164(5):739-52.
29. Emslie G, Kratochvil C, Vitiello B, et al. Treatment for adolescents with Depression Study (TADS): safety results. J Am Acad Child Adolesc Psychiatry. 2006;45(12):1440-55.
30. Thase ME. Treatment of major depression with psychotherapy or psychotherapy-pharmacotherapy combinations. Arch Gen Psychiatry. 1997;54(11):1009-15.
31. Guidi J, Fava GA, Fava M, et al. Efficacy of the sequential integration of psychotherapy and pharmacotherapy in major depressive disorder: a preliminary meta-analysis. Psychol Med. 2011;41(2):321-31.
32. Guidi J, Tomba E, Fava GA. The sequential integration of pharmacotherapy and psychotherapy in the treatment of major depressive disorder: a meta-analysis of the sequential model and a critical review of the literature. Am J Psychiatry. 2016;173(2):128-37.
33. Rothbaum BO, Astin MC. Integration of pharmacotherapy and psychotherapy for bipolar disorder. J Clin Psychiatry. 1997;58:68-75.
34. Cochran SD. Preventing medical noncompliance in the outpatient treatment of bipolar affective disorders. J Consult Clin Psychol. 1984;52(5):873-8.

35. Clarkin JF, Carpenter D, Hull J, et al. Effects of psychoeducational intervention for married patients with bipolar disorder and their spouses. Psychiatr Serv. 1998;49(4):531-3.
36. Frank E, Swartz HA, Boland E. Interpersonal and social rhythm therapy: an intervention addressing rhythm dysregulation in bipolar disorder. Dialogues Clin Neurosci. 2007;9(3):325-32.
37. Swartz HA, Rucci P, Thase ME, et al. Psychotherapy alone and combined with medication as treatments for bipolar II depression: a randomized controlled trial. J Clin Psychiatry. 2018;79(2):7-15.
38. Kaczkurkin AN, Foa EB. Cognitive-behavioral therapy for anxiety disorders: An update on the empirical evidence. Dialogues Clin Neurosci. 2015;17(3):337-46.
39. Rosa-Alcázar AI, Sánchez-Meca J, Gómez-Conesa A, et al. Psychological treatment of obsessive-compulsive disorder: a meta-analysis. Clin Psychol Rev. 2008;28(8):1310-25.
40. Chadda R, Chatterjee B. Need for psychosocial interventions: From resistance to therapeutic alliance. Indian J Psychiatry. 2018;60 (Suppl 4):S440-3.
41. Pettinati HM, Anton RF, Willenbring ML. The COMBINE Study: an overview of the largest pharmacotherapy study to date for treating alcohol dependence. Psychiatry (Edgmont). 2006;3(10):36-9.

CHAPTER 6

Update on Drug-assisted Psychotherapies

Pankaj Kumar, Rajeev Ranjan, Meha Jain

INTRODUCTION

Pharmacology and psychotherapy are majorly the two forms of treatment, which help in the reduction of symptoms of psychiatric illnesses. They have been used individually as well as in combination. The combination therapies have been found to be more effective in reducing symptoms and increasing quality of life of patients suffering from psychiatric illnesses. The drugs, since ancient times, have also been used to enhance psychotherapeutic healing. These drugs help in various ways such as diagnosing the problem, enhancing the therapeutic alliance, facilitating the production of memories, fantasies, and insights. This form of therapy is known as drug-assisted psychotherapy wherein clients undergo short, time-limited psychotherapy including some sessions enhanced by the acute action of a drug that has specific properties conducive to improving the efficacy of the psychotherapy. The drugs used for drug-assisted psychotherapy are mainly barbiturates, benzodiazepine, and psychedelics or hallucinogenic substances.

The drug-assisted therapy consists of 1–2 drug sessions while other drug-free sessions. These drug-free sessions are done before and after the drug sessions. The drug sessions are generally long for around 6–8 hours. The sessions are nondirective and patient driven. The client is allowed to talk freely during the drug sessions. It is important for the therapist to have the various counseling skills like reflection, active listening, and empathy to enhance the abreaction process. The therapist also gives suggestions like those given during the hypnotic process. Suggestions for problem solving, suggestions against alcohol use and remembering pleasant experiences are given. The process of drug-assisted psychotherapy is elucidated in **Figure 1**.

HISTORICAL PERSPECTIVE

Since ancient times, substances derived from plants like mushrooms, herbs such as nutmeg, anticholinergic plant derivatives, cannabis, and numerous other substances have been shown to have psychedelic effects **(Box 1)**. These substances have been used during the ancient times for healing, ceremonial, and recreational purposes.[1] The shamanic rituals performed in various cultures during those times used hallucinogenic plants for purposes of healing

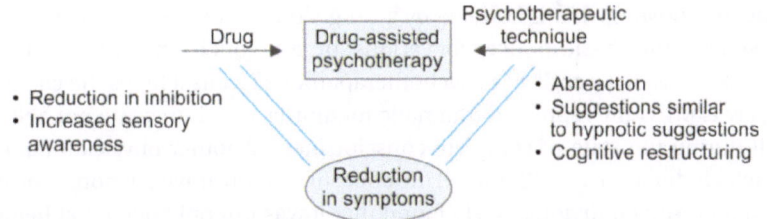

Fig. 1: The process of drug-assisted psychotherapy.

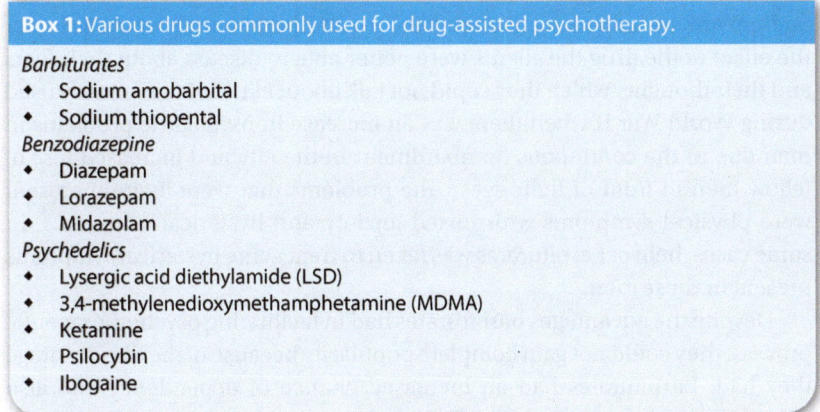

Box 1: Various drugs commonly used for drug-assisted psychotherapy.

Barbiturates
- Sodium amobarbital
- Sodium thiopental

Benzodiazepine
- Diazepam
- Lorazepam
- Midazolam

Psychedelics
- Lysergic acid diethylamide (LSD)
- 3,4-methylenedioxymethamphetamine (MDMA)
- Ketamine
- Psilocybin
- Ibogaine

and divination. These rites are performed by a shaman or a professional healer. Till date, many cultures still use such plants for therapeutic purposes such as Amazon basin in southwestern Mexico (where psychedelic mushrooms are used in healing rites) and peyote cactus is used in the Native American church services of Indians in the western United States.

Barbiturates were first synthesized by German Chemist Adolf von Baeyer in 1864.[2] They produce a variety of effects, from mild sedation to death, as these act as a central nervous system depressant. They have been widely used during and after World War II for "cathartic abreaction".[3] The administration of a barbiturate had disinhibiting effects on the client, which facilitated the process of catharsis or free expression of previously repressed traumatic memories. Some of the barbiturates used commonly for drug-assisted therapy during those times were phenobarbital, sodium amobarbital, sodium secobarbital, sodium pentobarbital, and sodium thiopental.

The first person to use intravenous barbiturates with clinical population was a physician named William Bleckwenn in 1930s. He used sodium amobarbital or sodium amytal for the treatment of neuropsychiatric disorders. This drug was first synthesized by the Lilly Company around 1927. He used this drug for "narco therapy" wherein the client is in a state of deep sleep or unconsciousness that is induced by a drug.[4] This condition is similar to that of general anesthesia induced for various surgeries but it is not that profound. This process of narcosis has psychotherapeutic effect as it helps the client to freely express the repressed traumatic memories which they are not able to tell during the state of complete consciousness. Another physician named Erich Lindemann in 1932 studied the effect of sodium amytal in both "normal and abnormal individuals".[5] He found that it was not only sleep that helped in improving the symptoms of psychiatric patients but it was also "a desire to communicate, a willingness to speak about very personal problems, an anticipation of future pleasant activities, and a feeling of relief and freedom".[5] Sodium amytal helped in enhancing the psychotherapeutic process as under the effect of the drug the clients were better able to discuss about their fears and their thoughts which they could not talk about earlier. It was mostly used during World War II when there was an increase in psychiatric problems in men due to the continuous bombardment in the city and increased loss of fellow men in front of their eyes.[6] The problems that were majorly present were physical symptoms with mixed anxiety and hysterical symptoms. In some cases, help of barbiturates was taken to treat acute hysterical symptoms present in these men.

Despite the advantages barbiturates had in facilitating psychotherapeutic process, they could not gain complete popularity because of the disadvantage they had. Barbiturates had an increased chance of dependency and also risk of death due to overdose.[7] Due to these shortcomings in the form of barbiturate dependence and significant death reports due to overdose, the USA and UK law restricted the use of barbiturates in 1960s.

Another set of drugs namely *benzodiazepines* appeared during the 1960s that overcame the shortcomings of the barbiturates. It was found to be a safe mode of treatment as compared to the barbiturates. Some of the benzodiazepines used are diazepam,[8] lorazepam,[9,10] and midazolam.[11] These benzodiazepines have been found to have similar therapeutic effects as barbiturates. They have been used for both diagnostic and therapeutic purposes. Very few articles are available on the benzodiazepine-assisted psychotherapy. This set of drug has mainly been used for the treatment of dissociative/conversion disorder, till date. It has been found to be effective in freely expressing the repressed memories of a traumatic event which may be too painful and anxiety provoking like sexual assault.

The term *psychedelic* was coined by Humphrey Osmond in 1957. It has been defined as the drugs that have "the capacity reliably to induce states of altered perception, thought, and feeling that are not experienced otherwise except in dreams or at times of religious exaltation".[12] These altered states are significantly different from a psychotic episode. For therapeutic purposes, they have been used in two ways. One method known as the psychedelic psychotherapy is where psychedelics are used in high doses for few sessions which create peak experiences thus enhancing the free expression process of psychotherapy.[13] Another method is the psycholytic method where they are used in smaller doses on a weekly or monthly basis, interspersed with talking therapy.[14] The various psychedelic drugs used are lysergic acid diethylamide (LSD), 3,4-methylenedioxymethamphetamine (MDMA), ketamine, psilocybin, and N,N-dimethyltryptamine (DMT).

Lysergic acid diethylamide is a semisynthetic compound, which was first synthesized by Swiss chemist, Albert Hofmann in 1938. The psychoactive effects of LSD were discovered in 1943.[15] Intake of LSD causes various changes in the thoughts, perception, memory, and mood of an individual. It has been used for treating various psychiatric disorders. By the 1960s, the misuse of LSD had started. The recreational and spiritual use of the drug had begun by then. Some of the famous clinicians to have misused LSD were Timothy Leary and Richard Alpert of Harvard University who had to be finally expelled from university for the same reason.[16] All of this created a lot of controversy for the use of LSD for purposes of psychotherapy. It eventually led United States to declare it illegal in 1966.[17] The Swiss Federal Office for Public Health in 1988 gave permission research for LSD assisted psychotherapy.

Another psychedelic that is being widely used is *MDMA*, which was first synthesized in 1914. It overcomes the shortcomings of LSD like presence of significant changes in perception and mood. It has been found to be a mild short-acting drug that helps in facilitating the psychotherapeutic process and temporarily reducing anxiety and depression. There has been a controversy about its use in clinical practice, as the Drug Enforcement Administration (DEA) has classified it as Schedule I in 1985. Various researches have been restarted in the last decade, which are proving its efficacy in facilitating the psychotherapeutic process.[18] It has been found to produce changes in mood, increases arousal and empathy. This increase in mood and empathy is a result of increase in serotonin and norepinephrine and dopamine which is induced by the intake of MDMA.[19] These changes help the patient to freely express the traumatic experiences without getting emotionally affected. Due to these effects of MDMA-assisted psychotherapy, it has been used for post-traumatic stress disorder (PTSD).

Along with increase in oxytocin, an elevated level of serotonin [5-hydroxytryptamine (5-HT)] has been reported post administration of MDMA. Serotonin is a major contributor to feelings like well-being and happiness, an increase in serotonin level diminishes negative response by increasing self-confidence along with reducing the stress and anxiety level which further helps in visiting past traumatic experience with a new perspective. The use of MDMA is debatable as there are various side effects

Psilocybin has been used since ancient times for healing purposes and in various religious rituals. It is available in the form of mushrooms which is known as teonanacatl meaning "god's flesh".[20,21] Its pictures have been found in various rock art in the Kimberly region of Australia and in the Kolo region of Eastern Tanzania indicating that psilocybin has been used for various shamanic rituals of those times.[22] Psilocybin-assisted psychotherapy has been used similar to that of other psychedelics. It has been used in treating various disorders.

PSYCHEDELIC-ASSISTED PSYCHOTHERAPY: A NEW APPROACH IN DRUG-ASSISTED PSYCHOTHERAPY

Psychedelics (potent psychoactive substance) are used in high doses for few sessions which create peak experiences thus enhancing the free expression used for therapeutic purpose. It is generally accompanied by before and after drug-free session which is called preparatory and integrative psychotherapy, respectively. Positive results are generally obtained with psychoactive substances and number of sessions generally varies as for example with ketamine 1–12 sessions are required, like that with MDMA three sessions, psilocybin and LSD two sessions, and with ibogaine only one effective session is enough.[23]

Key Steps of Different Psychedelic Psychotherapy

As initial steps, patients mostly listen to thought-provoking soothing music and subsequently they are encouraged to broader feeling and they are directed to memorize any soothing past event. They are generally told to engage in psychotherapy when they are feeling fresh and stress free.[24] Psychotherapeutic intervention varies in nature and frequency depending upon psychoactive substances. Sometimes they are engaged in only music like with ketamine and in others like MDMA, they generally go through multiple drug free sessions (different psychotherapy interventions are tried like transpersonal psychotherapy and cognitive behavior therapy). Between these two extreme points, limited numbers of sessions are tried with other psychoactive substance like psilocybin, LSD or ibogaine. Different strategies and methodologies have been tried with these psychoactive substances (both standardized psychotherapy and nonstandardized psychotherapy).

With different types and frequency of psychotherapy, interventions showed variable results with same psychotropic like ketamine studies with existential oriented psychotherapy for drug abuse[25] and cognitive behavioral therapy for depression (showed positive results).[26] In a nutshell, we can see psychedelic-assisted psychotherapy (PAP) can have more patient-oriented outcomes than existing therapy even for treatment-resistant patients. Outcomes of these studies are encouraging but still in preclinical trial.

Mechanism

Psychedelic-assisted psychotherapy is a specific drug-assisted intervention in which it induces trans-like state compared to direct action of psychoactive substance. When patient is properly intervened, it will induce meaningful experience to patient that will bring emotional, cognitive, and behavioral modification and hence they improve clinically. In treatment effect algorithm, PAP effect is more toward experience-based efficacy.

Diagnostic Value

Besides the therapeutic indications, PAP can also be used for diagnostic purpose, as PAP supports multidimensional diagnostic category. It is evident with following examples as ketamine and psilocybin with different pharmacological action can have same therapeutic effect in a single diagnosis like depression. On the other hand, single psychoactive substances like psilocybin have been used to treat two different conditions such as depression and drug abuse. Therefore it treats disorders with different diagnosis.

Further research in this category supports biopsychosocial approach[27] which actually is based on concept of set (personal experiences like belief, attitude, preferences, choices, motivation that represent psychological factors) and setting (generally defined as contextual/social/environmental factors).

Research Purpose

Psychedelic-assisted psychotherapy can be used for research purpose as it has a benefit that it can give desired result in short span of time in a particular research design. It also improves reliability of neuroimaging data which generally transfer into clinical application.

Explanatory

Psychedelic-assisted psychotherapy can be used as explanation of mental disorder and their treatment accordingly; for example, cathartic experience can be either positive or negative. PAP can have positive outcome for psychiatric illness if the theme which has come out from catharsis is tackled with proper protocol. Theme can be negative childhood experiences (neglect, abuse, deprivation and other adverse events of childhood) or stress at workplace, midlife crisis, and loneliness in elderly population.[28]

CLINICAL APPLICATIONS OF DRUG-ASSISTED INTERVIEWING (SEE TABLE 1)

Therapeutics

Barbiturates (Amobarbital)

Barbiturates are effective treatments for PTSD (traumatic neurosis), psychogenic paralysis, alcohol use disorder as an aversion therapy, somatoform disorder, anxiety neurosis, borderline personality disorder,

Table 1: Clinical application of psychotropics used in drug-assisted psychotherapy.		
Drugs	Diagnostics	Therapeutics
Barbiturates (Amobarbital)	• Catatonia (Organic vs. functional) • Confusion (Organic delirium vs. depressive pseudodementia) • Alcohol withdrawal vs. malingering • Conversion disorder • Dissociative disorder • Factitious disorder • Psychosis • Psychogenic amnesia	• Post-traumatic stress disorder (PTSD) • Psychogenic paralysis • Alcohol use disorder • Somatoform disorder • Anxiety neurosis • Borderline personality disorder • Conversion disorder • Catatonia
Benzodiazepine		• Dissociative amnesia • Dissociative fugue • Dissociative identity disorder
Psychedelics		
Ketamine		• Depression • Obsessive compulsive disorder (OCD) • PTSD • Suicide • Alcohol and cocaine use disorder
MDMA		• PTSD • Social anxiety in autistic adult • Anxiety in terminally ill patient/existential anxiety • Alcohol use disorder
Psilocybin		• Depression • Existential anxiety • Alcohol dependence • Cocaine and nicotine use disorder
LSD		• Existential anxiety

(MDMA: 3,4-methylenedioxymethamphetamine; LSD: lysergic acid diethylamide)

conversion disorder (as a narcosuggestion), and catatonia (Improvement in verbalization and alertness).

Benzodiazepines

Benzodiazepines are used for number of psychiatric disorders for therapeutic purpose in drug-assisted therapy. Major research evidence for dissociative amnesia (improved with lorazepam/diazepam-assisted interview), dissociative fugue (improved with lorazepam-assisted interview), and dissociative identity disorder (improved with lorazepam-assisted interview) in reported cases.

Psychedelics (Registered Phase 2 Clinical Trials using Psychedelics with Effect Size)

These substances are orally active but have different mechanisms of action. LSD and psilocybin effects depend on 5-HT2A agonism, MDMA inhibits monoamine transporters especially for serotonin, while ketamine is an NMDA (N-methyl-D-aspartate) antagonist and ibogaine nonspecifically binds to many receptors. Some reported therapeutic evidence for following four psychoactive substances, which are still in clinical trial phase:

1. *Ketamine* [Route of administration (oral, intranasal, IV); dose range (0.5–1.0 mg/kg oral, 0.2–0.5 mg/kg intranasal, 0.1–1.0 mg/kg IV); number of drug sessions (1–12)]: Effective in depression (effect size = 0.99–1.67), OCD (0.8), PTSD, suicide (0.67-0.84), and alcohol and cocaine use disorder.
2. *MDMA* [Route of administration (oral); dose range (62.5–187.5 mg); number of drug sessions (2–3)]: Effective in PTSD (1.17–1.24), social anxiety in autistic adult, anxiety in terminally ill patient or existential anxiety, and alcohol use.
3. *Psilocybin* [Route of administration (oral); dose range (10–40 mg); number of drug sessions (1–3)]: Effective in depression (2.0–3.1), existential anxiety (0.82–1.63), alcohol dependence (1.19–1.39), and cocaine and nicotine use disorder.
4. *LSD* [Route of administration (oral); dose range (200 μm); number of drug sessions (2)]: Evidence for existential anxiety (1.1–1.2) in terminally ill patients.

Diagnostic

Barbiturate (Amobarbital) Interviews

It is used in diagnostic interview for some psychiatric illness to differentiate from organic etiology, while in others, it serve as both diagnostic and therapeutic. For example, in catatonia, organic mutism has not improved while functional mutism has been found to improve. Organic delirium has not improved while depressive pseudodementia has improved with amobarbital interview. Alcohol withdrawal has also improved while malingering did not improve. Improvement has also been found in patients with conversion disorder, dissociative disorder, factitious disorder, psychosis, and psychogenic amnesia.

RESEARCH EVIDENCE FOR DRUG-ASSISTED PSYCHOTHERAPY

The drug-assisted psychotherapy has been used almost 90 years. However, the research evidence for drug-assisted psychotherapy has been predominantly in the form of case reports and case series. The controlled studies have been very few and have been conducted across heterogeneous clinical conditions. The published literature has been predominantly on the diagnostic and therapeutic uses of barbiturates.

The anecdotal reports suggest efficiency of amobarbital interviewing for variety of therapeutic applications. The commonly reported conditions are catatonia, conversion disorder, dissociation, factitious disorder, traumatic neurosis, somatoform disorder, etc.

Kraines (1967)[29] in his case series report had claimed success in treating over 1,000 patients with "depressive" or "neurotic reactions" with hypnotic suggestions under amobarbital narcosis. Solomon et al., 1971[30] in a report on case series of three patients with traumatic neurosis published that amobarbital facilitated therapeutic working through traumatic memories.

Hurwitz (1988)[31] in his report of five patients with conversion disorder who were given treatment of "narcosuggestion" (serial interview with intravenous amobarbital and methylphenidate) recommended that narcosuggestion was effective treatment for conversion disorder patients. Smith and colleague (1971)[32] in their case series of patients with alcoholism suggested that serial pentothal interviews in conjunction with aversion treatment are useful.

The controlled experiments regarding therapeutic benefits of amobarbital interviewing were published in the period from 1966 to 1977.

Hain and colleagues (1966)[33] published the triple blind controlled study on 49 patients diagnosed as psychoneurotic with different agents and saline as controlled. They reported no significant difference among agents in promoting emotional expression or recall during the drug-assisted interviewing. Amobarbital interviewing was associated with less emotional change than placebo, both during and after the interview.

In a follow-up study on re-analyzing the data to see relationship, between abreaction and subsequent clinical outcome, they reported that "abreaction" during interview did not correlate with symptom change. They negated the long held belief that abreaction is necessary for symptom change. In 1970, Smith and coworker demonstrated, from the same study, that there is powerful influence of the interviewer on many measures of interview outcome and quality.

Buckman et al. (1973)[34] published a double blind placebo controlled trial of different agents for drug-assisted interviewing with saline as control arm on 40 patients of "Psychoneurosis". No significant association was found between emotional expression and therapeutic benefits. They did find a significant correlation between de-suppression (talking about matters not usually discussed) and clinical improvement 24–48 hours after the interview but there was no significant difference among the drugs and placebo (saline) in such disclosure.

McCall and colleagues (1992)[35] in a double blind placebo controlled study on 20 patients with catatonia reported that amobarbital was significantly better than placebo (saline) in promoting verbal expression. In a follow-up study by retrospective chart review of same patients (1992), it was reported that response to amobarbital interview in catatonia patients had no predictive value for clinical course/prognosis. It was in contest to earlier reports, that response to amobarbital interview does predict the likelihood of response to ECT, antipsychotics or of spontaneous resolution of symptoms.

H Kaviranjan (1999),[36] in a survey of psychiatry literature regarding amobarbital interviewing (1966-97) revealed that there is only limited research evidence in support of diagnostic and therapeutic application of amobarbital interviewing in a variety of clinical situation. Most of the research evidence support is derived from case report and case series. The controlled studies failed to demonstrate superiority of amobarbital interview in variety of therapeutic and diagnostic uses. The only exception was catatonia where it was demonstrated to have significant superiority over placebo. Norma A Poole et al. (2010)[37] published a systematic review with meta-analysis on abreaction for conversion disorder in 2010. The review was conducted on all available research published in English on use of drug interviews for treating conversion/dissociative disorder. The most of the papers were case reports and case series. As reported in the paper, "the evidence suggests that drug interviews can be a useful treatment for individuals with both acute and treatment resistant conversion disorder although it is as yet unclear if the response is maintained in the long term". However, the study reported limitation of publication bias, quality of information, small study population, and generalizability of the findings.

The reported research papers regarding the therapeutic benefit of drug-assisted psychotherapeutics and benzodiazepines are only in the form of isolated case reports and case series. No systematic review in controlled design published study could be found during the literature survey in this area.

A novel approach in psychotherapy is "PAP" which implies professionally supervised use of ketamine, MDMA, LSD, psilocybin as part of elaborated psychotherapy programs. The most published article is for ketamine. The experimental intervention in almost 70 phase 2 trials for psychiatric disorder and two phase 3 trials for depression have shown safety and efficacy of ketamine. Most research published is for depression and also for OCD, PTSD, suicide, and alcohol and cocaine use disorders.

3,4-methylenedioxymethamphetamine is investigated in 17 phase 2 trials and was designated a breakthrough therapy for PTSD by the FDA.[38]

Lysergic acid diethylamide is the active substance in just two recent phase 2 trials for existential anxiety in the terminally ill. This is due to stigma surrounding large scale recreational use since the 1960s, with considerable political implications. Despite the dearth of trials, a recent meta-analysis with rigorous research from 60 years ago confirmed LSD also has important potential for alcohol use disorders.[39]

CURRENT STATUS

Drug-assisted psychotherapy has been used for approximately 90 years in the clinical practice for the range of psychiatric disorders. It was considered a very promising treatment in the early era of pre-psychopharmacological period, in 20th century (1930-60). With the advent of psychopharmacological agent in 1950s and subsequent research based understanding and increasing use of psychopharmacological agent, the use and preference for drug-assisted psychotherapy has been declining gradually. The published research evidence for it has failed to demonstrate its superiority in efficacy and utility in the clinical settings. There is no specific standard guideline or protocol for it. In spite of paucity of research evidence, it is used sparsely in isolated cases by clinician having selective interest and preference for this therapy. Psychedelic psychotherapy is a novel approach in drug-assisted psychotherapy, which appears promising and is in clinical trial stage. Among various agents being researched, MDMA appears most promising for PTSD, existential anxiety, and alcohol use disorders. There is also ethical and legal aspect for use of psychedelic-assisted psychotherapy which is a significant barrier for its use in routine clinical practice.

CONCLUSION

Drug-assisted psychotherapy is very old treatment approach for psychiatric disorder. It has been used across range of psychiatric disorder for diagnostic and therapeutic purpose for last 90 years. The origin of drug-assisted psychotherapy started with barbiturate era (1930-1960) which was later on replaced by benzodiazepines after 1960 due to equal efficacy and safer alternatives. Over the years, starting from late 1960s, there is a gradual decline in its use due to development of psychopharmacotherapeutic agents and better understanding of neurobiological basis on psychiatric disorder. The published scientific literature is predominantly uncontrolled studies in the form of case report and case series. The limited controlled studies have failed to demonstrate adequate evidence for its efficacy and utility till date.

In past few years, interest has been revived in research field in this technique in the form of psychedelic-assisted psychotherapy for anxiety disorder, PTSD, depression, substance use disorder etc. The preliminary findings are promising and further clinical trials are undergoing in large scale controlled study for its safety and efficacy. It is the appropriate time to reassess and explore the place of drug-assisted psychotherapy in clinical practice by extensive controlled research in this area and thereby reviving interest of clinicians and their training in drug-assisted psychotherapy.

REFERENCES

1. Fürst PT. Hallucinogens and Culture. San Francisco: Chandler & Sharp; 1976.
2. López-Muñoz F, Ucha-Udabe R, Alamo C. The history of barbiturates a century after their clinical introduction. Neuropsychiatric disease and treatment. 2005;1(4):329-43.
3. Lehmann HE. Before they called it psychopharmacology. Neuropsychopharmacol. 1993;8(4):291-303.
4. Bleckwenn WJ. Narcosis as therapy in neuropsychiatric conditions. JAMA. 1930;95(16):1168-71.
5. Lindemann E. Psychological changes in normal and abnormal individuals under the influence of sodium Amytal. Am J Psychiatry. 1932;88:1083-91.
6. Sargant W, Slater E. Acute war neuroses. The Lancet. 1940;(2):1-2.
7. Johns MW. Self-poisoning with barbiturates in England and Wales during 1959-74. Br Med J. 1977;1(6069):1128-30.
8. Ballew L, Morgan Y, Lippmann S. Intravenous diazepam for dissociative disorder: memory lost and found. Psychosomatics. 2003;44(4):346-7.
9. Ilechukwu ST, Henry T. Amytal interview using intravenous lorazepam in a patient with dissociative fugue. Gen Hosp Psychiatry. 2006;6(28):544-5.
10. Lee SS, Park S, Park SS. Use of lorazepam in drug-assisted interviews: two cases of dissociative amnesia. Psychiatry Investig. 2011 Dec 1;8(4):377-80.
11. Marcum JM. The use of midazolam with pulse oximetry in the drug-assisted interview. J Clin Psychiatry. 1996;57:111-3.
12. Jaffe JH. In: Gilman AG, Griffith RR (Eds). Goodman and Gilman's the Pharmacological Basis of Therapeutics. UK: Pergamon Press; 1990. p. 494.
13. Grof S. LSD psychotherapy. Pomona, CA: Hunter House Inc Publishers; 1980.
14. Leuner H. Halluzinogene. Bern, Switzerland: Hans Huber Verlag; 1981.
15. Hofmann A. How LSD originated. J Psychedelic Drugs. 1979;11(1-2):53-60.
16. Dass R, Metzner R, Bravo G. Birth of a psychedelic culture. Santa Fe, NM: Synergistic Press; 2010.
17. Grinspoon L, Bakalar JB. Psychedelic drugs reconsidered. New York: Lindesmith Center; 1997.
18. Oehen P, Traber R, Widmer V, et al. A randomized, controlled pilot study of MDMA (±3, 4-methylenedioxymethamphetamine)-assisted psychotherapy for treatment of resistant, chronic posttraumatic stress disorder (PTSD). J Psychopharmacol. 2013;27(1):40-52.
19. Liechti ME, Vollenweider FX. Acute psychological and physiological effects of MDMA after haloperidol pretreatment in healthy humans. Eur Neuropsychopharmacol. 2000;10(4):289-95.
20. Ott J, Bigwood J. Teonanacatyl. Hallucinogenic mushrooms of North America. Seattle, US: Madrona Publishers, Inc.; 1978.
21. Schultes RE, Hofmann A. Plants of the Gods: Origins of Hallucinogenic Use. New York: McGraw-Hill; 1979.
22. Pettigrew J. Iconography in Bradshaw b rock art: breaking the circularity. Clin Exp Optom. 2011;94(5):403-17.
23. Johnson MW, Richards WA, Griffiths RR. Human hallucinogen research: guidelines for safety. J Psychopharmacol. 2008;22(6):603-20.

24. Grof S. LSD Psychotherapy. Ben Lomond, CA: Multidisciplinary Association for Psychedelic Studies; 2008.
25. Krupitsky EM, Burakov AM, Dunaevsky IV, Romanova TN, Slavina TY, Grinenko AY. Single versus repeated sessions of ketamine-assisted psychotherapy for people with heroin dependence. J Psychoactive Drugs. 2007;39(1):13-9.
26. Wilkinson ST, Wright D, Fasula MK, Fenton L, Griepp M, Ostroff RB, et al. Cognitive behavior therapy may sustain antidepressant effects of intravenous ketamine in treatment-resistant depression. Psychotherapy and Psychosomatics. 2017;86(3):162-7.
27. Johnstone L. Psychological formulation as an alternative to psychiatric diagnosis. J Humanist Psychol. 2017;58:30-46.
28. Liechti ME, Dolder PC, Schmid Y. Alterations of consciousness and mystical-type experiences after acute LSD in humans. Psychopharmacol. 2017;234(9-10):1499-510.
29. Kraines SH. Sodium Amytal, hypnosis and psychotherapy. Int J Neuropsychiatry. 1967;3(3):248-56.
30. Solomon GF, Zarcone VP, Yoerg R, et al. Three psychiatric casualties from Vietnam. Archives of General Psychiatry. 1971;25(6):522-4.
31. Hurwitz TA. Narcosuggestion in chronic conversion symptoms using combined intravenous amobarbital and methylphenidate. The Canadian Journal of Psychiatry. 1988;33(2):147-52.
32. Smith JW, Lemere F, Dunn RB. Pentothal interviews in the treatment of alcoholism. Psychosomatics. 1971;12:330-1.
33. Hain JD, Smith BM, Stevenson I. Effectiveness and processes of interviewing with drugs. J Psychiatr Res. 1966;4(2):95-106.
34. Buckman J, Hain JD, Smith BM, et al. Controlled interviews using drugs. II. comparisons between restricted and freer conditions. Arch Gen Psychiatry. 1973;29:623-7.
35. McCall WV, Shelp FE, McDonald WM. Controlled investigation of the amobarbital interview for catatonic mutism. Am J Psychiatry 1992;149(2):202-6.
36. Kavirajan H. The amobarbital interview revisited: a review of the literature since 1966. Harv Rev Psychiatry. 1999;7(3):153-65.
37. Poole NA, Wuerz A, Agrawal N. Abreaction for conversion disorder: systematic review with meta-analysis. B J Psychiatry. 2010;197:91-5.
38. Kupferschmidt K. All clear for the decisive trial of ecstasy in PTSD patients. Science Magazine; 2017.
39. Krebs TS, Johansen PØ. Lysergic acid diethylamide (LSD) for alcoholism: meta-analysis of randomized controlled trials. J Psychopharmacology. 2012;26(7):994-1002.

CHAPTER 7

Current State of Management for Residual and Resistant Auditory Hallucinations and Delusions

Varun S Mehta, Smita N Deshpande

INTRODUCTION

As Waters put it—"auditory hallucinations are auditory perceptions that a person experiences in the absence of an external stimulus when awake".[1] Delusions were defined by Oyebode as "false judgements held with remarkable confidence and certitude, immune to any disapproval".[2] Both were known since early times and have been described in ancient Indian texts.[3] The International Pilot Study on Schizophrenia (IPSS) estimated that 70% of patients with schizophrenia experienced hallucinations, the most common being auditory and close to 60% had delusions.[4] Primary delusions are considered characteristic of schizophrenia; whereas secondary delusions, defined by their content or theme, are a part of various psychiatric disorders. The prevalence of schizophrenia is around 1% all over the world. A Finnish report on prevalence of schizophrenia, one of the most comprehensive to date, reported a rate of 0.87%.[5] However, prevalence rates may reportedly differ up to fivefold in different studies and population.[6]

Roughly 60 years after the introduction of chlorpromazine, antipsychotics still remain the primary mode of therapy in treating schizophrenia.[7] Delusions and hallucinations do improve with treatment of underlying disturbances in other psychiatric illnesses but not in schizophrenia as 30–40% remain nonresponders.[8] Even treatment responders may continue to experience delusions (17%) and hallucinations (10%) during the course of illness.[9] These "residual" and "unresponsive" delusions/hallucinations contribute to treatment resistance, a condition common to schizophrenia (treatment-resistant schizophrenia). The delusions, hallucinations, and disorganized thoughts together constitute the "positive symptom" domain[10] which is the center point of this discussion in treatment-resistant schizophrenia (TRS).

Persons affected with schizophrenia suffer from significant disability, including their capacity to maintain social bonds, sustainable employment, and independent living.[11] Cognitive impairment mediates many of the functional disabilities in schizophrenia.[12] In this chapter, we describe strategies for the management of residual and resistant delusions/hallucinations mainly in the context of TRS.

ASSESSMENT OF DELUSIONS AND HALLUCINATIONS

General measurement tools such as psychopathology rating scales are used to measure overall symptom severity. Delusions and hallucinations are multidimensional and understanding various dimensions such as conviction, insight, bizarreness, systemization, disorganization for delusions, and other related issues helps us understand them.[13] Commonly used rating scales, such as the "Psychotic Symptom Rating Scale" (PSYRATS), measure individual dimensions. PSYRATS is said to help quantify several multidimensional features of hallucinations and delusions.[14] Delusions and hallucinations are also measured using the "Positive and Negative Syndrome Scale (PANSS)"[15] for schizophrenia. Other standardized scales assess hallucinations and delusions independently **(Table 1)**.

Although rating scales do help us to measure symptom severity and response to treatment when used by trained and experienced evaluators, they are not conventionally used in day-to-day clinical treatment.

A "Clinician-Rated Dimensions of Psychosis Symptom Severity Scale" in the Diagnostic and Statistical Manual of Mental Disorders-5 (DSM-5) has been found to be useful to evaluate response to treatment.[18] The instrument is easy to administer and is available free for use.

TREATMENT STRATEGIES FOR REFRACTORY DELUSIONS AND HALLUCINATIONS

Classically, clinical drug treatment trials focused on overall changes in psychopathology rather than specific symptoms such as delusions or hallucinations. Hence there are no specific guidelines for the treatment of hallucinations or delusions alone. Even though medication does target these symptoms, indications are often disorder-specific. Apart from medications, noninvasive brain stimulation (NIBS) techniques and various psychological interventions[19,20] are used. While pharmacotherapy aims at symptom abolition, psychological therapies claim to address healing, recovery, and ultimately personal growth. NIBS is also said to currently help alleviate psychotic symptoms, but is usually used to augment other therapies.

Table 1: Some scales for measuring hallucinations and delusions.[16,17]	
Scales for hallucinations	*Scales for delusions*
• Beliefs about Voice Questions • Cognitive Assessment Schedule • Voice Compliance Scale • Power Differential Scale • Omniscience Scale • Risk of Acting on Commands Scale	• Dimensions of Delusional Experience • Belief Rating Scale • The Brown Assessment of Beliefs Scale • Delusion Assessment Scale • Conviction of Delusional Belief Scale • Simple Delusional Syndrome Scale • Peters Delusions Inventory

Pharmacotherapy

Oral Medication

Only antipsychotic drugs are said to comprehensively target delusions and hallucinations. Among them, clozapine is said to be the most efficacious for patients with treatment-resistant hallucinations and delusions.[8] An acceptable trial of clozapine requires trough serum levels between 350 ng/mL and 500 ng/mL[21] continuously for at least 12 weeks to gauge response. When favorable, the treatment should last at unchanged doses for at least a year or later still.[22]

Regular treatment at constant drug levels and dosages needs to continue for long, as the propensity to experience hallucinations may also depend on the individual's genetic makeup. This susceptibility lasts lifelong, and hence the need for prolonged treatment, or at least as long as side effects are tolerable. Maintenance treatment should continue at the same dosages as those which initially achieved symptom remission. This is most likely to achieve lowest rates of relapse.[23]

However, 40–70% of TRS patients may not respond to clozapine, implying that 12–20% of persons with schizophrenia are ultra-resistant[24] and may need still other augmentation strategies. A Cochrane review did propose that co-treatment with more than one antipsychotic could boost the clinical efficacy but quality of available evidence was weak.[25] The present evidence for the use of any nonantipsychotic augmentation strategy along with clozapine for treatment-resistant positive symptoms is mixed and of limited clinical utility.[8]

Depot Medication

Nonadherence to antipsychotic treatment is the most frequent reason for relapse of schizophrenia, including for hallucinations.[26] Long-acting injectable antipsychotics (LAIs) are important alternative or add-on to oral medication. Even though studies have found LAI superior to short-acting oral antipsychotics for relapse prevention and better social functioning,[27] studies on use of LAI alone, and their effectiveness in treatment-resistant symptoms are unavailable. In general, LAIs appear to be similar to one another in terms of efficacy and relapse prevention.[28]

Alternatives to Clozapine

Persons with schizophrenia may be unable to continue clozapine due to disabling side effects or unwillingness for blood monitoring. In some cases, alternative antipsychotics such as high dose olanzapine at 30–40 mg/day,[29] risperidone,[30,31] or ziprasidone[32] as monotherapy may be effective in patients unable to tolerate clozapine.

> **Box 1:** Psychological interventions for auditory verbal hallucinations.
> - Cognitive behavior therapy
> - Metacognitive therapy
> - Mindfulness-based therapy
> - Acceptance and commitment therapy
> - Experience-focused counseling
> - Hallucination-focused integrative treatment
> - Avatar therapy

Psychological Interventions

Psychological therapies developed for psychosis, mainly focus on treatment of refractory or positive symptoms such as delusions and hallucinations.[19] Clinicians may label auditory hallucinations as treatment resistant before trying psychological and other interventions. In clinical practice, both the treatment modalities have to be personalized. Different forms of psychological interventions have been used for drug-resistant auditory verbal hallucinations **(Box 1)**.

Cognitive Behavior Therapy

Among the available interventions, cognitive behavior therapy for psychosis (CBTp) has been the most discussed but was only low to moderately effective for auditory hallucinations and delusions.[19] It is said to be more effective for treating hallucinations[33] in moderately ill patients. CBTp aims to reappraise the meaning and purpose of hallucinations and delusions, thus improving the person's tolerance for these symptoms, rather than reduce their frequency and severity.[34] The shared goals of CBT are:[35]
- Cognitive conceptualization of psychotic symptoms
- Psychoeducation about the nature of the illness
- Establishment of a strong therapeutic alliance through collaborative empiricism
- Relapse prevention.

A combination of psychoeducation with supportive psychotherapy is probably better in improving daily functioning and self-esteem.

Metacognitive Therapy

A newer form of treatment, metacognitive therapy (MCT), was studied for treatment-resistant psychosis.[20] MCT encourages a person to develop a detached awareness of their thoughts with simultaneous control of their worries and ruminations, rather than confronting them about the thoughts and beliefs as in CBT.[36] This principle has been adapted for individuals with psychosis.

Mindfulness-based Interventions

Interventions using mindfulness are increasingly being used for psychosis.[37] Their essence lies in a nonjudgmental approach and attention to present moment experiences.[38] In mindfulness training, this skill is acquired through formal meditation practices and experiential exercises.[39] An individual brief (4-week) mindfulness intervention for persistent voices (iMPV) was developed with small to moderate effectiveness on reducing distressing auditory hallucinations.[40]

Avatar Therapy

Virtual therapy is in its very nascent stages as a treatment modality for persistent auditory hallucinations. Avatar therapy uses a nonimmersive virtual reality system to challenge the beliefs a person holds about the power of their "voices". Thus it helps them gain more control over these voices. The participants are asked to create an avatar of the entity that they believe is talking to them. They then engage in a dialogue with the avatar of their voice, which the therapist is able to control.[41]

Noninvasive Brain Stimulation Techniques

Repetitive transcranial magnetic stimulation (rTMS), transcranial direct current stimulation (tDCS), and electroconvulsive therapy (ECT) are employed for medication-resistant psychotic symptoms.[42]

Electroconvulsive Therapy

Used for over 70 years, ECT has a definite role as an add-on strategy for resistant-positive symptoms.[43] Various experts administered 3-4 sessions of ECT a week including a novel strategy using eight unilateral daily sessions of ECT.[44] Though ECT is commonly used in clinical practice for patients who have treatment-resistant positive symptoms, the clinical experience is supported only by open label and case reports/series. There are no new placebo controlled randomized trials since 2003, so the results are inconclusive regarding the role of ECT as an augmenting agent.[45]

Transcranial Magnetic Stimulation

Transcranial magnetic stimulation (TMS) is a technique in which a strong pulse of electrical current is sent through a coil. When given in a short time as multiple pulses, it is known as rTMS. Though various treatment paradigms have been used to target auditory hallucinations and positive symptoms, low frequency rTMS over the left temporoparietal region has been found to be the most effective.[46] We need to be cautious about the results as future studies may well show less favorable results than the initial well-controlled ones because rTMS is a relatively young treatment method.

Transcranial Direct Current Stimulation

Transcranial direct current stimulation is a NIBS technique. It acts by polarizing the neuronal membrane through use of a very low intensity electrical current. tDCS has mainly been used for refractory auditory hallucinations in schizophrenia. However, data on tDCS for medication-resistant symptoms is still sparse with small sample sizes and mixed results.[47]

CONCLUSION

Given the lack of high-quality options, augmentation strategies to clozapine should be individualized rather than taking a "one size fits all" approach. Even though ECT has been used for individuals with treatment-resistant delusions and hallucinations, it is not supported by convincing evidence. Some nonpharmacological modalities should be tried before labeling as treatment resistance. There is emerging evidence on the use of rTMS and tDCS in resistant hallucinations and delusions, but more data needs to be generated.

REFERENCES

1. Waters F (2014). Auditory hallucinations in adult populations. [online] Available from https://www.psychiatrictimes.com/schizophrenia/auditory-hallucinations-adult-populations/page/0/1 [Last accessed November, 2019].
2. Oyebode F. Pathology of perception. Symptoms of Mind. United Kingdom: Saunders Ltd; 2011.
3. Balsavar A, Deshpande SN. Hallucinations in the classical Indian system of Ayurveda: A brief overview. Indian J Psychiatry. 2014;56:325-9.
4. Sartorius N, Jablensky A, Korten A, et al. Early manifestations and first contact incidence of schizophrenia in different cultures. Psychol Med. 1986;16:909-28.
5. Perälä J, Suvisaari J, Saarni SI, et al. Lifetime prevalence of psychotic and bipolar I disorder in a general population. Arch Gen Psychiatry. 2007;64:19-28.
6. McGrath J, Saha S, Chant D, et al. Schizophrenia: a concise overview of incidence, prevalence, and mortality. Epidemiol Rev. 2008;30:67-76.
7. Kane JM, Correll CU. Past and present progress in the pharmacologic treatment of schizophrenia. J Clin Psychiatry. 2010;71:1115-24.
8. Buckley PF, Elkis H. Treatment-resistant schizophrenia. Psychiatr Clin N Am. 2016;39:239-65.
9. Schennach R, Riedel M, Obermeier M, et al. What are residual symptoms in schizophrenia spectrum disorder? Clinical description and 1-year persistence within a naturalistic trial. Eur Arch Psychiatry Clin Neurosci. 2015;265:107-16.
10. Kahn RS, Sommer IE, Murray RM, et al. Schizophrenia. Nat Rev Dis Primers. 2015;1:15067.
11. Harvey PD. Assessing disability in schizophrenia: tools and contributors. J Clin Psychiatry. 2014;75:e27.
12. Dark F, Cairns A, Harris A. Cognitive remediation: the foundation of psychosocial treatment of schizophrenia. Aust N Z J Psychiatry. 2013;47:505-7.

13. Pandarakalam JP. Pharmacological and non-pharmacological interventions for persistent auditory hallucinations in schizophrenia. BJMP. 2016;9:a914.
14. Haddock G, McCarron J, Tarrier N, et al. Scales to measure dimensions of hallucinations and delusions: the psychotic symptom rating scales (PSYRATS). Psychol Med. 1999;29:879-89.
15. Kay SR, Fiszbein A, Opler LA. The positive and negative syndrome scale (PANSS) for schizophrenia. Schizophr Bull. 1987;13:261-76.
16. Forgácová L. Delusion assessment scales. Neuropsychopharmacol Hung. 2008;10(1):23-30.
17. Peters ER, Joseph SA, Garety PA. Measurement of delusional ideation in the normal population: introducing the PDI (Peters et al. Delusions Inventory). Schizophr Bull. 1999;25(3):553-76.
18. American Psychiatric Association. Diagnostic and statistical manual of mental disorders. Arlington, VA: American Psychiatric Publishing; 2013.
19. Burns AM, Erickson DH1, Brenner CA. Cognitive-behavioral therapy for medication-resistant psychosis: a meta-analytic review. Psychiatr Serv. 2014; 65(7):874-80.
20. Hutton P, Morrison AP, Wardle M, et al. Metacognitive therapy in treatment-resistant psychosis: a multiple-baseline study. Behav Cogn Psychother. 2014;42:166-85.
21. Faden J, Citrome L. Resistance is not futile: treatment-refractory schizophrenia—overview, evaluation and treatment. Expert Opin Pharmacother. 2018;8:1-14.
22. Buchanan RW, Kreyenbuhl J, Kelly DL, Noel JM, Boggs DL, et al. Schizophrenia Patient Outcomes Research Team (PORT). The 2009 schizophrenia PORT psychopharmacological treatment recommendations and summary statements. Schizophr Bull. 2010;36:71-93.
23. Sommer IE, Slotema CW, Daskalakis ZJ, et al. The treatment of hallucinations in schizophrenia spectrum disorders. Schizophr Bull. 2012;38:704-14.
24. Siskind D, Siskind V, Kisely S. Clozapine response rates among people with treatment-resistant schizophrenia: data from a systematic review and meta-analysis. Can J Psychiatry. 2017;62:772-7.
25. Barber S, Olotu U, Corsi M, Cipriani A, et al. Clozapine combined with different antipsychotic drugs for treatment-resistant schizophrenia. Cochrane Database Syst Rev. 2017;23:CD006324.
26. Patel MX, de Zoysa N, Bernadt M, et al. A cross-sectional study of patients' perspectives on adherence to antipsychotic medication: depot versus oral. J Clin Psychiatry. 2008;69:1548-56.
27. Leucht C, Heres S, Kane JM, et al. Oral versus depot antipsychotic drugs for schizophrenia: a critical systematic review and meta-analysis of randomized long-term trials. Schizophr Res. 2011;127:83-92.
28. Correll CU, Citrome L, Haddad PM, et al. The use of long-acting injectable antipsychotics in schizophrenia: Evaluating the evidence. J Clin Psychiatry. 2016;77:1-24.
29. Citrome L, Kantrowitz JT. Olanzapine dosing above the licensed range is more efficacious than lower doses: fact or fiction? Expert Rev Neurother. 2009;9:1045-58.
30. Bondolfi G, Dufour H, Patris M, et al. Risperidone versus clozapine in treatment resistant chronic schizophrenia: a randomized double-blind study the risperidone study group. Am J Psychiatry. 1998;155:499-504.

31. Wahlbeck K, Cheine M, Tuisku K, et al. Risperidone versus clozapine in treatment resistant schizophrenia: a randomized pilot study. Prog Neuropsychopharmacol Biol Psychiatry. 2000;24:911-22.
32. Sacchetti E, Galluzzo A, Valsecchi P, et al. MOZART Study Group. Ziprasidone vs clozapine in schizophrenia patients refractory to multiple antipsychotic treatments: the MOZART study. Schizophr Res. 2009;113:112-21.
33. Van der Gaag M, Valmaggia LR, Smit F. The effects of individually tailored formulation-based cognitive behavioural therapy in auditory hallucinations and delusions: a meta-analysis. Schizophr Res. 2014;156:30-7.
34. Birchwood M, Trower P. Cognitive therapy for command hallucinations: not a quasi-neuroleptic. J Contemp Psychother. 2006;36:1-7.
35. Rector NA, Beck AT. Cognitive behavioral therapy for schizophrenia: an empirical review. J Nerv Ment Dis. 2012;10:832-9.
36. Wells A. Metacognitive Therapy for Anxiety and Depression. New York: Guilford Press; 2008.
37. Thomas N, Hayward M, Peters E, et al. Psychological therapies for auditory hallucinations (voices): current status and key directions for future research. Schizophr Bull. 2014;40:S202-12.
38. Kabat-Zinn J (1994). Whenever You Go There You Are. New York: Hyperion.
39. Strauss E, Sherman EMS, Spreen O. A Compendium of Neuropsychological Tests: Administration, Norms, And Commentary. New York: Oxford University Press; 2008.
40. Louise S, Rossell SL, Thomas N. The acceptability, feasibility and potential outcomes of an individual mindfulness-based intervention for hearing voices. Behav Cogn Psychother. 2018;9:1-17.
41. Rus-Calafell M, Garety P, Sason E, et al. Virtual reality in the assessment and treatment of psychosis: a systematic review of its utility, acceptability and effectiveness. Psychol Med. 2018;48:362-91.
42. Miyamoto S, Jarskog LF, Fleischhacker WW. New therapeutic approaches for treatment-resistant schizophrenia: a look to the future. J Psychiatr Res. 2014;58:1-6.
43. Porcelli S, Balzarro B, Serretti A. Clozapine resistance: augmentation strategies. Eur Neuropsychopharmacol. 2012;22:165-82.
44. Davarinejad O, Hendesi K, Shahi H, et al. A pilot study on daily intensive ECT over 8 days improved positive and negative symptoms and general psychopathology of patients with treatment-resistant schizophrenia up to 4 weeks after treatment. Neuropsychobiology. 2018;21:1-9.
45. Nieuwdorp W, Koops S, Somers M, et al. Transcranial magnetic stimulation, transcranial direct current stimulation and electroconvulsive therapy for medication-resistant psychosis of schizophrenia. Curr Opin Psychiatry. 2015;28:222-8.
46. Guo Q, Li C, Wang J. Updated review on the clinical use of repetitive transcranial magnetic stimulation in psychiatric disorders. Neurosci Bull. 2017;33:747-56.
47. Lee EHM, Chan PY, Law EYL, et al. Efficacy of transcranial direct current stimulation (tDCS) as a treatment for persistent hallucinations in patients with schizophrenia: a systematic review and meta-analysis. Schizophr Res. 2018;18:30413-4.

CHAPTER 8

Antiviral Therapy in Schizophrenia: Does It Work?

Smita N Deshpande, Konasale M Prasad, Vishwajit L Nimgaonkar

INTRODUCTION

Schizophrenia (SZ) is a common, disabling disorder. While many efficacious antipsychotic drugs (APDs) are available, they provide only symptomatic relief. Rational therapeutics dictates the use of drugs that counteract or negate etiologic factors. The etiology of SZ is uncertain, though a multitude of genetic and environmental factors have been proposed, suggesting that any individual putative factor is neither necessary nor sufficient to explain the etiology of SZ.[1] Much debate has centered on a viral etiology for SZ, but it has been difficult to arrive at a clear consensus.[2] Testing for beneficial effects of antiviral drugs is one way to address this debate;[3] indeed, several trials with antiviral drugs have been conducted among patients with SZ. We summarize those data herein.

ANTIVIRAL MEDICATIONS IN SCHIZOPHRENIA

Do Antipsychotic Drugs have Antiviral Properties?

Jones-Brando et al. (1997)[4] found that *in vitro*, two of nine metabolites of clozapine, an APD-exhibited antiviral activity against the human immunodeficiency virus type 1 (HIV-1). They suggested that inhibition of viral replication may be one of the mechanisms of antipsychotic effects of APDs.[4] They predicted that treatment with antivirus and anti-inflammatory medications could alleviate symptoms in some individuals with SZ.[5] This work provided the impetus for several investigations in which antiviral medications were tested for efficacy in SZ. If such drugs proved to be efficacious, they would provide a novel line of rational therapeutics. They could also help resolve the controversies surrounding the viral hypothesis of SZ genesis.

There are two key considerations for such studies:
1. It would be optimal to test antiviral medications only in patients with demonstrable viral infections. Optimally, the infection agent should be detectable in the patients' tissues and its levels should be monitored concomitantly with resolution of target features of SZ. As it is often difficult

to detect virions, particularly for neurotropic agents, most investigators have assayed antibodies to the virus in question.

2. It is difficult to treat most viral infections effectively, i.e. to eliminate virions completely from infected individuals. On the other hand, many antivirals are effective in inhibiting viral replication. While this level of efficacy may be sufficient in some situations, it can be a limitation for patients with SZ in whom viral infection has hypothetically already caused impairment in neuronal functions.

In the following section, we review treatment trials in which antivirals are tested for secondary prevention, i.e. inhibition of viral replication or clearance of viral loads in persons with SZ. These trials were conducted for the viruses of the *Herpesviridae* family, which includes more than 200 species. Among these, nine species which are given below are said to affect humans while the last two being carcinogenic: herpes simplex viruses (HSVs) types 1 and 2, varicella zoster virus, cytomegalovirus (CMV), roseoloviruses human herpesvirus-6 (HHV-6) (A and B) and HHV-7, Epstein–Barr virus (EBV), and Kaposi sarcoma-associated herpesvirus (HHV-8).[6]

TRIALS OF ANTIVIRALS FOR RESOLUTION OF SPECIFIC FEATURES OF SCHIZOPHRENIA

We are aware only of trials with acyclovir and its derivatives in this type of trial **(Table 1)**. Acyclovir and its derivative valacyclovir are potent antiviral agents as they inhibit replication of herpes simplex virus type 1 (HSV-1) virions in a highly specific manner, without altering replication of human deoxyribonucleic acid (DNA).[7] These drugs show few side effects and are used extensively for treating acute recurrence of HSV-1 infections in mucus membranes, the corneal surfaces, and in the brain. While they are highly efficacious for HSV-1, they are less effective for other herpes viruses such as CMV or EBV.

Acyclovir Treatment Trial for Epstein–Barr Virus Infection in Schizophrenia

In an early study, DeLisi et al. (1987)[8] conducted a small proof-of-concept trial on schizophrenic patients with elevated Epstein–Barr antibody titers. Only four patients were included, of whom two had elevated antibodies to HSV-1 and HSV-2 also. Participants received 4,000 mg/24 hours of oral acyclovir capsules in four divided doses for 6 weeks. The trial was preceded by use of a placebo for 2 weeks followed by a lower dose of acyclovir for 2 weeks, and placebo continuation even after the trial was over. The Brief Psychiatric Rating Scale (BPRS) was used for evaluation of beneficial effects. There was no statistically significant difference in total BPRS score, various symptom clusters, or physical symptoms between active and placebo periods. Although the sample was relatively small, it was one of the earliest trials of antiviral drugs in SZ.

Table 1: Clinical trials of adjuvant antiviral agents among patients with schizophrenia.

Reference	First author	Virus-targeted, drug	Type of trial	Sample	Evaluation	Results
Am J Psychiatry. 2003;160(12): 2234-6	Dickerson et al.	CMV, Valacyclovir	Open	Treatment nonresponsive outpatients with SZ, N = 65	PANSS, immunoassay for antibodies for "potentially neurotropic human herpes viruses"	Significant improvement in the psychiatric symptoms of individuals who were seropositive for cytomegalovirus, trend for more improvement on PANSS negative symptoms scale
Schizophr Res. 2009;107(2-3):147-9	Dickerson et al.	CMV, Valacyclovir	Double-blind	Outpatients with chronic SZ; N = 47	PANSS, immunoassay for CMV	Valacyclovir safe for patients. Persistent symptoms not significantly altered, but trend for more improvement on PANSS negative symptoms scale among CMV seropositive cases
Biol Psychiatry. 1987;22(2): 216-20	DeLisi et al.	EBV, Acyclovir	Before and after active drug	Outpatients and inpatients with SZ, N = 8	BPRS	No evidence for changes in symptoms with acyclovir
Schizophr Bull. 2013;39(4): 857-66	Prasad et al.	HSV-1, Valacyclovir	Randomized, double-blind controlled trial	HSV-1 seropositive outpatients with early course SZ; N = 24 total	PANSS, AIMS, BAS, Penn CNB domains	Patients treated with valacyclovir showed significant improvement in verbal memory, working memory, and visual object learning tasks of the CNB after 18-week trial. No significant change in psychotic symptoms
Schizophr Res. 2018;193: 161-7	Bhatia et al.	HSV-1, Valacyclovir	Randomized, double-blind placebo-controlled trial	HSV-1 seropositive outpatients with early course SZ intention to treat, N = 62; completers, N = 56	PANSS, AIMS, BAS, CNB domains	Valacyovir treated cases performed significantly better than those on placebo, on the accuracy index of emotion identification and discrimination domain of the CNB. There were no significant differences on any of the other domains of the CNB or for psychotic symptoms
Schizophr Res. 2019;206: 291-9	Breier et al.	HSV-1 (seropositive and seronegative patients included), valacyclovir	Randomized, placebo controlled double-blind multicenter efficacy study	HSV-1 seropositive outpatients with early course SZ, N = 170; HSV-1 positive N = 70; HSV-1 negative N = 96	PANSS, scales for clinical symptoms and activities of daily life, MATRICS consensus cognitive battery (MCCB)	No significant change in cognitive functions following valacyclovir in HSV-1 seropositive or seronegative groups. HSV-1 positive group more impaired at baseline than the seronegative group on letter number sequencing test, more positive symptoms with poorer quality of life

(AIMS: Abnormal Involuntary Movements Scale; BAS: Barnes Akathisia Scale, BPRS: Brief Psychiatric Rating Scale; CMV: cytomegalovirus; EBV: Epstein-Barr virus; HSV-1: herpes simplex virus type 1; MATRICS: Measurement and Treatment Research to Improve Cognition in Psychosis; PANSS: Positive and Negative Symptom Scale; Penn CNB: Pennsylvania Computerized Neurocogritive Battery; SZ: schizophrenia)

Valacyclovir Treatment Trials for Cytomegalovirus Infection in Schizophrenia

Two trials investigated the effect of antiviral agents on CMV with varying results. In the first trial, administering valacyclovir [1 g twice a day for 16 weeks to nonresponsive patients with SZ (N = 65)] resulted in significant improvement in clinical symptoms in patients seropositive for CMV but not for other herpes viruses.[9] In 2009, the same investigators[10] conducted a double-blind trial with CMV seropositive SZ patients (N = 24; valacyclovir 1 g twice daily for 16 weeks, against N = 23 on placebo for the same period). It was disappointing to find that there was no significant difference among active drug or placebo groups at the end of the trial. The authors noted the relatively low efficacy of valacyclovir against CMV. In addition, considerations such as sample size and chronicity of SZ might also have reduced the chances of detecting beneficial effects.

Valacyclovir Treatment for Persons with Schizophrenia Infected with Herpes Simplex Virus Type 1[11]

Herpes simplex virus type 1 causes primary infection through oropharyngeal or nasal mucosal surfaces. Following primary infection, which can be asymptomatic, it remains in a latent, predominantly inactive state in sensory ganglia, particularly the trigeminal ganglia. Though the human immune system mounts a robust response, primarily through increased production of immunoglobulin G (IgG) and immunoglobulin M (IgM) antibodies, virions cannot be eliminated from the latent state. Thus, HSV-1 causes lifelong infection and the prevalence of HSV-1 infection increases with age. HSV-1 commonly causes "cold sores" and less commonly it causes corneal infections that can lead to blindness. HSV-1 does cause encephalitis among immune-compromised individuals. Of note, it can cause subtle cognitive dysfunction among adults with no history of encephalitis.

Herpes simplex virus-1 exposure, but not exposure to five other herpes viruses, was associated with verbal memory deficits among infected men who suffered from SZ.[12] Other studies (including studies from India) have also reported cognitive impairments in patients with SZ who were exposed to HSV-1.[13-18] In a large sample (N = 1,308), infection with HSV-1 and CMV was associated with different types of cognitive impairments on the Trail Making Test, suggesting differential effects of the two viruses.[19] Verbal memory, vigilance, and processing speed were also affected.[19]

Herpes simplex virus-1 seropositive individuals may show structural alterations in their brains. Prasad et al. (2007)[13] investigated 30 patients in their first episode of SZ and 44 healthy subjects. They assayed sera for HSV-1 IgG antibody and conducted MRI scans. Patients had higher antibody titers (evidence of higher infection rates) and showed significant differences from controls in prefrontal gray matter. Patients exposed to HSV-1 showed decreased gray matter volume in dorsolateral prefrontal cortex (PFC) and anterior cingulate cortex compared to patients without serological evidence of HSV-1 exposure or normal controls. In a subsequent paper, the same investigators reported association of an exonic polymorphism of the major histocompatibility complexes (MHC) class I polypeptide-related sequence B (MICB), with both HSV-1 exposure status and reduced PFC volumes.[20] A longitudinal MRI study further strengthened these associations with the observation of temporal decline in the volume of posterior cingulate cortex over 1 year among first episode medication naïve SZ subjects but not in healthy controls.[11,21] A functional MRI study reported that HSV-1 + SZ subjects activated nonclassical working memory network with increased processing time but with no difference in accuracy of performance on n-back task.[22]

More significantly, HSV-1 exposure is associated with cognitive impairments in nonpsychiatric population as well (Indian samples—Bhatia et al. 2018,[23] US samples—Dickerson et al., 2008,[24] African Americans in the US—Watson et al., 2013,[16] and home dwelling elderly in Finland-Strandberg et al., 2003).[25] Longitudinal studies have also reported cognitive decline over time among HSV-1-exposed individuals (home dwelling elderly in Finland-Strandberg et al., 2003,[25] cases and controls in US—Prasad et al., 2011,[20] cases and controls in India—Bhatia et al., 2018[23]).

The associations between HSV-1 exposure and cognitive dysfunction can be detected even after correction for socioeconomic status. This is an important consideration, as HSV-1 infection is more common among individuals from lower socioeconomic strata. It is, therefore, reasonable to consider whether treating HSV-1-exposed persons could improve cognitive dysfunction or even prevent further decline in cognitive functions.

Randomized Controlled Trials of HSV-1 in Schizophrenia

To date, three randomized controlled trials (RCTs) have addressed this question. All of them have investigated adjunctive valacyclovir. It was considered appropriate to conduct the trials among persons with early course SZ, a group in which HSV-1-associated cognitive dysfunction has been noted repeatedly. As such individuals would benefit substantially from cognitive remediation, it was considered the appropriate group to test on ethical grounds. It is worthwhile to consider all three RCTs in detail because they illustrate several operational problems likely to be encountered in RCTs of other antiviral drugs.

The first RCT to study potential benefits of valacyclovir was conducted in the USA. This pilot, double-blind placebo-controlled RCT investigated a sample of HSV-1 seropositive SZ patients (total N = 24, N = 12 each in the adjunctive valacyclovir and placebo groups).[26] All participants were administered steady doses of antipsychotics for 1 month prior to, and during the RCT. Starting with valacyclovir 1 g orally twice daily for 2 weeks, the dose was increased to 1.5 g orally twice daily for the following 16 weeks. The primary outcome, cognitive functions, was evaluated using the Penn Computerized Neurocognitive Battery (CNB).[27] The Positive and Negative Symptom Scale (PANSS), Abnormal Involuntary Movements Scale (AIMS), Barnes Akathisia Scale (BAS), and detailed side effects checklist were also administered. Valacyclovir was well tolerated and there were no major side effects. The patients treated with valacyclovir, in comparison with the placebo treated group, showed significant improvements in verbal memory, working memory, and visual object learning tasks of the CNB at the end of the trial. Not unexpectedly, in view of the stable clinical state of participants at study entry, there were no significant changes in psychotic symptoms.

Following the interesting results from the US RCT, we undertook a similar RCT in India, in a group of early course (<7 years) patients with SZ. Like the US patients, the Indian patients were also on stable doses of APDs 1 month before and during the duration of the trial. Valacyclovir 1.5 mg twice daily was used. Evaluations were carried out using Hindi adaptations of the CNB and the same battery of other rating scales used in the US sample was administered to the Indian patients. Valacyclovir was well tolerated, with vomiting and nausea being the only significant side effects, not significantly more than controls. The final intention to treat (ITT) sample consisted of 62 patients (cases on valacyclovir 30; placebo 32), of which 56 participants completed the study (valacyclovir 25; placebo 31). Valacyclovir treated cases in the ITT sample as well as in the completer sample performed significantly better than those on placebo, on the accuracy index of emotion identification and discrimination domains of the CNB. There were no significant differences on any of the other domains of the CNB.

The VISTA study is the third evaluation of valacyclovir in relation to HSV-1 infected patients with SZ.[28] It was a 12-site multicenter study that compared valacyclovir (1.5 g twice daily) to placebo for a 16-week, double-blind efficacy study among 170 subjects with SZ: HSV-1 seropositive, N = 70 and HSV-1 seronegative, N = 96. The Measurement and Treatment Research to Improve Cognition in Psychosis (MATRICS) Consensus Cognitive Battery (MCCB)[29] was used to assess cognitive function.[30] The PANSS and other scales for clinical symptoms and activities of daily living were also administered. The HSV-1 seropositive group differed from the seronegative group at baseline with regard to several variables; they were significantly older, had a longer duration of illness (although duration <8 years was an inclusion criterion), included more women, they were more impaired on the letter-number sequencing test (an estimate of working memory), and they had higher scores on positive symptoms of SZ and had lower indices for quality of life. At the end of the trial, there were no significant changes in the working memory composite or the letter-number sequencing test of the MCCB after taking into account the HSV-1 serological status × treatment × time interaction. The HSV-1 seronegative group did not show significant changes, either. Nominally significant associations were noted but results did not withstand Bonferroni corrections for multiple comparisons.

Discussion of the Acyclovir/Valacyclovir Trials for HSV-1 Infections in Schizophrenia

The RCTs of valacyclovir demonstrated the feasibility of investigating the efficacy of antiviral drugs for SZ. The drug was well-tolerated, assuring safety. All three RCTs were conducted using similar diagnostic criteria and focused on patients with early course SZ to reduce the impact of chronicity on cognitive dysfunction. The Indian sample was adequately powered to test the results from the initial US study, with over 80% power to detect an effect size of 0.8, whereas the mean value for significant effect sizes from initial US sample[26] ranged from 0.34 to 1.14. The HSV-1 seropositive group in the VISTA trial had similar power to the Indian sample. The VISTA trial also included an additional group of HSV-1 seronegative patients that could be utilized to study whether any beneficial effects of valacyclovir were unrelated to its antiviral effects.

Notwithstanding these positive features, the Indian and the VISTA studies evidently did not detect beneficial effects of valacyclovir on the cognitive domains found to be improved with this drug in the initial US study. The lack of replication could be attributed to several factors. First, it should be noted that valacyclovir cannot eliminate HSV-1 virions from the human host, so any beneficial effects may have a limited duration. Second, the proportion of patients in each trial who were experiencing reactivation from latent infection was unknown. Arguably, this is the group of HSV-1 patients most likely to benefit from valacyclovir treatment.

While the lack of replication argues against further studies of valacyclovir in SZ, several important differences between the studies need to be kept in mind. The Indian RCT did not study verbal memory, a cognitive domain that showed substantial improvement in the pilot US study. The VISTA study did include a verbal memory task, but the MATRICS battery used in this RCT is not substantially correlated with the cognitive domains assessed with the CNB, the cognitive battery employed in the pilot US and Indian RCTs. Notably, the Indian RCT detected beneficial effects of valacyclovir on the emotion identification and discrimination domains, which were not evaluated in the VISTA trials.

The results from the Indian sample are plausible, for in an earlier sample from India we noted greater deterioration in the same domains among HSV-1 seropositive persons over a 1–2 years follow-up period, compared with a control group of persons who were HSV-1 seronegative at study entry.[23] Together, the results from the Indian studies suggest that there may be geographic differences in the pattern of HSV-1-associated cognitive dysfunction. For example, there could be differing strains of HSV-1 across different regions of the world.

Importantly, the data from the Indian studies challenge us to consider whether another RCT in India is warranted to test the HSV-1-associated dysfunction in the emotion identification and discrimination domains, which are considered to be an important component of social cognition.[31] Indeed, the studies of the Indian samples raise the challenging notion of RCTs of valacyclovir among HSV-1 seropositive persons *without* SZ.

CONCLUSION

There continue to be tantalizing reports implicating viral infections as risk factors for SZ, but it is difficult to conduct rigorous studies to test the viral hypothesis.[32] RCTs using antiviral drugs could provide a practical resolution for this debate. Reassuringly, the published reports indicate that such drugs neither exacerbate nor precipitate symptoms of mental illness. A central problem in this context is the relative paucity of effective drugs for most viral infections; the number of efficacious drugs that eliminate the viral target from the human host is even smaller. Viral infection may have led to irreversible changes in the brain which may not be affected by treatment; such a notion would argue strongly in favor of RCTs with a prophylactic goal.[28] All these considerations may explain why the published clinical trials have not provided irrefutable evidence of efficacy of antiviral therapy.

On the other hand, there is a growing body of evidence supporting structural and cognitive differences between HSV-1 seropositive and seronegative individuals, regardless of SZ status and even in the absence of a prior history of encephalitis.[33] The effects could be attributed to virus-induced neuronal damage, or indirectly through inflammatory cytokines generated by the host in response to infection. Because of the relatively high prevalence of HSV-1 infection, pursuing this line of research, including further RCTs, is a priority from a public health perspective.

REFERENCES

1. Gottesman II, Moldin SO. Schizophrenia genetics at the millennium: cautious optimism. Clin Genet. 1997;52(5):404-7.
2. Khandaker GM, Zimbron J, Lewis G, et al. Prenatal maternal infection, neurodevelopment and adult schizophrenia: a systematic review of population-based studies. Psychol Med. 2013;43(2):239-57.
3. Torrey EF. Stalking the schizovirus. Schizophr Bull. 1988;14(2):223-9.
4. Jones-Brando LV, Buthod JL, Holland LE, et al. Metabolites of the antipsychotic agent clozapine inhibit the replication of human immunodeficiency virus type 1. Schizophr Res. 1997;25(1):63-70.

5. Torrey EF, Leweke MF, Schwarz MJ, et al. Cytomegalovirus and schizophrenia. CNS Drugs. 2006;20(11):879-85.
6. Kukhanova MK, Korovina AN, Kochetkov SN. Human herpes simplex virus: life cycle and development of inhibitors. Biochemistry (Mosc). 2014;79(13):1635-52.
7. Elion GB. The biochemistry and mechanism of action of acyclovir. J Antimicrob Chemother. 1983;12(Suppl B):9-17.
8. DeLisi LE, Goldin LR, Nurnberger JI, et al. Failure to alleviate symptoms of schizophrenia with the novel use of an antiviral agent, acyclovir (Zovirax). Biol Psychiatry. 1987;22(2):216-20.
9. Dickerson FB, Boronow JJ, Stallings CR, et al. Reduction of symptoms by valacyclovir in cytomegalovirus-seropositive individuals with schizophrenia. Am J Psychiatry. 2003;160(12):2234-6.
10. Dickerson FB, Stallings CR, Boronow JJ, et al. Double blind trial of adjunctive valacyclovir in individuals with schizophrenia who are seropositive for cytomegalovirus. Schizophr Res. 2009;107(2-3):147-9.
11. Prasad KM, Watson AM, Dickerson FB, et al. Exposure to herpes simplex virus type 1 and cognitive impairments in individuals with schizophrenia. Schizophr Bull. 2012;38(6):1137-48.
12. Dickerson FB, Boronow JJ, Stallings C, et al. Association of serum antibodies to herpes simplex virus 1 with cognitive deficits in individuals with schizophrenia. Arch Gen Psychiatry. 2003;60(5):466-72.
13. Prasad KM, Shirts BH, Yolken RH, et al. Brain morphological changes associated with exposure to HSV1 in first-episode schizophrenia. Mol Psychiatry. 2007;12(1):105-13.
14. Shirts BH, Prasad KM, Pogue-Geile MF, et al. Antibodies to cytomegalovirus and Herpes Simplex Virus 1 associated with cognitive function in schizophrenia. Schizophr Res. 2008;106(2-3):268-74.
15. Prasad KM, Bamne MN, Shirts BH, et al. Grey matter changes associated with host genetic variation and exposure to herpes simplex virus 1 (HSV1) in first episode schizophrenia. Schizophr Res. 2010;118(1-3):232-9.
16. Watson AM, Prasad KM, Klei L, et al. Persistent infection with neurotropic herpes viruses and cognitive impairment. Psychol Med. 2013;43(5):1023-31.
17. Hamdani N, Daban-Huard C, Godin O, et al. Effects of cumulative Herpesviridae and *Toxoplasma gondii* infections on cognitive function in healthy, bipolar, and schizophrenia subjects. J Clin Psychiatry. 2017;78(1):e18-27.
18. Thomas P, Bhatia T, Gauba D, et al. Exposure to herpes simplex virus, type 1 and reduced cognitive function. J Psychiatr Res. 2013;47(11):1680-5.
19. Yolken RH, Torrey EF, Lieberman JA, et al. Serological evidence of exposure to herpes simplex virus type 1 is associated with cognitive deficits in the CATIE schizophrenia sample. Schizophr Res. 2011;128(1-3):61-5.
20. Prasad KM, Eack SM, Goradia D, et al. Progressive gray matter loss and changes in cognitive functioning associated with exposure to herpes simplex virus 1 in schizophrenia: a longitudinal study. Am J Psychiatry. 2011;168(8):822-30.
21. D'Aiuto L, Prasad KM, Upton CH, et al. Persistent infection by HSV-1 is associated with changes in functional architecture of iPSC-derived neurons and brain activation patterns underlying working memory performance. Schizophr Bull. 2015;41(1):123-32.

22. Roalf DR, Ruparel K, Gur RE, et al. Neuroimaging predictors of cognitive performance across a standardized neurocognitive battery. Neuropsychology. 2014;28(2):161-76.
23. Bhatia T, Wood J, Iyengar S, et al. Emotion discrimination in humans: Its association with HSV-1 infection and its improvement with antiviral treatment. Schizophr Res. 2018;193:161-7.
24. Dickerson F, Stallings C, Sullens A, et al. Association between cognitive functioning, exposure to herpes simplex virus type 1, and the COMT Val158Met genetic polymorphism in adults without a psychiatric disorder. Brain Behav Immun. 2008;22(7):1103-7.
25. Strandberg TE, Pitkala KH, Linnavuori KH, et al. Impact of viral and bacterial burden on cognitive impairment in elderly persons with cardiovascular diseases. Stroke. 2003;34(9):2126-31.
26. Prasad KM, Eack SM, Keshavan MS, et al. Antiherpes virus-specific treatment and cognition in schizophrenia: a test-of-concept randomized double-blind placebo-controlled trial. Schizophr Bull. 2013;39(4):857-66.
27. Gur RC, Ragland JD, Moberg PJ, et al. Computerized neurocognitive scanning: II. The profile of schizophrenia. Neuropsychopharmacology. 2001;25(5):777-88.
28. Breier A, Buchanan RW, D'Souza D, et al. Herpes simplex virus 1 infection and valacyclovir treatment in schizophrenia: Results from the VISTA study. Schizophr Res. 2019;206:291-9.
29. Kern RS, Nuechterlein KH, Green MF, et al. The MATRICS Consensus Cognitive Battery, part 2: Co-norming and standardization. Am J Psychiatry. 2008;165(2):214-20.
30. Nuechterlein KH, Green MF, Kern RS, et al. The MATRICS Consensus Cognitive Battery, part 1: Test selection, reliability, and validity. Am J Psychiatry. 2008;165(2):203-13.
31. Gur RC, Richard J, Hughett P, et al. A cognitive neuroscience-based computerized battery for efficient measurement of individual differences: Standardization and initial construct validation. J Neurosci Methods. 2010;187(2):254-62.
32. Xiao J, Prandovszky E, Kannan G, et al. *Toxoplasma gondii*: Biological parameters of the connection to schizophrenia. Schizophr Bull. 2018;44(5):983-92.
33. Nimgaonkar VL, Bhatia T, Mansour A, Wesesky M, Deshpande SN. Herpes simplex virus type-1 infection: associations with inflammation and cognitive aging in relation to schizophrenia. In: Khandaker G, Meyer U, Jones PJ (Eds). Neuroinflammation and Schizophrenia. Vol. 1. London: Springer; 2018.

CHAPTER 9

Nonpharmacological Therapies for Psychotic Disorders

Jahnavi Kedare, Ruksheda Syeda

INTRODUCTION

Psychotic disorders are characterized by common clinical features such as delusions, hallucinations, and behavioral problems like agitation, aggression, and negative symptoms. These disorders consist of a range of diagnoses from brief psychotic disorder to schizophrenia, schizoaffective disorder, and schizotypal personality disorder. Schizophrenia has always been a challenging disorder to treat because of the complex nature of its symptoms and its chronic and deteriorating course over a period of years.

Before 1950s, i.e. before the discovery of antipsychotic medication, psychoanalytic psychotherapy was the mainstay of treatment of schizophrenia. After antipsychotics came into use, there was an obvious shift in the focus of treatment from psychoanalysis to pharmacotherapy, as it led to improvement in core symptoms of schizophrenia and was cost-effective.

The second shift in management of severe mental illnesses came with deinstitutionalization. The care of the patients shifted to community settings and to families. Problems faced by family members while dealing with patients were recognized. The role of expressed emotions in family interactions also became clearer and hence family interventions were developed which mainly included educating the family members about the illness.

Manfred Bleuler did pioneering work in developing the concept of rehabilitation by engaging patients in meaningful occupations.[1]

Schizophrenia also causes social disability in patients. The onset of schizophrenia is very early, in adolescence, in most of the cases. They have a prolonged course of the disorder; have to be maintained on medications for years; medications themselves have a number of side effects and the illness and the medications lead to cognitive deficits too. Another problem in management of schizophrenia is treatment nonadherence which causes multiple relapses thus worsening the prognosis. All these factors lead to a number of issues. Their education and career decisions get affected by the illness; their peer, family, and social interactions are affected by the illness. They may face social isolation and alienation. The quality of life of the patient suffers.

Hence, the goal of the treatment of schizophrenia or any psychotic disorder cannot remain limited to alleviation of symptoms, that too mainly positive symptoms; but it has to focus on reintegrating the patient in the society. This cannot be achieved merely with pharmacotherapy.

The model of "recovery" helps in understanding this. Recovery has been defined by Patrick Corrigan in two ways. According to the first definition, recovery involves dealing with disabilities caused by serious mental illnesses and the outcome of successful coping is recovery. According to the second definition, creating hope, setting goals, and enabling a person with mental illness involves a process and signifies recovery. Pharmacotherapy with psychosocial interventions in combination leads to recovery.

The first step toward recovery is providing services in an atmosphere of hope. The National Institute for Health and Clinical Excellence (NICE) guidelines stress upon involving all the stakeholders including patients and caregivers; creating optimism in the minds of patients as well as caregivers. Now there is enough evidence to provide non-pharmacological interventions to patients of schizophrenia effectively. The concept of having optimistic atmosphere is an essential component of recovery.[2]

Toward Recovery[3]

- *Connectedness:* To establish social connections and relationships during the process of recovery, as young patients lose out on interpersonal relations during the illness.
- *Hope and optimism:* It is important to promote an optimistic outlook for recovery and a sense of hope for the future for the patients and their family.
- *Establishing and consolidating sense of identity:* To promote in the patient an identity not as a patient of psychosis but as friend, partner, worker or volunteer, sibling or team-mate is important.
- *Meaning and purpose in life:* To help patients get a sense of purpose in life and meaning for the future.
- *Empowerment:* To help patients understand their needs during recovery and to develop skills to fulfill the needs.

Thus, psychosocial interventions for psychotic illnesses are the need of the hour.

AIMS OF NONPHARMACOLOGICAL THERAPIES IN PSYCHOTIC DISORDERS[1]

The main aim of any intervention should be recovery and getting good quality of life for the patient.
- To improve clinical symptoms of schizophrenia, especially those not responding to medication. To decrease the distress associated with psychotic features
- To promote educational recovery

- To decrease depression and social anxiety which patients may develop because of the illness
- To help patients deal with cognitive deficits
- To establish support system and to promote family support
- To help in social integration by decreasing social disability.

Various nonpharmacological methods of interventions in schizophrenia and other psychotic disorders have been described. There is robust evidence for some interventions such as cognitive behavioral therapy (CBT), cognitive remediation, supported employment, and family interventions whereas compliance therapy, avatar therapy, art therapy, etc. still need further research.

PRINCIPLES OF NONPHARMACOLOGICAL THERAPIES[4]

- Psychosocial interventions and pharmacological management are complementary to each other.
- Engagement in therapy and having a good therapeutic relationship with the patient are the requirement of therapy for positive outcome.
- Outcome of therapy is symptom improvement, improvement in functioning, and improved quality of life.
- Defining immediate goals of treatment and long-term goals is essential. The treating psychiatrist involves the patient as well as the caregiver in the process.
- Adequate training of the staff carrying out the intervention is essential.
- Comorbid conditions such as substance use, anxiety, and depression need to be treated simultaneously.

NONPHARMACOLOGICAL THERAPIES FOR SCHIZOPHRENIA

Social integration of the patient suffering from schizophrenia is the ultimate goal of therapy in schizophrenia. This goal can be achieved by treating patient symptomatically, by having strategies for relapse prevention, and encouraging the patient in adaptive functioning. Not many patients achieve baseline functioning. Hence, combining both nonpharmacological and pharmacological treatments leads to maximum outcomes. **Table 1** summarizes various nonpharmacological therapies with their treatment outcomes. **Flowchart 1** gives an outline of psychotherapies used in psychotic disorders.[5]

Family Interventions

Clinical practice guidelines all over the world have described family interventions as the first recommendation.[4]

Treatment programs including family support lead to reduction in the rate of rehospitalization and lead to better social functioning.[5] Similar findings are observed in studies where psychoeducation is an integral part of the

Table 1: Nonpharmacological therapies with areas of improvement.

Therapies	Areas of improvement
Assertive community treatment (ACT)	Reduction in rates of homelessness and length of hospital stays
Cognitive behavioral therapy for psychosis (CBTp)	Decreases in both positive and negative symptoms and mood disturbances, and improved social functioning
Cognitive remediation	Improvements in cognition and psychosocial functioning
Family therapy/psychoeducation	Improvement in social functioning and family coping and empowerment
Peer support and self-help strategies	Enhancement of empowerment and ability to cope with the illness
Social skills training	Improvements in social functioning
Supported employment	Increases in employment rates, hours worked and wages earned. Gains in self-esteem and quality of life

Flowchart 1: Psychotherapies for psychosis.

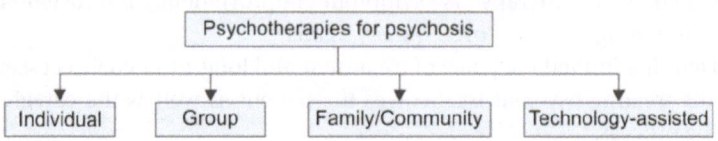

treatment.[6] Evidence shows that such interventions have long-term benefits lasting for more than 5 years.[7] Persons with a first episode of psychosis or recent onset of schizophrenia benefit the most with family psychoeducation. Family members also find psychoeducation to be useful in stress reduction, improving family relationships, dealing with various problems, and facing the responsibility of living with a person with schizophrenia in a better fashion.[8] Families also benefit from participating in multifamily psychoeducation groups. In addition to this, individual interventions may be supplemented to deal with specific issues. Problem-solving exercises are especially useful in this.[9]

There is strong evidence of supporting the role of family interventions as described in NICE and SIGN guidelines. They lead to a better outcome of the illness in terms of symptom reduction, relapses, hospitalizations, and social functioning. Family interventions improve the knowledge of caregivers regarding the illness thus leading to reduction in stress.[4]

Family intervention includes three components. The first component is establishing a therapeutic relationship with the family. During the first episode itself, if all the questions of the family members are addressed, the therapeutic alliance is quite successful. The second component involves educating about the nature of the illness. Several studies have found multifamily group interventions to be effective. This third component constitutes specialized therapeutic techniques for families.[10]

Family intervention addresses following issues:
- Communication skills
- Problem solving
- Psychoeducation
- Crisis management
- Relapse prevention.

Cognitive Behavior Therapy for Psychosis

There is strong evidence in favor of CBT to reduce symptoms, decrease number of hospitalizations and relapses, and also to improve depression. Beck used CBT for psychotic symptoms such as delusions in patients with schizophrenia as early as in 1952.[11]

Studies have shown that adjunctive treatment using cognitive behavioral therapy for psychosis (CBTp) can improve the effectiveness of pharmacotherapy.[12]

Individuals with schizophrenia:
- Draw conclusions based on very little information
- Lack insight about their rashness, and thus consider themselves indecisive
- On the one hand, are not sure whether they are drawing correct conclusions, but on the other hand feel sure about their misinterpretations
- Frequently have attributional biases
- Are often convinced of the accuracy of false recollections.[13]

Cognitive behavioral therapy for psychosis works on these areas.

Cognitive behavioral therapy may be considered when patients have shown partial response to antipsychotic medication, have persistent, distressing symptoms, and have symptoms of anxiety and/or depression. CBT can be started during the acute phase of the illness or during recovery phase; it can be given in outpatient as well as inpatient settings **(Flowchart 2)**.[4]

The CBTp therapist takes an approach of "collaborative empiricism", collaborating with the patient in a relationship of equality. The therapist tries to get an idea about their thoughts, emotions, and experiences.

Yulia Landa describes the CBTp process with the following elements:
- *Engagement*: Empathy, normalization of experiences, and managing ambivalence about therapy.
- *Assessment*: Detailed evaluation of the first episode/s using ABC assessment model and using narrations.

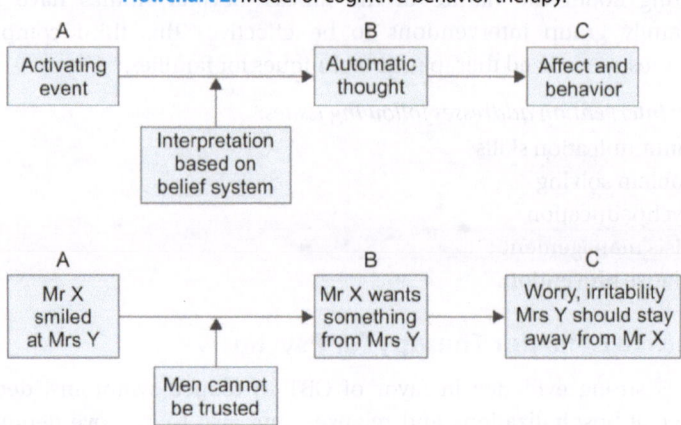

Flowchart 2: Model of cognitive behavior therapy.

- *Formulation*: Involves collecting details of current belief systems and the course of these beliefs in timeline. Formulation helps in understanding the patient's problem(s)/symptom(s).
- *Goals*: Treatment goals are decided on the basis of the formulation of problems faced by the patient.
- *Interventions*: Plan necessary interventions and evaluate their efficacy on the basis of reality testing, reasoning style, presence of automatic thoughts, etc.
- *Relapse work*: Cognitive styles of relapse, evaluation of these, individual patterns of relapse, and necessary interventions.

Metacognitive Training

Based on research about the cognitive processes and biases reported in persons with schizophrenia, Moritz and Woodward developed a novel psychotherapeutic approach called "metacognitive training" (MCT) based on three fundamental components. MCT aims at making patients aware of biases in their cognitions, which are related to their delusions and also at correcting these biases.[13] MCT has three components.

1. *Knowledge translation*: Explaining how cognitive biases may lead to formation of delusions.
2. *Specific exercises*: Aim at making patients aware that their cognitive biases lead to negative consequences.
3. *Alternative thinking strategies*: Help change cognitions so that cognitive biases disappear.[14]

One of the studies has shown that, individual MCT is more efficacious compared to group setting for patients with severe delusions.[15] A meta-analysis showed small to moderate effect sizes for efficacy of MCT on delusions and positive symptoms of schizophrenia.[16]

Cognitive Remediation

Patients of schizophrenia show a number of cognitive deficits. They suffer from attention difficulties, concentration and memory problems, problems in executive functions, information processing, or difficulties organization in thinking. Antipsychotics also lead to cognitive deficits. These deficits further lead to impairment in functioning and social interactions may cause trouble in education or in work and may lead to further social isolation and increasing disability leading to poorer outcomes.

Hence, cognitive remediation should be offered to patients with cognitive deficits. It is a behavioral training-based intervention with an aim to improve cognitive deficits such as information processing speed, attention, memory, executive function, etc.

Table 2 shows cognitive behavior therapies used in psychotic disorders with their group characteristics.

Compliance Therapy

According to Morken G et al., non-adherence rates in schizophrenia range from 37% to 74%.[17] Compliance therapy (Kemp and David) is a cognitive behavior intervention which includes components of psychoeducation, motivational interviewing, and other cognitive therapies. Some studies have shown that compliance therapy is successful in improving insight and compliance in the short-term.

Supported Employment Programs[4]

Vocational rehabilitation forms an important component of management as it helps the patient to live independently. Supported employment programs are available abroad. Occupational or educational activities, including prevocational training, are also useful. Nongovernmental organizations (NGOs) and voluntary organizations may also play a role in providing these.

Table 2: Cognitive remediation therapies.	
Cognitive remediation intervention	*Setting (Individual/Group)*
Integrated psychological therapy (IPT)	Group (6–8)
Integrated neurocognitive therapy (INT)	Group (6–8)
Cognitive remediation therapy (CRT)	Individual
Cogpack	Individual
Cognitive enhancement therapy (CET)	Group
Neuropsychological educational approach to remediation (NEAR)	Individual/Group (3–10)
Neurocognitive enhancement therapy (NET)	Individual/Group
Cognitive adaptation training (CAT)	Individual

Supported employment programs should include creating jobs catering to needs of the individual. Provision of support and availability of mental health services at the workplace should be ensured.

Social Skills Training[4]

Social skills training involves training in interpersonal skills such as conversational skills, making friends, facing job interviews, and assertiveness. This uses principles of learning through modeling, role-playing, and behavioral rehearsal. The technique involves giving a corrective but supportive feedback, and behavioral homework and practice so that the patient can use it in his or her social environment. Social skills training is more used in patients with negative symptoms.

Life Skills Training[4]

Life skills training includes practical aspects of day-to-day life such as dressing up, self-care, household work, and money matters. Life skills training programs consist of a thorough assessment, homework assignments, and feedback.

Patient Education[4]

Educating patients of schizophrenia spectrum disorders about the nature of their disorders, the onset, course, and treatment modalities available has also been found useful. Involving family members in this process is also useful. This helps patients in making informed decisions and empowers them.

Supportive Psychotherapy

Patients with more severe illness were found to tolerate supportive therapy better than insight-oriented therapy. It also improved outcome of illness in these patients.[18] Administering supportive psychotherapy in patients with schizophrenia is challenging and requires a knowledge about the course of the illness and the necessary skills for the therapy to be successful. A good therapeutic alliance between the doctor and the patient has better outcomes with improved compliance to treatment, symptom recovery (particularly negative symptoms), and social functioning.

Assertive Community Treatment

Stein and Test[19] described a community mental health treatment model known as assertive community treatment (ACT). This was especially useful in people with serious mental illness. The goal was to deinstitutionalize and integrate patients with serious mental illness in the society. It is based on the principles of providing integrated services in the community through outreach programs.[20]

NONPHARMACOLOGICAL THERAPIES IN FIRST EPISODE PSYCHOSIS

The focus of research in the last two decades has been on identifying people at risk of developing psychosis and progressing toward schizophrenia. The aim has been to reduce the duration of untreated psychosis so that the outcome of schizophrenia improves.

In many patients of schizophrenia a "prodrome" can be identified retrospectively. In recent years, the concept of "at risk mental state (ARMS)" has developed so that these individuals with a clinical high risk (CHR) are identified early and appropriate interventions are begun for them. Clear criteria have been laid down to identify three syndromal subgroups.[21]

1. *Attenuated positive symptom syndrome (APSS)*: It includes the emergence or worsening of disturbances in thought content, thought processes, or perceptual abnormalities not reaching the level of psychosis in the past year.
2. *Brief intermittent psychotic symptom (BIPS) syndrome*: It requires the presence of any one or more threshold positive psychotic symptoms (unusual thought content, suspiciousness, grandiosity, perceptual abnormalities, and disorganized communication), but these are too brief to meet diagnostic criteria for psychosis.
3. *Genetic risk and deterioration (GRD)*: This requires a combination of both genetic risk (i.e. either schizotypal personality disorder or a first-degree relative with a schizophrenia spectrum disorder) and functional decline.

PSYCHOSOCIAL INTERVENTIONS FOR CLINICALLY HIGH RISK INDIVIDUALS

Individual CBT should be offered to individuals with CHR. Family members may or may not be involved.[22]

If individuals at CHR have functional impairment or cognitive deficits, they may be given social skills training **(Box 1)**.[23,24]

Box 1: Cognitive behavior therapy for clinically high risk individuals.

- Enhancing the understanding of symptoms being experienced
- Challenging delusional thoughts and hallucinations
- Working on coping strategies regarding positive symptoms using techniques such as distraction and withdrawal
- Helping in establishing any relationship between symptoms and stress
- Teaching mastery and pleasure activities and cognitive restructuring of negative and self-defeating cognitions for depressive symptoms
- Teaching stress management techniques and assertiveness training.

First Episode Psychosis

First episode psychosis (FEP) is also an opportunity for early interventions, in the hope of improving the prognosis in these patients and at times even prevention of schizophrenia.

Psychosocial Interventions in FEP

These mainly include CBT.

Patients with FEP are encouraged to alternate ways of thinking and managing stress. Distress due to hallucinations or delusions is qualitatively similar to that caused by anxiety or depression. Hence, similar strategies are useful for these psychotic experiences too. These cognitive strategies include identifying triggers or precipitants, appraisal of the triggers, emotional, and behavioral responses to those and learning to modify them. Coping mechanisms such as normalizing, distraction, reality testing, self-talk, relaxation, acceptance, etc. should be taught to the patients.[25-27]

Two studies have examined the role of CBT in the acute phase—"the study of cognitive realignment therapy in early schizophrenia, or SoCRATES study[28] and the active cognitive therapy for early psychosis, or ACE project" **(Box 2)**.

Box 2: Studies for the role of cognitive behavior therapy.

SoCRATES model
Intense treatment during the acute phase: 15–20 hours within a 5-week treatment period, with booster sessions at 2 weeks, and 1, 2, and 3 months.
- Therapeutic engagement
- Detailed assessment of mental state and symptom dimensions
- Cognitive behavioral case formulation using the stress–vulnerability model to explain the biological and psychological basis
- Enlisting problems, deciding priorities according to associated distress
- Cognitive intervention by generating alternative hypotheses for abnormal beliefs and hallucinations, attempting to reduce distress associated with symptoms
- Continuous monitoring

Improvement in symptoms noted even at 18 months.

ACE project[28]
Providing cognitive therapy to young people in the acute phase of illness—maximum of 20 sessions of therapy over 14 weeks.
- Creating a hierarchy of presenting problems such as positive psychotic symptoms, comorbidities like anxiety, depression, negative symptoms, issues of identity
- Modules from the cognitively oriented psychotherapy for early (COPE) psychosis intervention
- Engagement into a therapeutic relationship
- Assessment of the patient in terms of his psychotic experience and explanation of the disorder
- *Adaptation*: Helping in recovery by reducing distress associated with altered self-perception post-psychosis and the possibility of ongoing vulnerability

---

(ACE:[28] Active Cognitive Therapy for Early Psychosis; SoCRATES: Study of Cognitive Realignment Therapy in Early Schizophrenia)

Other therapies described for treatment of schizophrenia include:
- Milieu therapy
- Psychodynamic psychotherapy
- Arts therapy
- Avatar therapy.

USE OF INFORMATION AND COMMUNICATION TECHNOLOGY

People's lives have changed in recent years because of tremendous developments in information technology (IT). IT has changed the way people take help and seek information about various health issues. People with psychosis are also making use of IT in a similar way (National Alliance on Mental Illness, 2011; Ennis, 2012; Aref-Adib, 2016; Firth, 2016).[29] This has encouraged the therapists to use information and communication technology (ICT) in this group. **Table 3** depicts the possible therapeutic benefits of using technology for therapy.[29]

Telepsychiatry

Telepsychiatry has been used effectively in mental health delivery, helping overcome barriers of access and affordability. Using various methods of videoconferencing, a physician in a remote place can seek expert opinion about a case, including an interview of the patient by the psychiatrist and provide diagnosis and medications. Telepsychiatry is especially handy for follow-up session. Mobile telepsychiatry units are equipped with a consultation room, videoconferencing gadgets, and a dispensing pharmacy making access easy.

Short Message Service (Text Message) Use

Telephone or short message service (SMS) exchanges with treating mental health professional may be useful. The aim of these exchanges will be to improve compliance to medication, helping in developing coping strategies,

Table 3: Use of technology and possible clinical benefits.	
Telepsychiatry	Access to care, compliance
SMS (text message) use	Compliance, support
Computer/web-based programs	Psychoeducation, interventions
Online counseling	Interventions
Smart device (phones and tabs) use	Routine care, tracking, support
Virtual reality (Avatar therapy)	Intervention
Augmented reality	Intervention
Therapeutic serious games	Motivation, compliance

and dealing with real-life problems faced by patients. This may improve the outcome of the disease; however, further research is needed in the field.[30]

Computer/Web-based Programs

A number of programs are available for patients and caregivers for various psychosocial interventions. Research has shown that web-based psychoeducation is useful. It is acceptable to patients and caregivers and is effective for people of various ages and stages of illness.[31]

Online Counseling

Cognitive behavioral therapy for psychosis is recommended to all schizophrenia spectrum disorder by NICE. CBTp can be offered online with trained counselors. Convenient scheduling and privacy improve treatment adherence. There are a few options available for cognitive rehabilitation therapies for cognitive deficits in psychosis. The use of computer software makes it easy to administer therapy through a variety of rewards, accurate feedback, and varying levels of complexities of tasks.[32] Amongst the interventions using ICT, computer-assisted cognitive remediation therapy (CACRT) has proven to be efficacious.[29]

Smart Devices (Phones and Tablets) Use

Smart phones are owned by many psychotic patients and more so by younger patients. Evidence suggests that people with psychosis increasingly own smartphones. Around 69% of patients with first-episode psychosis have an internet-enabled mobile device.[33] Several applications for psychosis have been developed, and results suggest that they are acceptable and feasible. Applications can help with routine care, medication tracker, low-level support, and CBT strategies for managing distress. Fitness applications are growing in popularity and these can be a more acceptable form of passive data collection while helping tackle obesity and cardiometabolic health.

Virtual Reality

Despite treatment, approximately 25% of people with psychotic conditions continue to experience hallucinations.[34]

Julian Leff in 2008 invented a new and innovative approach called Avatar therapy for auditory hallucinations. An audio-visual representation of the voice(s) is created. This represents the voice of the "persecutor". A face-to-face interaction between the patient and the voice of the "persecutor" is brought about through digital creations called "avatar". The therapist speaks in his own voice as well as in the voice of the "persecutor". The patient gradually establishes a relationship with the persecutor and gains control in it. After an initially promising pilot trial, Tom Craig and colleagues conducted a pilot study with "Avatar therapy" and have reported a reduction in auditory hallucinations.

Augmented Reality

O'Hanlon et al. in their review article on therapeutic use of technology in psychosis define augmented reality as "a perception of the real world that is augmented or supplemented by computer-generated stimuli. Computer-generated graphics and sounds are merged with objects and/or locations in the real world, and/or information in the form of text or speech is overlayed onto the user's visual field enhancing the real-world environment".[29] It has been proposed that this technology can be used in treatment of hallucinations and cognitive and social functioning. It could also be used in social rehabilitation or cognitive remediation therapy (CRT) with the help of providing reminders, instructions, etc.

Therapeutic Serious Games

Serious games are video games with a primary purpose other than pure entertainment. Techniques like daily "quests" and reward systems such as "boosters" or "extra lives" in a game—could be used as positive reinforcements in e-interventions for psychosis and these may improve adherence to these intereventions.[29] Therapeutic serious games in the form of "personalized fantasy gaming" have been used in study of cognitive training for adults with schizophrenia or schizoaffective disorder. It was found that this gaming helped in improving attention, motivation, and learning related to the cognitive task.[35]

Internet-based interventions are futuristic interventions and have the potential to provide cost-effective, nonstigmatizing, and ongoing support to people with psychosis.

There can be some disadvantages in internet-based interventions as it may increase social isolation, may not lead to a good therapeutic relationship, and at times wrong advice may be given in unmonitored groups. However, it must be remembered that these techniques may be popular in near future.[36]

NONPHARMACOLOGICAL BIOLOGICAL THERAPIES

Nonpharmacological biological therapies need to be discussed as they also form an important component of management of schizophrenia.

Electroconvulsive Therapy

Electroconvulsive therapy (ECT) has been recognized as an effective treatment option in the treatment of acute schizophrenia.[37] However, it is mainly indicated in treatment-resistant schizophrenia (TRS). It is considered as a treatment modality after an adequate trial with two different antipsychotics as well as clozapine when such treatment has proved to be ineffective or the patient has not been able to tolerate such treatment.[38] In such patients, a combination of ECT with pharmacotherapy can be useful.[39] Authoritative international guidelines do not generally recommend ECT for schizophrenia. Nevertheless, the American guidelines advocate the use of ECT as a first choice if fast clinical improvement is necessary or ECT was effective in a previous episode of the illness. The Royal College (UK) guidelines; however, suggest ECT in schizophrenia only in the fourth line, in TRS patients nonresponsive to clozapine. NICE guidelines allow ECT in schizophrenia only in acute, pharmacotherapy-resistant catatonia.[40] In several countries, particularly in the developing world, schizophrenia remains the first indication for ECT. According to Chanpattana et al., 36.5% of schizophrenia patients are treated with ECT in India[41] and in other studies, in some other countries including Thailand, Fiji Islands, Japan, Hungary, and the Chuvash Republic of the Russian Federation, ECT is mainly used in the treatment of schizophrenia. There may be efficacy of ECT in some clinical conditions loosely-linked schizophrenia particularly severe catatonia, NMS, and postpartum psychoses.[40]

Repetitive Transcranial Magnetic Stimulation

Application of low frequency repetitive transcranial magnetic stimulation (rTMS) at the junction of left temporal and parietal cortices may reduce resistant hallucinations. Daily prefrontal rTMS may lead to an improvement in negative symptoms of schizophrenia. Other neurostimulation methods have yet not been found to be useful in schizophrenia.[40]

Transcranial Direct Current Stimulation

The use of transcranial direct current stimulation (tDCS) is still in research stage, although there is some preliminary evidence that it may be useful in the treatment of auditory hallucinations and probably in negative symptoms.[10]

Vagus Nerve Stimulation

Recent functional magnetic resonance imaging (fMRI) studies showed the resting-state hyperactivity of the hippocampus to be predictive of poor cognition in schizophrenia patients.[42] Previous studies have also demonstrated increased hippocampal blood flow, blood volume, and hyperactivity during sensory processing in schizophrenia. This has led to a hypothesis that hippocampal hyperactivity may be a biomarker for cognitive deficits in the illness.[43] Reduced nicotinic and/or GABAergic signaling leading to loss of inhibitory signaling in the hippocampus results in sensory filtering deficits in psychosis.

Vagus nerve stimulation (VNS) studies have demonstrated decreased hippocampal activity (independent of the pathological state) of the patient.

VNS effects on neurotransmitters are:
- Increased release of norepinephrine
- Increased acetylcholine release
- Increased serotonin release affecting the hippocampal activity, and thus showing improvement in verbal recognition, attention, memory consolidation, and executive function.[44]

Despite its potential to improve cognition in schizophrenia, to our knowledge, no study has yet examined the clinical or physiological effects of VNS in patients with schizophrenia.[44]

CONCLUSION

The take-home message is that psychological interventions are gradually establishing themselves as effective treatments for psychotic symptoms. They also help in improving our understanding of the psychopathology of the illness. In our country clinicians perceive the need for nonpharmacological interventions of psychotic disorders. However, there are difficulties in providing these psychosocial interventions effectively. They are inadequacy of resources, lack of training, and time constraints. Various methods may be employed to overcome these problems, e.g. conducting group therapy sessions instead of individual sessions and using home-based paper-pencil tests for cognitive remediation instead of computer-based interventions. It is also important to include modules related to psychosocial interventions in the curriculum of mental health professionals.[45] An attitudinal change toward psychosocial interventions and an optimistic approach while treating patients with schizophrenia spectrum disorder will be the path toward recovery.

REFERENCES

1. Kuipers E, Yesufu-Udechuku A, Taylor C, et al. Management of psychosis and schizophrenia in adults: summary of updated NICE guidance. BMJ. 2014; 348:g1173.
2. Corrigan PW. Recovery from schizophrenia and the role of evidencebased psychosocial interventions. Expert Rev Neurother. 2006;6(7):993-1004.
3. Leamy M, Bird V, Le Boutillier C, et al. Conceptual framework for personal recovery in mental health: systematic review and narrative synthesis. Br J Psychiatry. 2011;199(6):445-52.
4. Norman R, Lecomte T, Addington D, et al. Canadian treatment guidelines on psychosocial treatment of schizophrenia in adults. Can J Psychiatry. 2017; 62(9):617-23.
5. Crismon L, Argo TR, Buckley PF. Schizophrenia. In: DiPiro JT, Talbert RL, Yee GC, Matzke GR, Wells BG, Posey LM (Eds). Pharmacotherapy: A Pathophysiologic Approach, 9th edition. New York: McGrawHill; 2014. pp. 1019-46.

6. Chien WT, Leung SF, Yeung FK, et al. Current approaches to treatments for schizophrenia spectrum disorders, part II: Psychosocial interventions and patientfocused perspectives in psychiatric care. Neuropsychiatr Dis Treat. 2013;9: 1463-81.
7. Sellwood W, Wittkowski A, Tarrier N, et al. Needsbased cognitive-behavioural family intervention for patients suffering from schizophrenia: 5year followup of a randomized controlled effectiveness trial. Acta Psychiatr Scand. 2007;116(9): 447-52.
8. Dixon LB, Dickerson F, Bellack AS, et al.; Schizophrenia Patient Outcomes Research Team (PORT). The 2009 schizophrenia PORT psychosocial treatment recommendations and summary statements. Schizophr Bull. 2010;36(1):48-70.
9. Breitborde NJ, Moreno FA, MaiDixon N, et al. Multifamily group psychoeducation and cognitive remediation for first-episode psychosis: a randomized controlled trial. BMC Psychiatry. 2011;11:9.
10. Galletly C, Castle D, Dark F, et al. Royal Australian and New Zealand College of Psychiatrists clinical practice guidelines for the management of schizophrenia and related disorders. Aust N Z J Psychiatry. 2016;50(5):410-72.
11. Beck AT. Successful outpatient psychotherapy of a chronic schizophrenic with a delusion based on borrowed guilt. Psychiatry. 1952;15(3):305-12.
12. Wykes T, Steel C, Everitt B, et al. Cognitive behaviour therapy for schizophrenia: effect sizes clinical models, and methodological rigor. Schizophr Bull. 2008;34(3): 523-37.
13. Jiang J, Zhang L, Zhu Z, et al. Metacognitive training for schizophrenia: a systematic review. Shanghai Arch Psychiatry. 2015;27(3):149-57.
14. Moritz S, Woodward TS. Metacognitive training in schizophrenia: from basic research to knowledge translation and intervention. Curr Opin Psychiatry. 2007; 20(6):619-25.
15. van Oosterhout B, Krabbendam L, de Boer K, et al. Metacognitive group training for schizophrenia spectrum patients with delusions: a randomized controlled trial. Psychol Med. 2014;44(14):3025-35.
16. Eichner C, Berna F. Acceptance and efficacy of metacognitive training (MCT) on positive symptoms and delusions in patients with schizophrenia: a meta-analysis taking into account important moderators. Schizophr Bull. 2016;42(4):952-62.
17. Morken G, Widen JH, Grawe RW. Non-adherence to antipsychotic medication, relapse and rehospitalisation in recent onset schizophrenia. BMC Psychiatry. 2008;8:32.
18. Gunderson JG, Frank AF, Katz HM, et al. Effects of psychotherapy in schizophrenia: II. Comparative outcome of two forms of treatment. Schizophr Bull. 1984; 10(4): 564-98.
19. Stein LI, Test MA. Alternative to mental health treatment. I. Conceptual model, treatment program, and clinical evaluation. Arch Gen Psychiatry. 1980;37(4): 392-7.
20. Bond GR, Drake RE. The critical ingredients of assertive community treatment. World Psychiatry. 2015;14(2):240-2.
21. Lecomte T, Abidi S, Garcia-Ortega I, et al. Canadian treatment guidelines on psychosocial treatment of schizophrenia in children and youth. Can J Psychiatry. 2017;62(9):648-55.

22. Addington J, Addington D, Abidi S, et al. Canadian treatment guidelines for individuals at clinical high risk of psychosis. Can J Psychiatry. 2017;62(9):656-61.
23. Ellis A. Rationalemotive therapy: research data that supports the clinical and personality hypotheses of RET and other modes of cognitive-behavior therapy. Couns Psychol. 1977;7(1):242.
24. Morrison AP, French P, Parker S, et al. Three-year follow-up of a randomized controlled trial of cognitive therapy for the prevention of psychosis in people at ultrahigh risk. Schizophr Bull. 2006;33(3):682-7.
25. Hughes A, Macneil C, Francey S, et al. Psychological Intervention: Why, How and When to use in Early Psychosis. Melbourne: Orygen (The National Centre of Excellence in Youth Mental Health); 2015.
26. Lewis S, Tarrier N, Haddock G, et al. Randomised controlled trial of cognitive behavioural therapy in early schizophrenia: Acute-phase outcomes. Br J Psychiatry Suppl. 2002;43:s917.
27. Haddock G, Lewis S. Psychological interventions in early psychosis. Schizophr Bull. 2005;31(3):697-704.
28. Haddock G, Tarrier N, Morrison AP, Hopkins R, Drake R, Lewis S. A pilot study evaluating the effectiveness of individual inpatient cognitive-behavioural therapy in early psychosis. Social Psychiatry and Psychiatric Epidemiology. 1999; 34(5):254-8.
29. O'Hanlon P, Aref-Adib G, Fonseca A, et al. Tomorrow's world: current developments in the therapeutic use of technology for psychosis. BJ Psych Adv. 2016;22(5):301-10.
30. Kasckow J, Felmet K, Appelt C, Thompson R, Rotondi A, Haas G. Telepsychiatry in the assessment and treatment of schizophrenia. Clin Schizophr Relat Psychoses. 2014;8(1):21-27A
31. van der Krieke L, Wunderink L, Emerencia AC, de Jonge P, Sytema S. E-mental health self-management for psychotic disorders: state of the art and future perspectives. Psychiatric Services. 2014;65(1):33-49.
32. Grynszpan O, Perbal S, Pelissolo A, Fossati P, Jouvent R, Dubal S, et al. Efficacy an specificity of computer-assisted cognitive remediation in schizophrenia: a meta analytical study. Psychol Med. 2011;41(1):163-73.
33. Stanmore E, Stubbs B, Vancampfort D, et al. The effectiveness of active video games on cognitive functioning in clinical and non-clinical populations: a meta-analysis of randomized controlled trials. Neurosci Biobehav Rev. 2017;78:34-43.
34. Aleman A, Larøi F. Insights into hallucinations in schizophrenia: novel treatment approaches. Expert Rev Neurother. 2011;11(7):1007-15.
35. ÁlvarezJiménez M, Gleeson JF, Bendall S, et al. Internetbased interventions for psychosis: a sneak-peek into the future. Psychiatr Clin North Am. 2012;35(3): 735-47.
36. Freeman CP (Ed). The ECT Handbook: The Second Report of the Royal College of Psychiatrists' Special Committee on ECT. London: Royal College of Psychiatrists; 1995.
37. Scott AI. College guidelines on electroconvulsive therapy: an update for prescribers. Adv Psychiatr Treat. 2005;11(2):150-6.
38. Gazdag G, KocsisFiczere N, Tolna J. The augmentation of clozapine treatment with electroconvulsive therapy. Ideggyogy Sz. 2006;59(78):261-7.

39. Gazdag G, Ungvari GS. Non-pharmacological biological therapies in schizophrenia. Neuropsychopharmacol Hung. 2011;13(4):233-8.
40. Chanpattana W, Kunigiri G, Kramer BA, et al. Survey of the practice of electroconvulsive therapy in teaching hospitals in India. J ECT. 2005;21(2):100-4.
41. Tregellas JR, Smucny J, Harris JG, et al. Intrinsic hippocampal activity as a biomarker for cognition and symptoms in schizophrenia. Am J Psychiatry. 2014; 171(5):549-56.
42. Tregellas JR. Neuroimaging biomarkers for early drug development in schizophrenia. Biol Psychiatry. 2014;76(2):111-9.
43. Vonck K, Raedt R, Naulaerts J, et al. Vagus nerve stimulation...25 years later! What do we know about the effects on cognition? Neurosci Biobehav Rev. 2014;45: 63-71.
44. Smucny J, Visani A, Tregellas JR. Could vagus nerve stimulation target hippocampal hyperactivity to improve cognition in schizophrenia? Front Psychiatry. 2015;6:43.
45. Kumar D. Psychosocial interventions in schizophrenia: a survey of clinical training and clinicians' opinions in India. Psychosis. 2018;10(1):22-37.

CHAPTER 10

Interventions for Personality Disorders

Ashlesha Bagadia

INTRODUCTION

Personality disorders (PD) are common but remain poorly understood in clinical practice, despite a large amount of work being done in this area over the last decade. Historically in India, personality disturbance would be brought to the attention of health professionals, only if the severity was high or if there was comorbidity. But as mental health awareness increases, peoples in the subcontinent are more likely to present to psychiatrists with behavioral disturbances resulting from a range of severity in personality disorders. Due to the pervasive and enduring nature of the disorder, and most marked disturbance in the interpersonal domain, people with personality disorder can often generate a lot of negative emotions in the treating psychiatrists. In this context, it is very important for us to better understand the psychopathology of these disorders and become aware of the evidence-based interventions that may help in our own clinical practice. This article will briefly outline personality and its dysfunction, then highlight interventions that can be broadly useful for personality disorders in general. More attention will be given to interventions and strategies that can be useful for borderline personality disorder, as it is the most common condition to present and often the most difficult to treat with traditional methods.

Personality can be understood as the integration of behavior patterns, determined by individual temperament, capacities, character, and internalized value systems. For a normal personality structure, three key aspects of life need to be organized to a reasonable level of functioning:[1]
1. A coherent sense of self and significant others which help in forming their core identity and affect interpersonal interactions.
2. A broad spectrum of affective response and regulation which can vary through a complex range of emotions without the loss of impulse control.
3. Presence of an integrated value system which is mature and internalized, not rigidly tied to nor likely to change frequently in response to external relations.

PERSONALITY DISORDER

Keeping the above in mind, personality disorder can be understood as a dysfunction in any or all of the above aspects, with most people lying on a continuum; ranging from being reasonably well-functioning exhibiting only traits or being at the severe end, affecting all capacity to function normally. Patients may also shift on the continuum, able to function through some aspects of their life except during crises when they move to the severe end, and revert back to baseline when the crisis is resolved.[2]

CLASSIFICATION

There are many systems that are used to classify personality disorders, with ongoing debates regarding the accuracy and applicability of these classifications. One of the most widely used is the categorical classification system that uses clear operational criteria defined by behavioral elements, as outlined in the Diagnostic and Statistical Manual of Mental Disorders-V (DSM-V) and International Classification of Diseases-10 (ICD-10) classification manuals: Cluster A—odd/eccentric: Paranoid, schizoid, and schizotypal; cluster B—dramatic: Antisocial, borderline, histrionic, and narcissistic; and cluster C—anxious/fearful: Avoidant, dependent, and obsessive/compulsive.[3]

Besides the categorical approach, ICD-11 suggests a dimensional perspective that should also be considered as it gives a quantitative understanding of severity and allows for inclusion of comorbidities and symptom overlap between the various categories. Patients may not present with a neat set of symptoms that fit into one category alone (For example, refer to the case in **Box 1**).

ASSESSMENT

An important start to management of personality disorder is a comprehensive assessment. A clinical interview with robust history taking can give valuable information that goes beyond diagnosis; it can help understand the

> **Box 1:** Case vignette.
>
> Miss CS is a 34-year-old woman who lives with her parents. She presented with mood swings and multiple conflicts in all her interpersonal interactions, stemming from her teenage years. She was married briefly and moved overseas with her husband, but reported to have become very suspicious of his nature, unable to trust him, and feeling like he is always putting her down. She ended up returning back home soon after and getting a divorce. Since then, any wedding in the family would upset her and she thought everyone was talking behind her back because she was a divorcee. She was querulous at work and not able to hold a job because she would easily get emotionally dysregulated and fight back angrily when she was questioned or reprimanded. She complained that even the smallest of problems would overwhelm her easily and had consistent thoughts of suicide. A careful history revealed many features of borderline personality disorder with a significant overlap with paranoid personality disorder, but not fulfilling the full criteria for a single personality disorder. There was no overt psychosis or evidence of other comorbid conditions.

motivation to seek help, rule out comorbidity, and help align the right treatment to the patient. It can give an opportunity to study the patient's interaction and response to the assessor and any reciprocal emotional response generated in the assessor, all of which can be helpful in understanding the diagnosis, engaging the patient, and setting the foundation for future therapeutic alliance. Apart from the standard interview schedule, some of the key points to remember during assessment are:

- Plenty of time should be set aside for the assessment interview. Often a series of interviews may be necessary; it is not recommended to confirm a diagnosis of personality disorder on a cross-sectional interview.
- Collateral from family members, friends, and significant others must be obtained and attempts must be made to educate and engage them in the treatment plan.
- The interview should include exploration of maladaptive behaviors, its effect on the individual and others, attitudes and relationships with others, and social functioning in all areas of the person's life over a prolonged period of time.[3]
- Apart from eliciting symptoms, questions should be targeted toward documenting the patient's own understanding of severity and what aspect of their life causes them the most distress. This can help in preparing collaborative treatment goals that are realistic and helpful.
- A comprehensive risk assessment should also be completed that covers risk of self-harm and harm to others, risks from comorbidities, and potential triggers that could lead to a crisis.
- Involving the patient in understanding their diagnosis and treatment options is proven to be beneficial. Clinicians are often reluctant to directly give patient a diagnosis of personality disorder, but evidence suggests that informing them and giving sound psychoeducation can itself help reduce their symptoms and improve long-term engagement.[4]

One of the limitations of a clinical interview is the reliability of the patients account; some may exaggerate their symptoms while others may minimize them. It is useful to support a clinical interview with an interview tool. There are many interview schedules, structured and semi-structured that have reasonable evidence in assessment of personality disorders.[3] However, they are time-consuming and are more likely to overdiagnose if used in isolation. Formalized interview schedules can be a barrier to developing a rapport and engaging the patient, so it should be used as an adjunct to, and not in place of, the clinical interview. Following are the interview schedules that can be used: International Personality Disorder Examination, Diagnostic Interview for DSM-IV Personality Disorders, Structured Interview for DSM-IV Personality Disorders, Structured Clinical Interview for DSM-IV Axis I Disorders, Personality Disorder Interview-IV, Personality Diagnostic Questionnaire, Standardized Assessment of Personality, Personality Assessment Schedule,

Schedule for Normal and Abnormal Personality, Personality Assessment Inventory, Minnesota Multiphasic Personality Inventory-II, Millon Clinical Multiaxial Inventory-III, Eysenck Inventory Questionnaire, NEO Five-Factor Inventory, Rorschach test, and Thematic Apperception Test.

GENERAL PRINCIPLES OF MANAGING PERSONALITY DISORDER

Several different service models are described in Western populations which may or may not be applicable to majority of the Indian clinicians. Psychiatrists often work in isolation and can be the sole practitioner looking after the patients and caring for their families. A divided functions approach where psychiatrists work along with psychologists and social workers is possible in an institutional setting or in a group practice.[5] Referral to a specialist team that exclusively works with personality disorder is less commonly available in India. Whatever the setting, some basic principles of managing personality disorder should be kept in mind as follows:

- *Treatment plan*: All patients should have a shared treatment plan which includes medication management, psychotherapy plan, crisis management, and access to acute inpatient care. Clearly outlined steps that will be taken during instances of self-harm or attempted suicide can reassure the patient, but also provide structure to the psychiatrist during crisis.
- *Engagement*: A considerable part of the initial phase of treatment should be spent on engaging the patient. It may involve helping them to stabilize social aspects of care, such as living arrangements and engaging families or addressing comorbid substance abuse or active mental illness. Attempts should be made to ensure that treatment is accessible and appointments are at times acceptable to both the patient and the treatment plan. Roles of each of the clinicians involved should be clearly defined, including what they will not be able to do (e.g. psychologist will not be involved in medication management, who will be the designated person to contact in crises, etc.). The initial part of the engagement should be spent on formulating their disorder and helping them to recognize and manage their frustration or impulsivity as it arises. A clear pathway to care during crisis is also crucial to engagement (Refer crisis plan in **Box 2**).
- *Consistency*: Providing consistent care to patients with challenging behaviors can be difficult. Limiting the care of the patient to only those people whose roles and tasks are clear that can reduce inconsistency (for example, clearly defining the role of the inpatient psychiatrist from that of the outpatient psychiatrist, designating therapy to a specific clinician, etc.). Steps should be taken to see if there are disagreements in the team that is contributing to the inconsistency or whether it is due

> **Box 2:** Crisis plan of Miss CS.
>
> - Demographic and contact details: ....
> - Contact details of next of kin: ....
> - Current self-harming behaviors: ....
> - Triggers/stressors: ....
> - Examples of crisis situations: ....
> - Current coping mechanisms: ....
> - Helpful people to contact in crises: ....
> - Specified clinician to be contacted in the times of crises: ....
> - Plan for support by phone during the crisis: (Designated clinician for crisis support, duration of each call, and designated time slots for the call)
> - Plan for time-limited hospital admission: (Encourage brief hospital stays only in the times of extreme crises)
> - Alternate crisis management plan: (Any other reasonable strategies that have helped the patient in the past)
> - List of helplines, nearby hospitals, and other resources that can be used in times of crises.

to the internal pathology of personality disorder which can often result in splitting between the different clinicians.[5] Often these patients would have had inconsistent care in their formative years, hence it becomes even more important to provide consistent care, which can also help in setting boundaries and sustaining engagement.

- *Constancy*: Patients with borderline personality disorder are most sensitive to changes in the professionals. It can reawaken feelings of loss, rejection, and abandonment. As far as possible, senior clinicians who are less likely to move between jobs, and have more experience with difficult patients, should take up long-term care of these patients. Even otherwise, clinicians should take extra care in reducing abrupt changes, abrupt termination, or unplanned handover to other clinicians.
- *Inpatient care*: Despite evidence suggesting that hospital admissions should be avoided at all costs for personality disorder, sometimes they can be the most effective way of managing a crisis. Other indications for hospital admissions are for a comprehensive assessment and diagnosis, managing comorbidity, reducing risk to others, and stabilizing medication. Bateman and Tyrer suggest some guidelines for inpatient care of personality disorders **(Box 3)**.[5]

> **Box 3:** Principles of admission to a general psychiatric ward of a PD patient.
>
> - Informal, with patient-determined admission and discharge
> - Organized around specific goals agreed between the patient, psychiatrist, and nursing staff
> - Arranged with the clear agreement of nursing staff
> - Brief, time-limited, and goal-determined—the patient may be discharged if the goals of admission are not met

Medication Management

There is a significant role of pharmacotherapy for management of personality disorder, but often it is limited to addressing behavioral clusters and comorbidities. There is no robust evidence for any particular medication that is directly indicated for treatment of specific personality disorder and psychiatrists must use their clinical judgment to prioritize the problem area that needs to be addressed first. Borderline personality disorder is the most studied for pharmacotherapy as these patients are more likely to seek medications.[6] Whereas those with schizoid or schizotypal, personality resist drug therapy so there is limited evidence in their management. One of the major factors to bear in mind is access to medication for those with suicidal ideas. Shorter duration of prescriptions with weekly pickup from their pharmacy, or supervised access with the help of family members, is encouraged.

Antidepressants

Selective serotonin reuptake inhibitors (SSRIs) are the most researched and commonly prescribed in borderline personality disorder. Apart from treating comorbid depression or anxiety, there is also evidence to suggest a reduction in aggression, irritability, mood instability, and self-harming behaviors after treatment with SSRIs. Although there are also reports of SSRIs causing an increase in suicidal thoughts, which must be kept in mind while prescribing these drugs.

Mood Stabilizers

These are also commonly prescribed and help manage emotional dysregulation, irritability, impulsivity, and recurrent depression. Lithium is often used to reduce suicidality and aggressive or assaultative behavior.[7,8] Small studies show some efficacy with the use of carbamazepine and sodium valproate.

Antipsychotics

Although the direct evidence of efficacy in personality disorders is very limited, regular use of atypical antipsychotics is also advised in reducing paranoid thoughts, impulsivity, and other psychotic symptoms.[9] Doses of the antipsychotics are usually lower than those used for severe mental disorders, except when indicated by severity of the psychosis.

Substance Abuse

Appropriate treatment for substance withdrawal, treatment of cravings, and maintaining substitution should be undertaken as indicated. Benzodiazepines should be prescribed judiciously and only restricted to intermittent use, as there is a high risk of misuse and dependency and some evidence of increased risk of disinhibition. There is no evidence to prove its efficacy in management of personality disorders.

Psychotherapy

Psychotherapy remains the fundamental intervention to address the psychopathology in personality disorder. Most of the advances in psychotherapy in the last 2 decades have been in the management of borderline personality disorder. Traditional psychotherapy relied on long-term engagement, dynamic interpretations of object relations, allowing for internal fantasies is usually highly speculative and based on therapist experience. Over the years, there has been a move from speculative to explorative, time-limited, and structured therapies. Therapies are goal-directed and focused on reducing dysfunctional behaviors. Therapies that are effective remain focused and moved from exploring pathology to developing resilience. Outlined below are key principles of some of the therapies with the most successful outcomes in management of borderline personality disorder.

Dialectical Behavior Therapy

Developed by Marsha Linehan, originally for women who self-harm, dialectical behavior therapy (DBT) evolved into a comprehensive program as a skill-based therapy for borderline personality disorder.[10,11]

Theoretical framework: Based on biosocial theory, Linehan suggested that patients are born with a genetic vulnerability, which, when coupled with an invalidating social environment can lead to the development of personality disorder. She defined invalidating environments as those where communication of private experiences are met by erratic, inappropriate, and extreme responses such as in cases of physical, sexual, and emotional abuse, neglect, substance abuse in the caregiver, perfectionism—overemphasis on control and high expressed emotion. Effects of invalidating environment can be not having any labels for emotional experiences; patients learn self-invalidation; extreme displays are very strongly rewarded; emotional inhibition is encouraged; reduced sense of self; impaired problem-solving skills and poor distress tolerance; unrealistic goals, and expectations. Linehan used principles of change through cognitive behavioral therapy (CBT) and added elements of acceptance and mindfulness, this creating a dialectic between acceptance and change which is the central tenet of DBT.

Principles of therapy: Therapy is divided into two stages: Stage 1 is focused on social skills training that helps to reduce self-harming behaviors, therapy-interfering behaviors, and increase behaviors that improve quality of life. Stage 2 is focused on addressing longer-term goals such as reducing post-traumatic stress disorder (PTSD), increasing self-respect, and achieving

> **Box 4:** Case vignette.
>
> A 19-year-old TS presented with self-harming behavior in the form of cutting and severe mood swings, since she started failing in her 12th standard examinations repeatedly over the last 3 years. She was described as a bright student who could not cope with the excess pressure from school and family to constantly perform well. Family was supportive and caring, but there was no room for being "emotionally weak". Through individual DBT, using mindfulness, she was able to start regulating her emotions, she used distress tolerance skills to use alternate methods of managing distress, and stopped self-harming. Interpersonal skills helped her to communicate better with her parents and talk about her aims and goals more realistically

life goals. A comprehensive DBT model includes engagement in individual as well as group therapy for 1–2 years.[12] Group therapy is used to educate the patients in social skills through four modules:
1. Emotional regulation
2. Distress tolerance
3. Interpersonal interaction
4. Mindfulness.

Individual therapy is used to reinforce these skills and reduces self-harming behaviors. Some of the key strategies used in DBT are behavioral chain analysis of self-destructive behavior, looking at alternative more adaptive behaviors, solution analysis, and validation techniques (Refer to case example in **Box 4**).

Mentalization-based Therapy

Developed by Anthony Bateman and Peter Fonagy, mentalization-based therapy (MBT) is an amalgamation and further development of elements of psychodynamic principles and structured therapy.[13]

Theoretical framework: The borderline pathology is conceptualized as emerging from disruption in attachment systems in early years. Children develop internal working models through initial attachment systems. Secure attachment leads to better self-soothing and self-regulating of emotions; a good enough caregiver reflects on infants intentions accurately and does not overwhelm the infant. Consistent secure care enables the child to understand others emotions and learn from them: through contingent marked mirroring (basis for affect regulation). Disorganized/insecure attachment leads to patients vacillating between intimacy and autonomy and a limited ability to understand their own mental states and those of others.

Normal mentalizing: Mentalization is a realistic perception of our own mental functioning. The ability to consider what is happening in the *mind* of the other and not just focus on behaviors, with an appreciation of changeability. It is the ability to adequately reflect on past, present, or future events, with regulated emotions.

Nonmentalizing modes: Patients with personality disorder are more likely to lose their reflective functioning and slip into nonmentalizing modes which are specifically defined in MBT as:
- Psychic equivalence (thoughts are held with the conviction of being the only reality, intolerance to alternate perspectives *she always neglects me*, or *this is the only way I will be able to calm down*).
- Pretend mode (no bridge between inner world and outer reality; endless inconsequential talk of thoughts and feelings but linked with emptiness and dissociation).
- Teleological stance (ability to consider the mind of others through physical constructs, only actions with physical impact are perceived to affect the mental state, self-harming, or reliance on medication to self-soothe).

Principles of therapy: Evidence suggests a combination of individual and group therapy along with psychiatric support for at least 12-18 months has the most favorable outcome for patients.[13] The central aim is to enable the patients to identify when they are not mentalizing and to increase their reflective functioning capacity. Using narratives of examples from their own life events therapy is first focused on regulation of arousal, followed by identification of nonmentalizing modes, empathic validation, and targeted interventions aiming to restore mentalizing.

There is emerging evidence for MBT in treatment of antisocial personality disorder and other mental disorders (Refer to **Box 5**).

Schema-focused Therapy

Developed by Jeffrey Young combining principles of CBT, gestalt therapy, and psychoanalytical object relations.[14]

Theoretical framework: Patients with personality disorders develop maladaptive schema, identification of which can help change the behavior patterns. If a patient's basic emotional needs (connection, mutuality, reciprocity, flow, and autonomy) are not met in childhood, then schemas, coping styles, and modes (mind states) can develop in a dysfunctional

---

Box 5: Case vignette.

A 27-year-old BR had been struggling with alcohol dependence since the last 6 years, after the passing of her mother. She had a poor relationship with her since childhood and was unable to process the range of thoughts and emotions following her demise. Apart from managing the alcohol dependence, therapy was used to explore breakdown in her mentalization whenever she interacted with people who triggered her attachment insecurity and the conflicting emotions that were emerging in response to her mother's death. Through MBT, she was able to hold the conflicting emotions together and appreciate their changeability, which in turn helped her to be more reflective the next time she felt threatened.

maladaptive manner leading to the personality disorder.[14] Changing cognitive patterns linked to the schema can develop adaptive patterns of behavior. Schemas are defined into five main domains, which are further expanded into more narrow schemas:
1. Disconnection/rejection
2. Impaired autonomy/performance
3. Impaired limits
4. Other directness
5. Overvigilance/inhibition.

Modes are defined as momentary mind states triggered by unpleasant or threatening stimuli. Young, Klosko, and Weishaar defined 10 modes, grouped into four categories:
1. Child modes *(vulnerable child, angry child, impulsive/undisciplined child, and happy child)*
2. Dysfunctional coping modes *(compliant surrenderer, detached protector, and overcompensator)*
3. Dysfunctional parent modes *(punitive parent* and *demanding parent)*
4. Healthy adult mode.

Principles of therapy: Schema-focused therapy (SFT) uses three basic techniques—(1) cognitive, (2) experiential, and (3) behavioral. Experiential techniques expand on Gestalt therapy using empty chair techniques and other forms of psychodrama. The aim is to identify the dysfunctional schema and guides the patient to developing more mature behavioral schemas. SFT is delivered in individual and group therapy format for 1–2 years duration.

Transference-focused Psychotherapy

Developed by Otto Kernberg and his team, this is fundamentally structured around a psychoanalytical and object relations framework.[15]

Theoretical framework: Kernberg suggested that a break in object relations at an early age leads to patients holding unreconciled and contradictory representations of self and significant others. This leads to a split between positive and negative image of self.

Principles of therapy: Transference-focused psychotherapy (TFP) is also highly structured delivered as twice weekly therapy, where the split sense of self is reintegrated using transference and countertransference to understand the splits. Once they are able to internalize stable object relations, they are able to have a more coherent sense of self, better regulate their emotions, and also improve their external relationships. Although studied more extensively for treatment of borderline personality disorder, TFP has also been manualized for treatment of narcissistic personality disorder, but more research needs to be done to determine its efficacy.

> **Box 6:** Principles to enhance therapeutic alliance with PD patients.
>
> - Patients want to improve
> - They are doing the best they can
> - They need to do better, try harder, and be more motivated to change
> - Patients may not have caused all their problems but they have to solve them any way
> - Their lives are unbearable as they are currently being lived
> - They need to learn new behaviors in relevant context
> - Treatment should be administered as a real relationship between equals
> - Principles of behavior are universal affecting therapists no less than patients
> - Therapists need support
> - Therapists can fail
> - Therapy can fail even when therapists do not.

Traditional psychodynamic therapy and psychoanalysis remain as therapies that can help integrate the self in patients with personality disorders and there is still robust evidence for therapeutic communities, which may be difficult to implement in a low-resource setting, but has sustained outcomes in the community. The initial phase of dysregulation and disengagement seems to be better managed with the abovementioned structured therapies.[16]

Self-care for psychiatrists: Apart from assessing the treatability of the patient, clinicians should also assess their ability to take on challenging patients, especially when they are highly dysregulated or engaging in high-risk behaviors. Some principles that can help empathize and improve therapeutic alliance with patients are outlined in **Box 6**.[11]

Working with personality disorders is a lengthy process and can be very challenging. Clinicians should ideally be supported by regular supervision and group discussions with peers and team members. Being genuine and honest in therapy can reduce the feeling of constantly walking on eggshells. Clinicians should plan for ways to manage their own anxiety during confrontations. There should be space and time for personal reflection or therapy, which can help manage conflicting feelings of guilt and anger.

With the new interventions showing better outcomes and an improved prognosis, managing patients with personality disorder need no longer be something that is dreaded in clinical practice. It can help reduce the overall burden of care on the society and be rewarding to the practitioner.

CONCLUSION

Personality disorders are common but remain mostly inconspicuous, undetected, and poorly understood. It is often associated with other co-morbid psychiatric disorders. They are poorly responsive to standard modes of therapeutic interventions, even though they are responsible for lot of suffering to self and also others in the immediate social milieu. This provides the rationale for a separate discourse and independent evaluation of therapeutic options for personality disorders. Managing a case of personality disorder would require and stretch almost all the therapeutic skills that a psychiatrist may possess along with taking help of from allied mental health professional, making a shared treatment plan and observing the principles of engagement, consistency and constancy. Drugs and psychotherapy, both are required. In fact psychotherapy itself has evolved substantially in the process of trying to make it suitable for patients of personality disorder. These patients need to be taken care of not only to reduce the suffering of the individual but also to reduce the burden of care on the society.

REFERENCES

1. Yeomans FE, Clarkin JF, Kernberg OF. Transference-Focused Psychotherapy for Borderline Personality Disorder: A Clinical Guide. Washington: American Psychiatric Association Publishing; 2015.
2. Tyrer P, Reed GM, Crawford MJ. Classification, assessment, prevalence, and effect of personality disorder. Lancet. 2015;385:717-26.
3. Banerjee PJM, Gibbon S, Huband N. Assessment of personality disorder. Adv Psychiatr Treatment. 2009;15:389-97.
4. Biskin RS, Paris J. Diagnosing borderline personality disorder. CMAJ. 2012;184: 1789-94.
5. Bateman AW, Tyrer P. Services for personality disorder: organisation for inclusion. Adv Psychiatr Treatment. 2004;10:425-33.
6. Tyrer P, Bateman AW. Drug treatment for personality disorders. Adv Psychiatr Treatment. 2004;10:389-98.
7. Tyrer P. Drug treatment of personality disorder. Psychiatr Bulletin. 1998;22:242-4.
8. Davison SE. Principles of managing patients with personality disorder. Adv Psychiatr Treatment. 2002;8:1-9.
9. Walker C, Thomas J, Allen TS. Treating impulsivity, irritability, and aggression of antisocial personality disorder with quetiapine. Int J Offender Ther Comp Criminol. 2003;47:556-67.
10. Linehan M. Cognitive-behavioral Treatment of Borderline Personality Disorder. New York: Guilford Press; 1993.
11. Salsman NL, Linehan MM. Dialectical-behavioral therapy for borderline personality disorder. Primary Psychiatr. 2006;13:51-8.
12. Linehan M. DBT® Skills Training Manual. New York: Guilford Publications; 2014.
13. Bateman A, Fonagy P. Handbook of Mentalizing in Mental Health Practice. Washington: American Psychiatric Publishing; 2012.
14. Young JE, Klosko JS, Weishaar ME. Schema Therapy: A Practitioner's Guide. New York: Guilford Press; 2003.
15. Kernberg OF. Psychotherapeutic treatment of borderline patients. Psychother Psychosom Med Psychol. 1995;45:73-82.
16. Kernberg OF. New developments in transference focused psychotherapy. Int J Psychoanal. 2016;97:385-407.

CHAPTER 11
Critical Overview of Polypharmacy Debate

Sai Spoorthy Mamidipalli, Sai Krishna Tikka, Mohd Aleem Siddiqui

INTRODUCTION

The problem with the psychiatric classificatory systems is that they are still based on identification of symptom clusters to label a particular diagnosis. These diagnostic categories have overlapping symptoms, syndromes and thus lack validity.[1] Psychiatrists are not still fortunate enough because these syndromes and symptoms cannot be reduced to single biological markers based on the existing research.[2]

Psychiatrists often land up in treating these disorders with more than one medication as they target the symptoms and this practice of prescribing multiple medications in a broader sense is termed "polypharmacy."[3] Though considered irrational by most clinicians, it is a double-edged sword particularly in psychiatric illnesses. The problem with the drugs currently used in the management of these disorders is that of their limited action at receptor sites, adverse effect profile, and limited efficacy.[4]

DEFINITION AND CLASSIFICATION

Polypharmacy in the context of psychiatric disorders has been defined differently by different authors. The lack of consistency in the definition is based on two factors, one is the number of medications to be considered and the second is the diagnosis. However, the most agreed upon definitions about polypharmacy are—the process of combining two or more psychiatric medications in a given patient, or using two or more medication with similar pharmacological action to treat the same condition.[4]

Briefly, polypharmacy is classified into:
- Minor, moderate, and major
- Validated, empirical, and irrational
- Same-class, multi-class, adjunctive, augmentative, and total
- Therapeutic and counter-therapeutic.

For description of these classifications for polypharmacy, please refer to Nizamie and Tikka (2015).[5]

We try to emphasize the evidence base available for polypharmacy practices in various psychiatric disorders while providing a framework to limit the use of polypharmacy just when it seems irrational.

DEPRESSION

Only 42–46% of individuals with major depressive disorders, who receive treatment, achieve remission, approximately 30% of them will not remit even after adequate trials of multiple antidepressants.[6]

The STAR*D (Sequenced Treatment Alternatives to Relieve Depression) trial and American Psychiatric Association Practice guidelines suggest that patients in several phases of treatment resistance show improvement with combination or augmentation therapies.[7] Though some trials showed that combination therapy with two antidepressants was more effective than monotherapy,[8,9] the Combining Medications to Enhance Depression Outcomes Study did not find any differences between monotherapy and combination therapy.[10] These trials are not free of limitations—insufficient duration and lower doses of monotherapy agents.[11]

Various synergists are used in the treatment of depression in combination with an antidepressant. As per a review done by Tundo et al., 2015,[12] aripiprazole has the highest degree of evidence from controlled studies. As per this review, other antipsychotics (APs) such as quetiapine, olanzapine (with fluoxetine) showed favorable results in combination. These findings were in contrast to that of another review[13] which suggested that there was no difference in efficacy between different APs used for augmentation.

Bauer et al., 2010[14] in their meta-analysis found significantly greater response rate in the lithium group. However, Connolly and Thase (2011)[15] question its generalizability stating lithium is only effective for use in combination with tricyclic antidepressants (TCAs). Though clinicians prefer to use lithium conveniently for augmentation purposes, available evidence is contradictory.[16] While trials on pindolol have failed to replicate positive effects, there is no consensus of the role of buspirone, mifepristone, and methylphenidate. The effect of estrogen augmentation seems to be more limited to women in menopausal age group.[17]

The use of combination of TCAs and monoamine oxidase inhibitors (MAOIs) is not encouraged due to the risk of serotonin syndrome. Despite the multiple options in the treatment of resistant depression, the evidence base for effectiveness is available only for a few drugs and use of other drugs in combination therapies will add to adverse effects and placebo response.

SCHIZOPHRENIA

Even in the CATIE (Clinical Antipsychotic Trials of Intervention Effectiveness) trial, it was noted that before entering into the study most patients were on polypharmacy.[18] Despite the development of second generation APs with their unique "intramolecular polypharmacy" the unmet needs for these patients remain high.

In patients with schizophrenia, practice guidelines too do not indicate combination treatments except while switching from one to another. Even the Texas Medication Algorithm[19] project proposes the use of AP polypharmacy at stage 4, after failure of monotherapy with three APs.

Clozapine is the most common AP for which the studies on combination therapy are available. A meta-analysis by Correll et al., 2009[20] suggested the efficacy of clozapine plus another AP drug. Inclusion of small number of trials, variable study methods, lack of data on adverse effects, and studies limited to specific geographic region limit the generalizability of the findings.

In non-clozapine AP polypharmacy and multiple studies have suggested favorable results for either adding aripiprazole or switching to it from olanzapine, risperidone, and quetiapine only with respect to the improvement in metabolic parameters but not related to efficacy.[21,22]

Summarizing the data from the meta-analysis by Galling B et al., 2017,[23] the difference in efficacy between monotherapy and combination therapy was only restricted to low-quality studies but was not seen in high-quality studies.

None of the existing studies suggests any positive evidence for combination therapy with antidepressants or benzodiazepines. Among mood stabilizers (MS) randomized controlled data is available for valproate and carbamazepine, but not for lithium.[24-26] Augmentation agents such as beta-blockers, anti-inflammatory agents, antidepressants, and glutamatergic agents did not show much benefit in schizophrenia patients.[20]

BIPOLAR DISORDERS

The use of more than one MS is considered appropriate early in the course of treatment of bipolar disorder.[6] The need for the polypharmacy is almost equal in both acute and maintenance phases, because of the need for rapid symptom reduction in the former and prevention of relapse, treatment of residual symptoms in the latter.

Mania

Most treatment guidelines recommend monotherapy as the first option, and reserve combination therapy, for when patients do not respond to monotherapy.

A meta-analysis done by Ogawa et al., 2014[27] found out that in patients who did not respond to the first agent (MS or AP), combination/augmentation of MS and AP was more effective than either drug alone but was associated with more side effects. Such effects were demonstrated for haloperidol, olanzapine, risperidone, and quetiapine when administered as cotherapy compared with monotherapy with lithium or valproate.[28]

Bipolar Depression

Though antidepressants are most frequently prescribed, evidence-based recommendations are inconclusive. So far fluoxetine has the best evidence in combination with olanzapine. Although some guidelines recommend the use of selective serotonin reuptake inhibitors or bupropion in combination with antimanic agents as first-choice treatment, others do not. None of the guidelines recommends use of antidepressants beyond acute phase.[29]

Controlled trials of antidepressant treatment have drawn inconsistent conclusions of some showing effectiveness and some no benefit compared to monotherapy.[30]

The categories of evidence for pharmacological treatment of acute bipolar depression as per meta-guidelines[31] are mentioned in **Table 1**.

Prophylaxis

Combination treatment and polypharmacy are the most common choices concerning relapse prevention. Positive placebo-controlled randomized controlled trials (RCTs) exist for combination treatments of MS—valproate

Table 1: Evidence level for various combinations in bipolar depression.	
Combination/Augmentation treatments	*Category of evidence*
Olanzapine + Fluoxetine	B
Lamotrigine + Lithium	B
Modafinil + Ongoing treatment	B
N-acetylcysteine + Lithium or Valproate	B
Sertraline + Lithium or Valproate	C
Tranylcypromine + Ongoing treatment	C
Venlafaxine + Lithium or Valproate	C
L-thyroxine + Ongoing treatment	C
Topiramate + Lithium or Valproate	C
Zonisamide + Lithium or Valproate	C
Imipramine + Lithium	D
Inositol + Lithium or Valproate	D
Omega-3 fatty acids + Lithium or Valproate	D
Paroxetine + Lithium or Valproate	D
Bupropion + Lithium or Valproate	D
Gabapentin + Ongoing treatment	D
B: Limited positive evidence from controlled studies; C: Evidence from uncontrolled studies; D: Inconsistent results	

+ lithium,[32] valproate or lithium, with all atypical APs that have a license for bipolar maintenance treatment—aripiprazole, quetiapine, risperidone, and ziprasidone.[33]

Real world patients are virtually impossible to capture in a guideline whose focus is the efficacy of a given combination treatment. These limitations should be kept in mind when interpreting data of randomized controlled combination maintenance studies.[33]

ANXIETY DISORDERS

Combination of both pharmacological and nonpharmacological treatments shows superior efficacy in the treatment of anxiety disorders overall. However, the response rates are highly variable and majority patients suffer from residual symptoms.[34] Combination therapy with antidepressants and benzodiazepines is effective only in the initial 4 weeks in several anxiety disorders.[35-38] Augmentation with drug from different class is broadly supported by research suggesting the involvement of multiple neurotransmitters in anxiety disorders. **Table 2** outlines evidence for combination/augmentation agents in various anxiety disorders.[35,39]

Table 2: Treatment of resistant anxiety disorders.		
Disorder	*Drugs used in augmentation/combination*	*Evidence*
Obsessive compulsive disorder	Antipsychotics (Haloperidol > Risperidone > Quetiapine > Olanzapine)	Positive evidence from controlled studies
	Lithium + Clomipramine Thyroxine + Clomipramine Buspirone	Limited evidence
	SRI + Morphine	Inconsistent
	Pindolol + SSRI + L-tryptophan	Uncontrolled studies
Generalized anxiety disorder	SSRI + Atypical antipsychotic (Olanzapine/Risperidone)	Limited positive from controlled studies
Panic disorder	SSRI + Pindolol SSRI's + TCAs SSRI's + Olanzapine Valproate + Clonazepam	Positive Limited positive from uncontrolled studies
Post-traumatic stress disorder	SSRI + Prazosin SSRI + Olanzapine SSRI + Risperidone Imipramine + Clonidine SSRI + Gabapentin	Limited positive Limited positive Inconsistent Limited positive evidence from uncontrolled studies
Social anxiety	Paroxetine + Pindolol	Limited negative evidence from controlled studies
	SSRI + Buspirone	Limited positive evidence from uncontrolled studies

(SRI: serotonin reuptake inhibitor; SSRI: selective serotonin reuptake inhibitor; TCAs: tricyclic antidepressants)

SUBSTANCE USE DISORDERS

Alcohol Use Disorders

All the anticraving agents in the treatment of alcohol dependence such as naltrexone, acamprosate, and baclofen have shown only low-medium efficacy in reducing drinking as per recent systematic reviews and meta-analysis.[40,41] Some evidence suggests disulfiram use in combination with either acamprosate or naltrexone as a second-line treatment.[42] Though clinicians follow the technique of combining acamprosate and naltrexone in patients with failed treatment with either drug alone, a recent COMBINE trial; however, failed to prove that combination was better.[43]

Apart from relapse prevention, in the treatment of alcohol withdrawal delirium/hallucinosis, combination therapies have been tried. APs were used in combination with benzodiazepines for acute agitation in alcohol withdrawal delirium and related psychosis, no data from randomized-controlled studies is present.[44]

Opioid Use Disorders

The combination with highest evidence in the treatment of opioid use disorders is that of buprenorphine–naloxone as a substitution therapy. Though recent RCTs have shown the efficacy of combination is similar to methadone, it has superior efficacy compared to naltrexone.[45,46] Combination of buprenorphine plus naloxone and methadone plus lofexidine has also been used in detoxification for opioid dependence.[47] In patients who present in opioid intoxicated state and having comorbid benzodiazepine use, combining naloxone and flumazenil was significantly effective.[48] Combining clonidine and naltrexone for rapid detoxification is considered safe and effective.[49]

GERIATRIC POPULATION

Polypharmacy is a rule rather than exception in elderly population. They are vulnerable to morbidity and mortality due to age-related pathophysiological changes, comorbidity, changing pharmacokinetics and pharmacodynamics, and increased susceptibility to side effects.[50] The main addition to the updated version of the Beers criteria was the inclusion of section on drug-drug interaction.[51] The society recommends strongly against the use of TCAs, paroxetine, short- and intermediate-acting benzodiazepines alone or in combination in elderly patients. First- and second-generation APs are to be avoided in dementia or delirium unless nonpharmacological management fails or is not possible and there is risk of harm to self or others. This was due to the increased risk of cerebrovascular accident, greater cognitive decline, and mortality in these patients.

Controlled trials in dementia were done to look for the efficacy of combination of memantine with various cholinesterase inhibitors and galantamine. But the results from these studies have been inconclusive. There is some negative evidence from open studies on the effect of donepezil and gingko biloba combination.[52-54]

CHILD POPULATION

The use of pharmacological agents in this subgroup has been increasing amidst low effectiveness. The number of FDA (Food and Drug Administration)-approved drugs considered to be safe and effective in children are methylphenidate, dextroamphetamine, imipramine, sertraline, fluoxetine, and fluvoxamine.

Regarding polypharmacy, American Academy of Child and Adolescent Psychiatry supports judicious use of combined medications, keeping such use to clearly justifiable clinical circumstances.[55] In children, same-class polypharmacy is rare, and multi-class polypharmacy is used, but the data is limited. To date, the worldwide prevalence of psychiatric polypharmacy in children and adolescent population is 2-9-27%. Antidepressants are the most commonly coprescribed drugs followed by attention deficit and hyperactivity disorder (ADHD) medications, APs, MSs, and benzodiazepines.[56] Recent report as per Olashore et al., 2017[57] showed rates as high as 29.2%.

In children and adolescents diagnosed with bipolar disorder and ADHD, combining methylphenidate with lithium or valproate seemed to improve ADHD symptoms compared to combining it with aripiprazole.[57]

RATIONALIZATION OF POLYPHARMACY

Zigman et al., 2012[58] have suggested certain strategies for reduction of irrational polypharmacy **(Box 1)**.

Werder and Preskorn, 2007[59] suggested adding TIDE approach to SAIL protocol[60] (**S**imple drug regimens, know **A**dverse effects, use drugs with clear **I**ndications, and keep a **L**ist of all medications) to avoid negative consequences of polypharmacy.

Thorough evaluation of the patient's clinical and drug history is of utmost importance and clinicians should assess the compliance before going ahead

---

Box 1: Strategies for reduction of irrational polypharmacy.

- Avoiding pharmacodynamic redundancy
- Avoiding multifunctional medications
- Avoid pharmacokinetic interactions
- Avoid pharmacodynamic interactions
- Avoid inadequate dosing
- Avoid incomplete clinical assessment and judgment issues.

with polypharmacy in poor responders. Measures such as the Naranjo nomogram may be used to assess the causality of adverse effects. It is also important to note that the chances of precipitating idiosyncratic reactions are increased exponentially when practicing polypharmacy.[61]

Polypharmacy justification checklist was developed by Dr Clif Tennison. It is a 38-item checklist which targets nine domains (see review by Nizamie and Tikka, 2015).[6]

INDIAN CONTEXT

The available Indian studies show rates of polypharmacy ranging from 9% to 73%.[62,63] Because of the restriction of these studies to a particular geographical area generalizability of these findings is questionable. Indian psychiatric society has formulated certain guidelines for combination therapies in various disorders. Some comments are made on these treatment regimens due to lack of clear-cut recommendations **(Table 3)**.

Table 3: Data on polypharmacy regimens in the Indian Psychiatric Society Treatment Guidelines.		
Year	Disorder	Existing evidence and comments
2017	Schizophrenia[64]	• Adjunctive medications recommended: Lithium carbonate, antidepressants, benzodiazepines, and anticonvulsants • Recommend these drugs for use with proper rationale and shortest possible duration—limited efficacy • Combination antipsychotics—reserved for clozapine non-responders
2017	Depression[65]	• Strategies for treatment non-response • Augmentation first (Lithium > Thyroid > Stimulants > Buspirone) • Combination therapy—second antidepressant from a different class • An SSRI combined with a TCA/Bupropion—SSRI • TCA with MAO inhibitor, in severe resistant cases
2017	Bipolar disorder[66]	• Mania • Lithium or valproate plus an antipsychotic suggest greater efficacy than with these agents alone • Depression • Use of antidepressants along with mood stabilizers is superior to use of mood stabilizer alone; bupropion—lowest risk of switch • Paroxetine to be avoided • Maintenance phase • Severe cases—combination of valproate and lithium • Reassess continued use of antipsychotic in patients on mood stabilizer + antipsychotic combination • Discontinue antidepressants once depression remits • Combination therapy only for patients who have not responded to monotherapy

Contd...

Contd...

Year	Disorder	Existing evidence and comments
2014–15	Alcohol use disorders[67]	Data from animal studies suggest: Combination of disulfiram + naltrexone, acamprosate + naltrexone are more effective than monotherapy
2014–15	Opioid use disorders[67]	• In the management of withdrawal, medications such as clonidine, benzodiazepines, NSAIDs or a combination • Rapid detoxification: Naloxone in combination with clonidine and/benzodiazepines • Buprenorphine and naloxone combination utilized for maintenance therapy
2018	Dementia[68]	• Nonavailability of agents with robust effectiveness and issues related to tolerability • Combination of donepezil and memantine—approved for moderate to severe Alzheimer's dementia • Combination therapy should be individually tailored • Trials of low dose antipsychotics (risperidone, quetiapine, olanzapine), mood stabilizers (divalproex, carbamazepine), and SSRIs for behavioral symptoms—but limited effectiveness
2017	Elderly depression[69]	• Options for augmentation/combination strategies same as that of adult depression • Limited studies evaluating efficacy • Lithium preferred • Some data supports aripiprazole augmentation to venlafaxine
2018	Psychosis in elderly[70]	• If agitation is severe enough to cause harm to self/others—combination of benzodiazepines and the typical/atypical antipsychotics • Refractory cases may be tried on a combination of clozapine + amisulpride, lithium augmentation, citalopram + methylphenidate, modafinil + fluoxetine or mirtazapine, dexamethasone plus any antidepressant
2008	Depression in children and adolescents[71]	Recommendation for adults with TRD applicable
2008	ADHD[72]	Combined pharmacotherapy only to be used when at least two agents (methylphenidate and dexamphetamine) fail

(ADHD: attention deficit and hyperactivity disorder; MAO: monoamine oxidase; NSAID: nonsteroidal anti-inflammatory drugs; SSRI: selective serotonin reuptake inhibitor; TCA: tricyclic antidepressant; TRD: treatment-resistant depression)

CONCLUSION

A traditional view that polypharmacy should always be considered irrational is fast changing. It should be used in a judicious way based on clinical judgment as most patients with psychiatric disorders do not improve completely with monotherapies. But clinicians need to be active in monitoring the adverse effects, minimizing the number of drugs as and when needed for patients on polypharmacy. Evidence needs to be weighed against the clinical demand of individual patient to opt for polypharmacy.

REFERENCES

1. Prakash OM. Poly-pharmacy in psychiatry: a debatable contemporary practice? Not much evidence. Afr J Psychiatry (Johannesbg). 2011;14(5):410.
2. Möller HJ, Seemüller F, Schennach-Wolff R, et al. History, background, concepts and current use of comedication and polypharmacy in psychiatry. Int J Neuropsychopharmacol. 2014;17(7):983-96.
3. Freudenreich O, Kontos N, Querques J. Psychiatric polypharmacy: a clinical approach based on etiology and differential diagnosis. Harv Rev Psychiatry. 2012;20(2):79-85.
4. Kukreja S, Kalra G, Shah N, et al. Polypharmacy in psychiatry: a review. Mens Sana Monogr. 2013;11(1):82-99.
5. Nizamie SH, Tikka SK. Rational polypharmacy in psychiatry. In: Badria FA (Ed). Evidence-based Strategies in Herbal Medicine, Psychiatric Disorders and Emergency Medicine. Rijeka, Croatia: InTech Publishers; 2015. pp. 75-99.
6. Frye MA, Ketter TA, Leverich GS, et al. The increasing use of polypharmacotherapy for refractory mood disorders: 22 years of study. J Clin Psychiatry. 2000;61(1): 9-15.
7. Si T, Wang P. When is antidepressant polypharmacy appropriate in the treatment of depression? Shanghai Arch Psychiatry. 2014;26(6):357-9.
8. Nelson JC, Mazure CM, Jatlow PI, et al. Combining norepinephrine and serotonin reuptake inhibition mechanisms for treatment of depression: a double-blind, randomized study. Biol Psychiatry. 2004;55(3):296-300.
9. Blier P, Ward HE, Tremblay P, et al. Combination of antidepressant medications from treatment initiation for major depressive disorder: a double-blind randomized study. Am J Psychiatry. 2010;167(3):281-8.
10. Rush AJ, Trivedi MH, Stewart JW, et al. Combining medications to enhance depression outcomes (CO-MED): acute and long-term outcomes of a single-blind randomized study. Am J Psychiatry. 2011;168(7): 689-701.
11. Rush AJ. Combining antidepressant medications: a good idea? Am J Psychiatry. 2010;167(3):241-3.
12. Tundo A, de Filippis R, Proietti L. Pharmacologic approaches to treatment resistant depression: evidences and personal experience. World J Psychiatry. 2015;5(3):330-41.
13. Nelson JC, Papakostas GI. Atypical antipsychotic augmentation in major depressive disorder: a meta-analysis of placebo-controlled randomized trials. Am J Psychiatry. 2009;166(9):980-91.
14. Bauer M, Adli M, Bschor T, et al. Lithium's emerging role in the treatment of refractory major depressive episodes: augmentation of antidepressants. Neuropsychobiology 2010;62(1):36-42.
15. Connolly KR, Thase ME. If at first you don't succeed: a review of the evidence for antidepressant augmentation, combination and switching strategies. Drugs. 2011;71(1):43-64.

16. Moret C. Combination/augmentation strategies for improving the treatment of depression. Neuropsychiatr Dis Treat. 2005;1(4):301-9.
17. Liu P, He FF, Bai WP, et al. Menopausal depression: comparison of hormone replacement therapy and hormone replacement therapy plus fluoxetine. Chin Med J (Engl). 2004;117(2):189-94.
18. Chakos MH, Glick ID, Miller AL, et al. Baseline use of concomitant psychotropic medications to treat schizophrenia in the CATIE trial. Psychiatr Serv. 2006;57(8):1094-101.
19. Argo TR, Crismon ML, Miller AL, Moore TA, et al. Texas Medication Algorithm Project Procedural Manual: Schizophrenia Algorithm. Austin, TX: Texas Department of State Health Services; 2008.
20. Correll CU, Rummel-Kluge C, Corves C, et al. Antipsychotic combinations vs monotherapy in schizophrenia: a meta-analysis of randomized controlled trials. Schizophrenia Bull. 2009;35(2):443-57.
21. Stroup TS, McEvoy JP, Ring KD, et al.; Schizophrenia Trials Network. A randomized trial examining the effectiveness of switching from olanzapine, quetiapine, or risperidone to aripiprazole to reduce metabolic risk: Comparison of antipsychotics for metabolic problems (CAMP). Am J Psychiatry. 2011;168(9):947-56.
22. Kane JM, Correll CU, Goff DC, et al. A multicenter, randomized, double-blind, placebo controlled, 16-week study of adjunctive aripiprazole for schizophrenia or schizoaffective disorder inadequately treated with quetiapine or risperidone monotherapy. J Clin Psychiatry. 2009;70(10):1348-57.
23. Galling B, Roldán A, Hagi K, et al. Antipsychotic augmentation vs. monotherapy in schizophrenia: Systematic review, meta-analysis and meta-regression analysis. World Psychiatry. 2017;16(1):77-89.
24. Leucht S, McGrath J, Kissling W. Lithium for schizophrenia. Cochrane Database Syst Rev. 2003;(3):CD003834.
25. Leucht S, Helfer B, Dold M, et al. Carbamazepine for schizophrenia. Cochrane Database Syst Rev. 2014;(5):CD001258.
26. Schwarz C, Volz A, Li C, et al. Valproate for schizophrenia. Cochrane Database Syst Rev. 2008;(3):CD004028.
27. Ogawa Y, Tajika A, Takeshima N, et al. Mood stabilizers and antipsychotics for acute mania: a systematic review and meta-analysis of combination/augmentation therapy versus monotherapy. CNS Drugs. 2014;28(11):989-1003.
28. Grande I, Vieta E. Pharmacotherapy of acute mania: monotherapy or combination therapy with mood stabilizers and antipsychotics? CNS Drugs. 2015;29(3):221-7.
29. Vieta E, Valentí M. Pharmacological management of bipolar depression: acute treatment, maintenance, and prophylaxis. CNS Drugs. 2013;27(7):515-29.
30. Sidor MM, Macqueen GM. Antidepressants for the acute treatment of bipolar depression: a systematic review and meta-analysis. J Clin Psychiatry. 2011;72(2):156-67.
31. Grunze H, Vieta E, Goodwin GM, et al.; WFSBP Task Force on Treatment Guidelines for Bipolar Disorders. The World Federation of Societies of Biological Psychiatry (WFSBP) Guidelines for the Biological Treatment of Bipolar Disorders: Update 2010 on the treatment of acute bipolar depression. World J Biol Psychiatry. 2010;11(2):81-109.

32. Geddes JR, Goodwin GM, Rendell J, et al.; BALANCE Investigators and Collaborators. Lithium plus valproate combination therapy versus monotherapy for relapse prevention in bipolar I disorder (BALANCE): A randomised open-label trial. Lancet. 2010;375(9712):385-95.
33. Grunze H, Vieta E, Goodwin GM, et al.; WFSBP Task Force on Treatment Guidelines for Bipolar Disorders. The World Federation of Societies of Biological Psychiatry (WFSBP) guidelines for the biological treatment of bipolar disorders: Update 2012 on the long-term treatment of bipolar disorder. World J Biol Psychiatry. 2013;14(3):154-219.
34. Pallanti S, Hollander E, Bienstock C, et al.; International Treatment Refractory OCD Consortium. Treatment non-response in OCD: Methodological issues and operational definitions. Int J Neuropsychopharmacol. 2002;5(2):181-91.
35. Delini-Stula A, Holsboer-Trachsler E. Treatment strategies in anxiety disorders—an update. Ther Umsch. 2009;66(6):425-31.
36. Bandelow B, Zohar J, Hollander E, et al. World Federation of Societies of Biological Psychiatry (WFSBP) guidelines for the pharmacological treatment of anxiety, obsessive-compulsive and post-traumatic stress disorders—first revision. World J Biol Psychiatry. 2008;9(4):248-312.
37. Pollack MH, Simon NM, Worthington JJ, et al. Combined paroxetine and clonazepam treatment strategies compared to paroxetine monotherapy for panic disorder. J Psychopharmacol. 2003;17(3):276-82.
38. Goddard AW, Brouette T, Almai A, et al. Early coadministration of clonazepam with sertraline for panic disorder. Arch Gen Psychiatry. 2001;58(7):681-6.
39. Ipser JC, Carey P, Dhansay Y, et al. Pharmacotherapy augmentation strategies in treatment-resistant anxiety disorders. Cochrane Database Syst Rev. 2006;(4):CD005473.
40. Palpacuer C, Duprez R, Huneau A, et al. Pharmacologically controlled drinking in the treatment of alcohol dependence or alcohol use disorders: a systematic review with direct and network meta-analyses on nalmefene, naltrexone, acamprosate, baclofen and topiramate. Addiction. 2018;113(2):220-37.
41. Jonas DE, Amick HR, Feltner C, et al. Pharmacotherapy for adults with alcohol use disorders in outpatient settings: a systematic review and meta-analysis. JAMA. 2014;311(118):1889-900.
42. Soyka M, Kranzler HR, van den Brink W, et al. The World Federation of Societies of Biological Psychiatry (WFSBP) guidelines for the biological treatment of substance use and related disorders. Part 2: Opioid dependence. World J Biol Psychiatry. 2011;12(3):160-87.
43. Anton RF, O'Malley SS, Ciraulo DA, et al.; COMBINE Study Research Group. Combined pharmacotherapies and behavioural interventions for alcohol dependence: The COMBINE study: a randomized controlled trial. JAMA. 2006;295(17):2003-17.
44. Mayo-Smith MF, Breecher LH, Fischer TL, et al.; Working Group on the Management of Alcohol Withdrawal Delirium, Practice Guidelines Committee, American Society of Addiction Medicine. Management of alcohol withdrawal delirium. An evidence-based practice guideline. Arch Intern Med. 2004;164(13):1405-12.
45. Lee JD, Nunes EV Jr, Novo P, et al. Comparative effectiveness of extended-release naltrexone versus buprenorphine-naloxone for opioid relapse prevention

(X:BOT): a multicentre, open-label, randomised controlled trial. Lancet. 2018;391(10118):309-18.
46. Hser YI, Evans E, Huang D, et al. Long-term outcomes after randomization to buprenorphine/naloxone versus methadone in a multi-site trial. Addiction. 2016;111(4):695-705.
47. Law FD, Diaper AM, Melichar JK, et al. Buprenorphine/naloxone versus methadone and lofexidine in community stabilisation and detoxification: arandomised controlled trial of low dose short-term opiate-dependent individuals. J Psychopharmacol. 2017;31(8):1046-55.
48. Megarbane B, Buisien A, Jacobs F, et al. Prospective comparative assessment of buprenorphine overdose with heroin and methadone: Clinical characteristics and response to antidotal treatment. J Subst Abuse Treat. 2010;38(4):403-7.
49. Kleber HD, Weiss RD, Anton RF Jr, et al.; Work Group on Substance Use Disorders; American Psychiatric Association; Steering Committee on Practice Guidelines. Treatment of patients with substance use disorders, second edition. American Psychiatric Association. Am J Psychiatry. 2007;164(4 Suppl 5):5-123.
50. Mortazavi SS, Shati M, Keshtkar A, et al. Defining polypharmacy in the elderly: a systematic review protocol. BMJ Open. 2016;6(3):e010989.
51. By the American Geriatrics Society 2015 Beers Criteria Update Expert Panel. American Geriatrics Society 2015 Updated Beers Criteria for Potentially Inappropriate Medication Use in Older Adults. J Am Geriatr Soc. 2015;63(11): 2227-46.
52. Ihl R, Frölich L, Winblad B, et al.; WFSBP Task Force on Treatment Guidelines for Alzheimer's Disease and other Dementias. World Federation of Societies of Biological Psychiatry (WFSBP) guidelines for the biological treatment of Alzheimer's disease and other dementias. World J Biol Psychiatry. 2011;12(1): 2-32.
53. Dantoine T, Auriacombe S, Sarazin M, et al. Rivastigmine monotherapy and combination therapy with memantine in patients with moderately severe Alzheimer's disease who failed to benefit from previous cholinesterase inhibitor treatment. Int J Clin Pract. 2006;60(1):110-8.
54. Yancheva S, Ihl R, Nikolova G, et al.; GINDON Study Group. Ginkgo biloba extract EGb 761(R), donepezil or both combined in the treatment of Alzheimer's disease with neuropsychiatric features: a randomised, double-blind, exploratory trial. Aging Ment Health. 2009;13(2):183-90.
55. Kowatch RA, Sethuraman G, Hume JH, et al. Combination pharmacotherapy in children and adolescents with bipolar disorder. Biol Psychiatry. 2003;53(11): 978-84.
56. Comer JS, Olfson M, Mojtabai R. National trends in child and adolescent psychotropic polypharmacy in office-based practice, 1996-2007. J Am Acad Child Adolesc Psychiatry. 2010;49(10):1001-10.
57. Olashore AA, Rukewe A. Polypharmacy among children and adolescents with psychiatric disorders in a mental referral hospital in Botswana. BMC Psychiatry. 2017;17(1):174.
58. Zigman D, Blier P. A framework to avoid irrational polypharmacy in psychiatry. J Psychopharmacol. 2012;26(12):1507-11.

59. Werder SF, Preskorn SH. Managing polypharmacy: walking the fine line between help and harm. Curr Psychiatry. 2003;2(2):24-36.
60. Lee RD. Polypharmacy: a case report and new protocol for management. J Am Board Fam Pract. 1998;11(2):140-4.
61. Trumic E, Pranjic N, Begic L, et al. Idiosyncratic adverse reactions of most frequent drug combinations longterm use among hospitalized patients with polypharmacy. Med Arch. 2012;66(4):243-8.
62. Devi P, Amarjeeth R, Sushma M, et al. Prescription patterns of psychotropic drugs in hospitalized schizophrenic patients in a tertiary care hospital. Calicut Med J. 2007;5:e3.
63. Sawhney V, Chopra V, Kapoor B, et al. Prescription trends in schizophrenia and manic depressive psychosis. J K Sci. 2005;7(3):156-8.
64. Grover S, Chakrabarti S, Kulhara P, et al. Clinical Practice Guidelines for Management of Schizophrenia. Indian J Psychiatry. 2017;59(Suppl 1):S19-33.
65. Gautam S, Jain A, Gautam M, et al. Clinical Practice Guidelines for the management of Depression. Indian J Psychiatry. 2017;59(Suppl 1):S34-50.
66. Shah N, Grover S, Rao GP. Clinical Practice Guidelines for Management of Bipolar Disorder. Indian J Psychiatry. 2017;59(Suppl 1):S51-66.
67. Basu D, Dalal PK. Overview of IPS Guidelines 2014. In: Basu D, Dalal PK (Eds). Clinical Practice Guidelines for the Assessment and Management of Substance Use Disorders. New Delhi: Indian Psychiatric Society; 2014. pp. 1-12.
68. Shaji KS, Sivakumar PT, Rao GP, et al. Clinical Practice Guidelines for Management of Dementia. Indian J Psychiatry. 2018;60(Suppl 3):S312-28.
69. Avasthi A, Grover S. Clinical practice guidelines for management of depression in elderly. Indian J Psychiatry. 2018;60(Suppl 3):S341-62.
70. Gautam S, Jain A, Gautam M, et al. Clinical practice guideline for management of psychoses in elderly. Indian J Psychiatry. 2018;60(Suupl 3):S363-70.
71. Awasti A. Treatment of depression in children and adolescents. Indian Psychiatric Society Treatment Guidelines; 2008.
72. Gautam S, Batra L, Gaur N, Meena PS. Clinical practice guidelines for the assessment and treatment of attention-deficit/hyperactivity disorder. Indian Psychiatric Society Treatment Guidelines. Indian Psychiatric Society Treatment Guidelines; 2008.

CHAPTER 12

Cosmetic Psychopharmacology

Vishal Indla, Chethan Basavarajappa, Indla Ramasubba Reddy

INTRODUCTION

Happiness is one of the central themes around which life revolves. With the advent of busy lives and many man-made diseases and destruction of the natural habitat and resultant calamities, this happiness has long sunken into the abyss. From time immemorial, we have been using mood-altering agents, such as alcohol and opiates in the pursuit of happiness.[1] We have drugs such as cocaine, heroin, lysergic acid diethylamide (LSD), and 3,4-methylenedioxymethamphetamine (MDMA/ecstasy) which increase happiness but they are all habituating and they disrupt the link between "feelings of happiness and our actions and experiences in the world".[2] Does the modern medicine aid in this pursuit of the Holy Grail?

The basic purpose of medicine is to heal the sick, not turn healthy people into superhumans and Gods. But what about doctors treating other conditions that are not technically illnesses? For example, minoxidil and hair transplant for baldness; cosmetic surgery for people unhappy with their nose, lips, and looks; acne treatment for self-conscious teenagers; gastric bypass surgery for obesity; abortion in an unmarried girl; immunizations, etc. In the last 50 years, plastic surgery has evolved into cosmetic surgery. Plastic surgery began as a set of reconstructive procedures aimed at restoring a person's appearance. Cosmetic surgery in contrast to plastic surgery aims at enhancing person's appearance. Viagra and similar drugs for sexual satisfaction have become lifestyle agents rather than therapeutic agents.

Is it wrong to change the personality for the better of human "enhancement" through psychopharmacology? Some future psychotropics especially antidepressants may offer the possibility of altering personality traits, both inborn and acquired traits. But do they raise the mood from a normal state to an enhanced state? If such a drug is found, is such treatment good for the society? The goal of medicine should not only be the relief of suffering, but also enhancing the quality of life. A person who is shy may want to become confident or an introvert person may want to become more social. If medications can help in this aspect, should it be denied? Patient's autonomy should be protected and promoted as the patient is the arbiter of his own suffering. Here, distinction should be made between health and illness, clinical illness, and cosmetic. While cosmetic surgery affects the self indirectly, cosmetic psychopharmacology affects manifestations of the self directly. In fact, this is not new to us at all. Dentistry changed its public image after collaboration with Colgate toothpaste for a public education campaign which promoted the idea of dental checkup. This campaign changed the nature of dental practice in India. Since then, dentistry has moved from restorative to preventive. The success of this transition is well-known. People get routine dental checkups rather than waiting for toothache to appear.[3]

Such a paradigm in the field of mental health was brought about by Peter Kramer in his 1993 best seller "Listening to Prozac" in which he used "cosmetic psychopharmacology". It refers to the use of psychoactive substances to bring out fruitful changes in individuals without a clinical diagnosis, not suffering from any subclinical conditions or any form of psychopathology.[4,5] Cosmetic psychiatry is the enhancement of cognitive, behavioral, and emotional processes in persons who do not suffer from illness or disease.[6]

IMPORTANCE OF COSMETIC PSYCHOPHARMACOLOGY

Public tends to view psychiatrists narrowly, associating us chiefly with our expertise in mental illness and not associating us with positive mental health and well-being. As long as public view us as doctors for treating only mentally ill, the stigma of mentally ill and our profession would continue. In reality, psychiatrists can promote coping and wellness in addition to diagnosing and treating mental illness.

But, we have been doing this by adding almost every human emotion to the diagnostic array and treating it. Benzodiazepines and barbiturates were once considered as "pill for every mental ill".[7] Soon after its release in 1988, fluoxetine also attained this status. With drugs like amphetamines, the increase in number of reported cases of attention deficit hyperactivity disorder (ADHD) and associated controversies have further fuelled the public's fear of our overinclusiveness. Whether this is cosmetic or therapeutic is debated till today.[8]

ETHICAL CONSIDERATIONS

There are many questions that need to be answered or at least understood before we proceed further.
- Who defines a condition is in need of treatment?
- Who defines suffering, doctor or client?
- Suffering is a subjective experience and who decides how much suffering is enough and tolerable?
- Who determines whether and how enhancement is used?
- Does patients' impression of the quality of their lives always correspond directly to biomarkers and symptoms of disease?

The society is moving away from the paternalistic attitude of health professionals toward rights perspective, thereby the answers to the above questions are moving toward the clients themselves. But, it should also be kept in mind that the society might also be guided by various forces working behind the curtains. A significant percentage of all patients who visit a psychiatrist have no diagnosable mental illness. They are labeled as "worried well" or "the discontent".[9] To identify the discontent and the mentally ill, one can use the following perspectives: "diseases, dimensions of personality, behaviors, and life stories". This would be a useful tool in assessing a patient's problems.[9,10] Diseases can be treated by medications, personality disorders, and behaviors that need both medications and therapy. The problems arising out of life stories would probably not need medications although therapy would help them. The diagnosis of the discontent is by exclusion of the first three perspectives.[9] Let us see some examples of the fourth perspective.

Mr A, a 22-year-old final MBBS student, requests methylphenidate for final examinations. There is no history of ADHD or learning disabilities. No active medical problems. No history of drug-seeking behavior or substance abuse or psychosis. There is no family history of substance abuse or psychosis. If this young man comes to your outpatient department (OPD), would you prescribe him methylphenidate or a modafinil to help him concentrate better for his examination, even though he does not meet diagnostic criteria for a mental disorder?

Ms B, a 30-year-old female, is usually shy and dull regardless of the environment she is in. She wants to be as outgoing as some of her friends and come out of the gloomy mood she is always in. She always thinks pessimistic. She does not qualify for dysthymia and does not have enough time for therapy sessions. She requests medications to help alleviate the problem. What about prescribing antidepressants for her?

Mr C is a salesman in a car showroom. He too goes through ups and downs in his mood as others. But even these normal mood swings would be costly for him in his job where he needs to be constantly optimistic and cheerful. He believes that medicines will improve his personality and help him become more effective in his job.

These examples constitute the cosmetic use of an antidepressant as none of the above has a clinical diagnosis. Regarding Mr C, who thought medicine will help him sell more cars, without any symptom of disorder, most psychiatrists would refuse his request for any medications and consider his problem to be cosmetic. But, what about a woman who wants a breast reduction surgery to improve her career as a club dancer? Would her request be refused as well? Not likely, because most doctors would see the physical and the psychological benefits of such a procedure for a professional dancer. There is a social and medical acceptance conferred upon these practices and why not for people like Mr C. As Erica Rangel in her journal discussion side effects before any class so that we can learn better? Would we pay more for efficient pilots or doctors or lawyers who are taking a medication that make them more alert? Would we take a medicine to selectively dampen disturbing memories?[15] If the concern is the side effects of medications, which medical drug in the market is there without side effect? If we would wish to take medications for cosmetic purposes in the above examples, how can we respond to the clients when they turn to us as the gatekeepers in their pursuit of happiness?

But, these enhancing drugs may keep us away from our "true self". Would governments give "happy pills" free to the masses to keep them happy, so that they may not be motivated to do something against the government if their rights started to disappear; the way the governments distribute freebies in today's society!

When psychiatric disorders are treated with drugs, the creative impulse often associated with mania or depression may decline. Many artists who need treatment resist it as they think that the treatment may alter their creativity. Many notable personalities like Albert Einstein, Winston Churchill, Salvador Dali, and Thomas Alva Edison probably had ADHD traits, viz. impulsivity and a disorganized life. Would they have achieved what they have if they were treated?[16] Medicines may help us, but as Moreno notes, "there are still lots of hills to climb, and they are pretty steep".[17] Gadgets have immensely enhanced our ability to cope with difficult tasks. That does not mean that life's struggles have disappeared. Life awaits with the next ones. Human life involves a roller coaster of ups and downs. To feel the fullest extent of happiness, one must suffer as well; it is the experience of being human.

Again discerning judgment is necessary to alter nature, it might help you think more clearly and pray more effectively. True healing needs a mixture of medical, psychological, and spiritual strategies. Those who desire altered states will find the drug and those who do not want to alter their sense of "who they are" will ignore the availability of the drug. The government should stay out of it, letting our own ethical and moral sense guide us through the new enhancement landscape.

Any system in the society either political or health care develops from one stage to another. Healthcare system also gradually moved from curative, then to preventive, and now to promotional sectors.

For example, in the past people were seeing a doctor when they get chickenpox, but now every child is getting vaccinated for prevention of these diseases. At present, the healthcare system is moving even from preventive to promotional aspects, for example, taking vitamin E for improving muscle mass, regular exercise, or liposuction to reduce abdominal fat, etc. The important quality of a good politician or a leader is not only to maintain law and order, but also to work for the welfare and well-being of his people.

As stated by Corneliu E Giurgea, it is important to remember that "man is not going to wait passively for millions of years before evolution offers him a better brain".[14] Now the time has come to decide whether we want evolution or revolution!

REFERENCES

1. Rangel EK. Cosmetic psychopharmacology and the goals of medicine. Virtual Mentor. 2007;9(6):428-32.
2. Cerullo MA. Cosmetic psychopharmacology and the President's Council on Bioethics. Perspect Biol Med. 2006;49(4):515-23.
3. Reddy IR. Making psychiatry a household word. Indian J Psychiatry. 2007;49(1):10-8.
4. Kramer PD. Listening to Prozac. New York: Viking Press; 1993.
5. Bjorklund P. Can there be a 'cosmetic' psychopharmacology? Prozac unplugged: the search for an ontologically distinct cosmetic psychopharmacology. Nurs Philos. 2005;6(2):131-43.
6. Studyslide (2008). Cosmetic Psychiatry. [online] Available from http://studyslide.com/doc/719676/cosmetic-psychiatry [Last accessed December, 2019].
7. Stein DJ. The bioethics of cosmetic psychopharmacology. S Afr Psychiatry Rev. 2005;8:50-1.
8. Silverman BC, Treisman GJ. Attention-deficit disorder at the crossroads of cosmetic and therapeutic psychiatry. Johns Hopkins Adv Stud Med. 2006;6(1):13-5.
9. Kheriaty AD. Cosmetic drugs for mental makeovers: antidepressants and our discontents. In: Kheriaty AD (Ed). Continuity + Change: Perspectives on Science and Religion. Philadelphia: Elsevier; 2006.
10. McHugh P, Slavney P. The Perspectives of Psychiatry, 2nd edition. Baltimore: Johns Hopkins; 1988.
11. Reformed Church in America. Cosmetic Surgery for the Soul? Perspectives. J Reformed Thought. 2000;15(4):15-6.
12. Parens E. Enhancing Human Traits: Ethical and Social Implications. Washington: Georgetown University Press; 1998.
13. The Free Library (2003). The battle for your brain: science is developing ways to boost intelligence, expand memory, and more. But will you be allowed to change your own mind? [online] Available from https://www.thefreelibrary.com/The+battle+for+your+brain%3A+science+is+developing+ways+to+boost...-a096644874 [Last accessed December, 2019].
14. Gazzaniga MS. Shaping the smart brain with drugs. In: Gazzaniga MS (Ed). The Ethical Brain: The Science of Our Moral Dilemmas. New York: Harper Perennial; 2005. pp. 71-84.
15. Chatterjee A. Cosmetic neurology: the controversy over enhancing movement, mentation, and mood. Neurology. 2004;63(6):968-74.
16. Baker S (2009). Are Smart Drugs the Answer to Bad Moods—and a Bad Economy? [online] Available from http://discovermagazine.com/2009/apr/02-are-smart-drugs-the-answer-to-bad-moods-and-bad-economy [Last accessed December, 2019].
17. Center for Cognitive Liberty and Ethics (2003). Battle for Your Brain, neuroethics, Fukiyama, enhancement of neuroscience. [online] Available from http://www.cognitiveliberty.org/neuro/bailey.html [Last accessed December, 2019].

18. DBEssays (2014). Cosmetic psychopharmacology essay research paper: the controversies. [online]. Available from http://dbessays.com/essay/365817-cosmetic-psychopharmacology-essay-research-paper-the-controversies [Last accessed December, 2019].
19. Oliver B, Molewijk E, van Oorschot R. New animal models of anxiety. Eur Neuropsychopharmacol. 1994;4(2):93-102.
20. Sobo S. Psychotherapy perspectives in medication management. Psychiatr Times. 1999;16:23-5.
21. Gelfin Y, Gorfine M, Lerer B. Effect of clinical doses of fluoxetine on psychological variables in healthy volunteers. Am J Psychiatry. 1998;155(2):290-2.
22. Knutson B, Wolkowitz OM, Cole SW, et al. Selective alteration of personality and social behavior by serotonergic intervention. Am J Psychiatry. 1998;155(3):373-9.

CHAPTER 13

Nutraceuticals in Psychiatry

Kabir Garg

INTRODUCTION

There is an increasing recognition that food habits and nutritional intake are related to mental health and morbidity.[1,2] This is compounded by a peculiar situation in current times where the type of energy-dense, highly processed, and mass-produced food being consumed worldwide, has resulted in a large percentage of population to be overfed and undernourished at the same time,[3] further worsened by increasing substance use, lifestyle habits, and increase in stress. On the positive side though, there is also an increasing interest in exploring food supplements for treatment of different disorders.[4] It goes without saying that the burden of mental and behavioral disorders in the world is high and recent literature continues to confirm that.[5] It is, however, worth noticing that the traditionally defined pharmaceutical approach has provided only a moderate amelioration of this burden,[3] and despite the best efforts to innovate and continued development of pharmacological frontiers, the burden of mental disorders is expected to keep on increasing.[5] Among these, the major ones are depressive disorders and anxiety disorders.[5,6] The morbidity and chronicity of illnesses, along with other factors such as poor quality of life, increasing recognition among the general public, and limitations of pharmacological agents are increasing the demand for alternative treatments, and mental health services users are no different to this phenomenon.[7,8]

The word "nutraceuticals" very evidently fuses "nutrition" and "pharmaceuticals". They can be defined as "food components or active principles present in aliments which have positive effects for health and quality of life, including preventing or treating disorders".[7,9] Over the years, continued research and development has yielded specific food components isolated and synthesized for their ameliorative and treating properties.[7]

There is, however, always a legal gray area about the mental health effects of nutrients and where does one draw the line between food and drug.[1] Traditionally, the definitions of food and drugs have been dependent on the intended use of the product rather than the component, i.e. whether the product was meant for reducing hunger and providing nourishment versus whether it was to be used for treatment or prevention or modification of illness process, thus the morning cup of coffee is regulated as food but an equivalent tablet of caffeine is classified as drug.[1] Overall, a majority of such available products are unregulated on account of being considered as dietary supplements, while some of the drugs from natural derivates are classified and marketed as drugs, subject to the same levels of testing and monitoring as other medications.[7]

In this paper, we will have a look on the prevalent and upcoming nutraceutical agents that are being used for improving mental health conditions.

MOOD DISORDERS

Perhaps the most widely identifiable nutraceutical is St John's Wort. It has been used traditionally to treat a number of physical and mental health conditions.[10] A probable reason for it to be used historically in mental illnesses is the fact that it was known to be carried to battlegrounds for protection against evil, and mental illnesses have long been associated with evil spirits.[7] It is widely available in market today and in some countries, such as Germany, enjoys an identity equivalent to traditional antidepressants.[11] *Hypericum perforatum* is not a single molecule, rather it represents a mixture of potentially multiple active chemical constituents.[7] The commercially available preparations are derived from air-dried young buds and flowers that are chopped and soaked in ethanol.[12] There are multiple, identified, and proposed neuropharmacological actions of the extract. It has been demonstrated to have a mild selective serotonin reuptake inhibitor (SSRI) like effect and to have mild sigma receptor affinity, catechol-O-methyltransferase (COMT) inhibition, and possible gamma-amino butyric acid (GABA) enhancement.[13] It, however, does not cross the blood–brain barrier. Thus, an alternate proposed working mechanism involves inhibition of monocyte interleukin 6 and 1β production, thus reducing the production of cortisol, which is known to mediate the neurochemistry of depression.[14] It is noticeable that the commercial preparations contain multiple essential oils, flavonoids, and other active compounds which may be a compounding factor.[12] The evidence for its efficacy in literature is quite equivocal. While there are a number of European papers that find it superior to placebo, they have been questioned on their methodology and soundness,[7] others have found it to be nonsuperior to placebo.[15,16] The Cochrane review on the matter, while acknowledged the contradictory findings, noted that with inclusion of large trials, hypericum extract has a "modest effect" comparable to the standard antidepressants and attempt to treat mild-to-moderate depression with the tested preparations is justified.[17] It is important as every preparation and possibly every batch of the preparation is nonuniform.[7] St John's Wort is considered to be well tolerated with only a small number of the service users identifying to have side effects, usually gastrointestinal (GI) upset, fatigue, and photodermatitis, and these are reported in lower numbers than other antidepressants.[18] It should be noted, however, that it has cytochrome P450 induction properties.[19,20] It is a potential problem where the extract is available in the food stores for service users to take without bringing this to the notice of the physicians as there can be a number of interactions.[17] The usual recommended doses are 900–1,800 mg daily of the entire herb, starting with 300–600 mg daily oral, and increasing every 1–2 weeks.[7]

Perhaps the other most common over-the-counter aliment for management of depression is S-adenosylmethionine (SAMe). It has been known for a long time and there is a sizeable amount of literature present.[7] Meta-analyses have concluded that it may have a role in treatment of depression[21] and may provide an effect size against placebo which is comparable to standard antidepressant drugs.[22] As it is involved in biochemical reactions in the pathways of monoamine formations, it has the potential to increase the availability of these neurotransmitters, an action similar to conventional antidepressants.[23] Furthermore, an action involving blockade of monoamine uptake is also proposed.[7] The starting doses are usually 400–800 mg daily and up to 1,600 mg daily. As it has a short half-life (1.5 hours), multiple (3–4) divided doses are necessary.[24] Usually well tolerated, higher doses are associated with gastric upset and nausea. There have been reports of neuropsychiatric side effects including increasing anxiety and manic switch.[25] The biochemistry and working of SAMe is closely associated with Vitamin B group. People diagnosed with major depressive disorder have been demonstrated to have folate[26] and vitamin B_{12}[27] deficiencies. They have a common proposed mechanism of action involving formation of SAMe.[26] They also have a modulator effect on action of SSRIs.[27,28] Folate has been thus used as an adjunctive to antidepressant treatment in doses of up to 500 μg. It is fairly well tolerated but may cause vitamin B_{12} deficiencies, interference with anticonvulsant and even seizures at high doses.[29] For vitamin B12, deficiency states have been known to be associated with many psychiatric sequelae, and milder deficiencies have been associated with depression.[30] It is advisable to have B_{12} level estimations and supplementation in certain patient populations such as elderly, malnourished, and people with bariatric surgeries.[31] Inositol (vitamin B_8) is another member of vitamin B family that has been used in depression and anxiety disorders. In a small study, inositol has been separated from placebo in patients of major depression at 4 weeks.[32] Other studies, however, have failed to demonstrate any significant benefits either alone or as adjunctive.[33,34] The proposed mechanism is through desensitization of serotonin and monoamine receptors and it has been found to be well tolerated in doses up to 18 g/day.[7] At present there are no conclusive results. Its role has been studied in cases of obsessive-compulsive disorder (OCD) and panic disorders, and positive results have been reported.[35]

Recently, a combination of SAMe with inositol has been patented for use in depression and panic disorders[36] with a possibility of addition of St John's Wort in future.[7]

Omega-3 fatty acids (OFA) are one of the building blocks of the fats in the body. The most commonly recognized OFAs are—linolenic acid, eicosapentaenoic acid (EPA), and docosahexaenoic acid (DHA).[3] Fatty acid deficiencies and dysregulations have been identified to be correlated with mood disorders, especially depression over last decades.[37] Deficiencies of the OFAs have been associated with proinflammatory states similar to ones found in cardiovascular and depressive disorders,[38] increasing ratio of arachidonic acid to EPA have been demonstrated to have a correlation with severity of depression.[39] Animal studies have demonstrated that OFA deficiency has effect on serotonin and dopamine transmissions[40] and similar to St John's Wort, reduction of proinflammatory cytokines and further downstream reduction of cortisol production have also been reported.[38,41] Furthermore, mood stabilizer like actions, on inhibition of protein kinase C[42] and suppression of phosphatidylinositol-associated second messenger activity,[43] have also been identified. Studies in major depressive disorders have shown positive results as compared to placebo when used as an adjunctive.[40,44,45] The doses used in these positive studies ranged from 1 g to 2 g of EPA per day or higher doses in combination with DHA.[37] The picture is more equivocal in bipolar disorder; recent Cochrane review found positive result from one study as an adjunctive in depression but no efficacy in manic symptoms could be found.[46] The report by the Committee on Research on Psychiatric Treatments of the American Psychiatric Association (APA) recommends that psychiatric patients should not opt for OFAs supplementation in place of established psychiatric treatments.[37] Both groups identified a need for larger placebo-controlled trials to be able to demonstrate significant effect sizes. Adjunctive treatment may be suitable for specific patient groups that are particularly sensitive to side effects of conventional antidepressants (pregnant and lactating women, elderly, people with comorbid physical conditions, etc.).[7] They have been found to be generally well-tolerated. The side effects are generally associated with higher doses and include GI distress and breath odor.[7] There is also a potential for thinning of blood and prolonged bleeding in patient populations taking warfarin.[47] No major interactions with psychiatric medications or switch potential have been demonstrated.[48]

Cucurmin is no stranger to Indian households. Turmeric's use as medicine is long known and has been passed down through generations. Animal models and human studies have shown significant antidepressant properties.[49] Placebo-controlled study showed significant reduction in depression rating scores after 6 weeks of 1,000 mg daily supplementation of curcumin; they also recorded a reduction in the pro-inflammatory cytokine levels.[50]

ANXIETY DISORDERS

As noted above, inositol has been noted to have positive results in anxiety states. In addition, *St John's Wort* has been postulated to be of use based on its GABA modulation and benzodiazepine receptor agonism properties.[51] It has been studied in social anxiety and OCD where no significant results were found; however, positive results were found in case reports of patients of generalized anxiety disorders.[52] Although melatonin supplements have been long used for insomnia and jet lag, researchers have been able to identify anxiolytic properties in patients of nicotine withdrawal in doses of up to 0.3 mg.[53] Kava (*Piper methysticum*) is a historically well-known plant and has been traditionally used in certain cultures as a beverage during ceremonies.[7,51] It has been progressively gaining popularity in the developed world owing to its relaxing and anxiogenic properties. The active moiety as the "kava-lactone" that has been found to modulate GABA binding and increasing the available GABA sites.[54] It also possibly inhibits norepinephrine uptake.[55] Meta-analyses of placebo-controlled trials of kava in anxiety disorders have found positive effects of kava in these patient populations.[56,57] The usual dose is recommended to be 60–120 mg of the pyrone daily. If using the tea from root, it is recommended to be taken 2–3 times daily. A very important aspect, however, is the high risk of liver damage,[10] which has led to it being banned in multiple countries.[51] Attempts at refining the extract have not yielded much benefits and close hepatic monitoring is still required. There is also a potential risk of delirium as it increases the effects of other central nervous system (CNS) depressants such as barbiturates, alcohol, and benzodiazepines.[7] Due to these associated risks, it is not recommended to be an anxiety treatment despite demonstrating benefits.[51]

Valerian's (Valeriana Officinalis) use has been well-documented in cultures spanning the American and European continents. Traditionally, in folk medicine, the root is made into a tea and liquid elixir formulations for different ailments. It is also used as a beverage and flavoring substance. Its proposed mechanism of action involves sesquiterpenoids that reduce sleep latency.[58] A root extract, valerenic acid, has been demonstrated to impede the breakdown of GABA[59] and to enhance GABA neurotransmission.[60] It has primarily been used in treatment of anxiety and sleep disorders, and recommended doses are 300–600 mg extract up to three times a day.[7] In addition, it has been proposed for treatment of conditions such as headaches, dysmenorrhea, and abdominal pain.[7] The predominant side effects are associated with CNS depression and sedation and similar to kava, it potentiates other CNS depressants.[61] There have been proposals of formulations involving valerian, St John's wort, and other herbs for help with smoking cessation.[62] This is, however, subject to skepticism as none of these herbs have been identified to have any effects on the reward pathways.[7]

A subspecies of passionflower *Passiflora incarnata* has been found to have anxiolytic actions, although the active moiety or the mechanism of action is yet to be clearly identified.[7] Like other plants discussed in this article, it also has well-documented use in folk medicine for its anxiolytic, sedative, and antispasmodic properties.[63,64] Currently, it is available in multiple formations including capsules, powders, tablets, and drops. Its use for indications including nervousness, insomnia, and anxiety are indicated by the Federal Health Agency of Germany and the British Herbal Compendium.[51,65] The only clinical trial using *passionflower* in anxiety compared it with oxazepam and found it to be equally efficacious and having significantly less functional impairments.[66] Therapeutic doses are 500–1,000 mg up to three times a day.[7] It is well tolerated and mild side effects include sedation, dry mouth, and constipation.[67] It has been noticed to increase the potency of Hypericum perforatum, decreasing the required dose for antidepressant action.[68]

PSYCHOSES

Despite ongoing efforts, the only effective treatment for psychoses is antipsychotics although it is well-known that current antipsychotic agents afford little to no respite in negative and cognitive symptoms of psychotic disorders, and this has been a driving factor for exploration of alternative drugs, including nutraceuticals.[69] OFAs are perhaps one avenue that is progressively gaining momentum.[49] This is fueled in part by demonstration of abnormalities in myelination in brains of people with schizophrenia and OFAs being important for the same. Clinical studies have found that augmentation of treatment with up to 2 g of EPA provides positive results in symptom reduction.[70,71] Perhaps owing to its multifarious actions on the CNS as noted above, researchers have found that they may reduce the risk of pathogenesis and morbidity associated with psychoses in high-risk individuals.[72] In continuation of its demonstrated anti-inflammatory properties and antidepressant action, curcumin has been shown to reduce the serious side-effects of anti-psychtics[73] and its role has been proposed for management of orofacial-dyskinesia.[74] N-acetylcysteine (NAC) has been studied as an adjunctive and found to have reduction in positive symptoms and an overall improvement in the functioning of individuals.[75] The proposed mechanism involves production of glutathione which has been found to be deficient in brains of people with schizophrenia.[49] Similar increase in glutathione has been observed with cucurmin.[76] Studies involving vitamins B and D have shown positive trends but the effect sizes are small and any recommendations are still wanting for conclusive studies.[49] Identified herbal extracts with potential benefits include *Bacopa monniera* which has been demonstrated to reduce dopamine levels in frontal cortex[77] and *Ficus platyphylla*.[78] It is notable that ongoing research continues in multiple herbal and traditional aliments but no conclusive results are available yet.[49]

OTHERS

Ginkgo biloba is probably one of the more widely known nutraceuticals. Its use has been documented in Asian cultures for millennia and it has witnessed a progressive surge in its popularity. While the most popular use for memory problems is associated with aging, the studies on the topic have been found to have multiple methodological issues and thus are far from being considered conclusive.[79] Additional studied uses involve administration to people on antidepressants to mitigate the sexual side effects; the quality of evidence is, however, poor as it is limited to open labels and case reports.[80] It is not free from its share of side effects though the leaf of the herb may cause allergic reactions and high doses have been found to increase bleeding tendency and confusional states.[81] This risk increases if taken with other antiplatelet drugs.[82]

CURRENT CHALLENGES AND FUTURE DIRECTIONS

As noted in the above text, there are multiple food derivatives and nutraceuticals that are available for use in different conditions, albeit with equivocal evidence. There has been an increasing popularity of nutraceuticals for management of psychiatric conditions since the end of the last millenia. This has led to creation of dedicated departments for research and regulations of such products in multiple countries.[7] As discussed above, they are mostly food derivatives and thus free from regulations of conventional pharmaceutical agents, but it is usually illegal for any manufacturer to claim effectiveness for any illness, and only in limited cases, can manufacturers claim effectiveness in certain symptoms.

One of the important differences between pharmaceuticals and nutraceuticals is that the latter are exempted from the need for efficacy to be established in a stringent manner similar to drugs, which in turn means that the currently available data is not as conclusive as with drugs.[83] There is also a lack of quality control that results in manufacturers marketing products that may not have—(1) correct amount of the active ingredient, (2) contamination with additional products, (3) substitution of one compound with another, and (4) adulterations with heavy metals, steroids, etc. among other difficulties. This is significant as these factors open up possibilities of not only de novo side effects but also of interactions with other drugs an individual may be on and quite often physicians omit asking service users about them taking any of these.[83] Even if they were to be aware, there are hardly any concrete or consistent known interaction patterns with pharmaceuticals.[84] Furthermore, the shelf lives of these products are largely unknown and some herbal preparations have been shown to oxidize rapidly, making one wonder if the supplements are even potent while they are being taken.[7] All this is compounded by the general perception that equates "natural" or "herbal" with being good and devoid of side effects, prompting self-medication further aided by the over-the-counter availability of these agents.[85] It should be remembered that a majority of drugs are in fact isolated, purified, characterized, and synthesized from plant sources and they have identified side effects, quite often serious ones.[86]

As mental health disorders and morbidity are unique when it comes to issues such as consent and treatment choices, the rising popularity and public perception of terms like "herbal" and "natural" should be offset against sound scientific research and prudent clinical and politicolegal decisions. This does not take away anything from the importance of exploring novel and innovative agents to manage symptoms and side effects in psychiatric illnesses with least possible adverse effects and restrictions. These agents also hold a potential for reducing the stigma that goes hand in glove with mental illnesses and psychiatric treatment, as these are agents closer to "foods" that are perceived normal.[7] It should be remembered that a large number of people without any illnesses use these agents and further research needs to be directed at answering questions such as what is needed, by whom, and in what doses.[3] It is also advisable to direct efforts at convincing legislators and decision makers to improve food quality, and promote healthier lifestyles.[87] All these efforts are components of nutritional medicine that should be promoted further in the area of mental health.

REFERENCES

1. Young SN. Clinical nutrition: 3. The fuzzy boundary between nutrition and psychopharmacology. CMAJ. 2002;166(2):205-9.
2. O'neil A, Quirk SE, Housden S, et al. Relationship between diet and mental health in children and adolescents: a systematic review. Am J Public Health. 2014;104(10):e31-42.
3. Sarris J, Logan AC, Akbaraly TN, et al.; International Society for Nutritional Psychiatry Research. Nutritional medicine as mainstream in psychiatry. Lancet Psychiatry. 2015;2(3):271-4.
4. Wu P, Fuller C, Liu X, et al. Use of complementary and alternative medicine among women with depression: results of a national survey. Psychiatr Serv. 2007;58(3):349-56.
5. Whiteford HA, Degenhardt L, Rehm J, et al. Global burden of disease attributable to mental and substance use disorders: Findings from the Global Burden of Disease Study 2010. Lancet. 2013;382(9904):1575-86.
6. Murray CJ, Lopez AD; World Health Organization. The Global Burden of Disease: A Comprehensive Assessment of Mortality and Disability from Diseases, Injuries, and Risk Factors in 1990 and Projected to 2020: Summary. Harvard School of Public Health, World Health Organization, World Bank; 1996.
7. Chiappedi M, de Vincenzi S, Bejor M. Nutraceuticals in psychiatric practice. Recent Pat CNS Drug Discov. 2012;7(2):163-72.
8. Burg MA, Hatch RL, Neims AH. Lifetime use of alternative therapy: a study of Florida residents. South Med J. 1998;91(12):1126-31.

9. Brower V. Nutraceuticals: poised for a healthy slice of the healthcare market? Nat Biotechnol. 1998;16(8):728-31.
10. Schatzberg AF, DeBattista C. Manual of Clinical Psychopharmacology. American Psychiatric Pub; 2015.
11. Linde K, Ramirez G, Mulrow CD, et al. St John's wort for depression—an overview and meta-analysis of randomised clinical trials. BMJ. 1996;313(7052):253-8.
12. Wagner H, Bladt S. Pharmaceutical quality of hypericum extracts. J Geriatr Psychiatry Neurol. 1994;7(Suppl 1):S65-8.
13. Bennett DA Jr, Phun L, Polk JF, et al. Neuropharmacology of St. John's wort (Hypericum). Ann Pharmacother. 1998;32(11):1201-8.
14. Thiele B, Brink I, Ploch M. Modulation of cytokine expression by hypericum extract. J Geriatr Psychiatry Neurol. 1994;7(Suppl 1):S60-2.
15. Hypericum Depression Trial Study Group. Effect of Hypericum perforatum (St John's wort) in major depressive disorder: A randomized controlled trial. JAMA. 2002;287(14):1807-14.
16. Fava M, Alpert J, Nierenberg AA, et al. A double-blind, randomized trial of St John's wort, fluoxetine, and placebo in major depressive disorder. J Clin Psychopharmacol. 2005;25(5):441-7.
17. Linde K, Berner MM, Kriston L. St John's wort for major depression. Cochrane Database Syst Rev. 2008;(4):CD000448.
18. Woelk N, Burkard G, Grunwald J. Evaluation of the benefits and risks of the hypericum extract LI-160 based on a drug-monitoring study with 3250 patients. Nervenheilkunde. 1993;12(6A):308-13.
19. Markowitz JS, Donovan JL, DeVane CL, et al. Effect of St John's wort on drug metabolism by induction of cytochrome P450 3A4 enzyme. JAMA. 2003;290(11):1500-4.
20. Whitten DL, Myers SP, Hawrelak JA, et al. The effect of St John's wort extracts on CYP3A: a systematic review of prospective clinical trials. Br J Clin Pharmacol. 2006;62(5):512-26.
21. Williams AL, Girard C, Jui D, et al. S-adenosylmethionine (SAMe) as treatment for depression: a systematic review. Clin Invest Med. 2005;28(3):132-9.
22. Bressa GM. S-adenosyl-l-methionine (SAMe) as antidepressant: meta-analysis of clinical studies. Acta Neurol Scand Suppl. 1994;154:7-14.
23. Bottiglieri T, Hyland K, Reynolds EH. The clinical potential of ademetionine (S-adenosylmethionine) in neurological disorders. Drugs. 1994;48(2):137-52.
24. Najm WI, Reinsch S, Hoehler F, et al. S-adenosyl methionine (SAMe) versus celecoxib for the treatment of osteoarthritis symptoms: A double-blind cross-over trial. [ISRCTN36233495]. BMC Musculoskel Disord. 2004;5:6.
25. Carney MW, Chary TK, Bottiglieri T, et al. The switch mechanism and the bipolar/unipolar dichotomy. Br J Psychiatry. 1989;154(1):48-51.
26. Fava M, Borus JS, Alpert JE, et al. Folate, vitamin B12, and homocysteine in major depressive disorder. Am J Psychiatry. 1997;154(3):426-8.
27. Hintikka J, Tolmunen T, Tanskanen A, et al. High vitamin B12 level and good treatment outcome may be associated in major depressive disorder. BMC Psychiatry. 2003;3:17.

28. Papakostas GI, Petersen T, Lebowitz BD, et al. The relationship between serum folate, vitamin B12, and homocysteine levels in major depressive disorder and the timing of improvement with fluoxetine. Int J Neuropsychopharmacol. 2005;8(4):523-8.
29. Shane B. Folate and vitamin B12 metabolism: Overview and interaction with riboflavin, vitamin B6, and polymorphisms. Food Nutr Bull. 2008;29(Suppl 2):S5-19.
30. Shorvon SD, Carney MW, Chanarin I, et al. The neuropsychiatry of megaloblastic anaemia. Br Med J. 1980;281(6247):1036-8.
31. Coppen A, Bolander-Gouaille C. Treatment of depression: Time to consider folic acid and vitamin B12. J Psychopharmacol. 2005;19(1):59-65.
32. Levine J, Barak Y, Gonzalves M, et al. Double-blind, controlled trial of inositol treatment of depression. Am J Psychiatry. 1995;152(5):792-4.
33. Levine J, Mishori A, Susnosky M, et al. Combination of inositol and serotonin reuptake inhibitors in the treatment of depression. Biol Psychiatry. 1999;45(3):270-3.
34. Nierenberg AA, Ostacher MJ, Calabrese JR, et al. Treatment- resistant bipolar depression: A STEP-BD equipoise randomized effectiveness trial of antidepressant augmentation with lamotrigine, inositol, or risperidone. Am J Psychiatry. 2006;163(2):210-6.
35. Saeed SA, Bloch RM, Antonacci DJ. Herbal and dietary supplements for treatment of anxiety disorders. Am Fam Physician. 2007;76(4):549-56.
36. Seneci A, Giovannone D, Zio C. Compositions for Oral Use Based on S-adenosylmethionine and a Process for their Preparation. Google Patents; 2010.
37. Freeman MP, Hibbeln JR, Wisner KL, et al. Omega-3 fatty acids: Evidence basis for treatment and future research in psychiatry. J Clin Psychiatry. 2006;67(12):1954-67.
38. Stoll AL, Locke CA. Omega-3 fatty acids in mood disorders: a review of neurobiological and clinical actions. In: Mischoulon D, Rosenbaum J (Eds). Natural Medications for Psychiatric Disorders: Considering the Alternatives. Philadelphia: Lippincott Williams & Wilkins; 2002. pp. 13-34.
39. Adams PB, Lawson S, Sanigorski A, et al. Arachidonic acid to eicosapentaenoic acid ratio in blood correlates positively with clinical symptoms of depression. Lipids. 1996;31(Suppl):S157-61.
40. Su KP, Huang SY, Chiu CC, et al. Omega-3 fatty acids in major depressive disorder. A preliminary double-blind, placebo-controlled trial. Eur Neuropsychopharmacol. 2003;13(4):267-71.
41. Simopoulos AP. Omega-3 fatty acids in inflammation and autoimmune diseases. J Am Coll Nutr. 2002;21(6):495-505.
42. Mirnikjoo B, Brown SE, Kim HF, et al. Protein kinase inhibition by omega-3 fatty acids. J Biol Chem. 2001;276(14):10888-96.
43. Kinsella JE. Lipids, membrane receptors, and enzymes: Effects of dietary fatty acids. JPEN J Parenter Enteral Nutr. 1990;14(Suppl 5):200S-17S.
44. Peet M, Horrobin DF. A dose-ranging study of the effects of ethyl-eicosapentaenoate in patients with ongoing depression despite apparently adequate treatment with standard drugs. Arch Gen Psychiatry. 2002;59(10):913-9.

45. Nemets B, Stahl Z, Belmaker RH. Addition of omega-3 fatty acid to maintenance medication treatment for recurrent unipolar depressive disorder. Am J Psychiatry. 2002;159(3):477-9.
46. Montgomery P, Richardson AJ. Omega-3 fatty acids for bipolar disorder. Cochrane Database Syst Rev. 2008;(2):CD005169.
47. Kremer JM. n-3 Fatty acid supplements in rheumatoid arthritis. Am J Clin Nutr. 2000;71(Suppl 1):349S-51S.
48. Parker G, Parker K. Which antidepressants flick the switch? Aust N Z J Psychiatry. 2003;37(4):464-8.
49. Holloway JB. The role of herbal and nutraceutical supplementation in the amelioration of schizophrenia and schizoaffective symptomology. Scientia et Humanitas. 2016;6:95-114.
50. Lopresti AL, Maes M, Maker GL, et al. Curcumin for the treatment of major depression: a randomised, double-blind, placebo controlled study. J Affect Disord. 2014;167:368-75.
51. Kinrys G, Coleman E, Rothstein E. Natural remedies for anxiety disorders: Potential use and clinical applications. Depress Anxiety. 2009;26(3):259-65.
52. Davidson JR, Connor KM. St. John's wort in generalized anxiety disorder: Three case reports. J Clin Psychopharmacol. 2001;21(6):635-6.
53. Zhdanova IV, Piotrovskaya VR. Melatonin treatment attenuates symptoms of acute nicotine withdrawal in humans. Pharmacol Biochem Behav. 2000;67(1):131-5.
54. Yuan CS, Dey L, Wang A, et al. Kavalactones and dihydrokavain modulate GABAergic activity in a rat gastric-brainstem preparation. Planta Med. 2002;68(12):1092-6.
55. Seitz U, Schüle A, Gleitz J. [3H]-monoamine uptake inhibition properties of kava pyrones. Planta Med. 1997;63(6):548-9.
56. Pittler MH, Ernst E. Kava extract versus placebo for treating anxiety. Cochrane Database Syst Rev. 2003;(1):CD003383.
57. Witte S, Loew D, Gaus W. Meta-analysis of the efficacy of the acetonic kava-kava extract WS1490 in patients with non-psychotic anxiety disorders. Phytother Res. 2005;19(3):183-8.
58. Bent S, Padula A, Moore D, et al. Valerian for sleep: a systematic review and meta-analysis. Am J Med. 2006;119(12):1005-12.
59. Ortiz JG, Nieves-Natal J, Chavez P. Effects of Valeriana officinalis extracts on [3H] flunitrazepam binding, synaptosomal [3H]GABA uptake, and hippocampal [3H] GABA release. Neurochem Res. 1999;24(11):1373-8.
60. Benke D, Barberis A, Kopp S, et al. GABAA receptors as in vivo substrate for the anxiolytic action of valerenic acid, a major constituent of valerian root extracts. Neuropharmacology. 2009;56(1):174-81.
61. Abebe W. Herbal medication: potential for adverse interactions with analgesic drugs. J Clin Pharm Ther. 2002;27(6):391-401.
62. Valencia G, DeLaRosa DM. Formulations Containing Borojo. Google Patents; 2009.
63. Dhawan K, Kumar S, Sharma A. Anxiolytic activity of aerial and underground parts of Passiflora incarnata. Fitoterapia. 2001;72(8):922-6.
64. Lakhan SE, Vieira KF. Nutritional and herbal supplements for anxiety and anxiety-related disorders: systematic review. Nutr J. 2010;9:42.

65. Bradley P. British Herbal Compendium: A Handbook of Scientific Information of Widely used Plant Drugs, Volume 2. British Herbal Medicine Association; 2006.
66. Vazirian M, Khazaeli A, Naghavi H, et al. Passionflower in the treatment of generalized anxiety disorder: A double-blind ANF randomized trial with oxazepam; 2002.
67. Bourin M, Bougerol T, Guitton B, et al. A combination of plant extracts in the treatment of outpatients with adjustment disorder with anxious mood: Controlled study versus placebo. Fundam Clin Pharmacol. 1997;11(2):127-32.
68. Fiebich BL, Knörle R, Appel K, et al. Pharmacological studies in an herbal drug combination of St. John's Wort (Hypericum perforatum) and passion flower (Passiflora incarnata): In vitro and in vivo evidence of synergy between Hypericum and Passiflora in antidepressant pharmacological models. Fitoterapia. 2011;82(3):474-80.
69. Brown HE, Roffman JL. Vitamin supplementation in the treatment of schizophrenia. CNS Drugs. 2014;28(7):611-22.
70. Peet M. Eicosapentaenoic acid in the treatment of schizophrenia and depression: rationale and preliminary double-blind clinical trial results. Prostaglandins Leukot Essent Fatty Acids. 2003;69(6):477-85.
71. Emsley R, Myburgh C, Oosthuizen P, et al. Randomized, placebo-controlled study of ethyl-eicosapentaenoic acid as supplemental treatment in schizophrenia. Am J Psychiatry. 2002;159(9):1596-8.
72. Smesny S, Milleit B, Schaefer MR, et al. Effects of omega-3 PUFA on the vitamin E and glutathione antioxidant defense system in individuals at ultra-high risk of psychosis. Prostaglandins Leukot Essent Fatty Acids. 2015;101:15-21.
73. Trebatická J, Ďuračková Z. Psychiatric disorders and polyphenols: can they be helpful in therapy? Oxid Med Cell Longev. 2015;2015:248529.
74. Bishnoi M, Chopra K, Kulkarni SK. Protective effect of Curcumin, the active principle of turmeric (Curcuma longa) in haloperidol-induced orofacial dyskinesia and associated behavioural, biochemical and neurochemical changes in rat brain. Pharmacol Biochem Behav. 2008;88(4):511-22.
75. Minarini A, Ferrari S, Galletti M, et al. N-acetylcysteine in the treatment of psychiatric disorders: current status and future prospects. Expert Opin Drug Metab Toxicol. 2017;13(3):279-92.
76. Lavoie S, Chen Y, Dalton TP, et al. Curcumin, quercetin, and tBHQ modulate glutathione levels in astrocytes and neurons: Importance of the glutamate cysteine ligase modifier subunit. J Neurochem. 2009;108(6):1410-22.
77. Jash R, Chowdary KA. Ethanolic extracts of Alstonia Scholaris and Bacopa Monniera possess neuroleptic activity due to anti-dopaminergic effect. Pharmacognosy Res. 2014;6(1):46-51.
78. Chindo BA, Kahl E, Trzeczak D, et al. Standardized extract of Ficus platyphylla reverses apomorphine-induced changes in prepulse inhibition and locomotor activity in rats. Behav Brain Res. 2015;293:74-80.
79. Birks J, Grimley Evans J. Ginkgo biloba for cognitive impairment and dementia. Cochrane Database Syst Rev. 2009;(1):CD003120.
80. Taylor MJ, Rudkin L, Hawton K. Strategies for managing antidepressant-induced sexual dysfunction: Systematic review of randomised controlled trials. J Affect Disord. 2005;88(3):241-54.

81. Bent S, Goldberg H, Padula A, et al. Spontaneous bleeding associated with Ginkgo biloba: a case report and systematic review of the literature. J Gen Intern Med. 2005;20(7):657-61.
82. Zink T, Chaffin J. Herbal 'health' products: What family physicians need to know. Am Fam Physician. 1998;58(5):1133-40.
83. Crone CC, Gabriel G. Herbal and nonherbal supplements in medical-psychiatric patient populations. Psychiatr Clin North Am. 2002;25(1):211-30.
84. Markowitz JS, von Moltke LL, Donovan JL. Predicting interactions between conventional medications and botanical products on the basis of in vitro investigations. Mol Nutr Food Res. 2008;52(7):747-54.
85. Eisenberg DM, Davis RB, Ettner SL, et al. Trends in alternative medicine use in the United States, 1990-1997: Results of a follow-up national survey. JAMA. 1998;280(18):1569-75.
86. Borghi C, Cicero A, Forti GC, et al. Nutraceutici e Alimenti Funzionali in Medicina Preventiva. Bologna: Bononia University Press; 2011.
87. Tripathi A, Garg K, Javed A. Prevention in Psychiatry: A Narrative Review of Conceptual Basis and Current Status. Advances in Psychiatry. Springer; 2019. pp. 577-94.

CHAPTER 14

Therapeutic Role of Sleep and Exercise in Management of Health

Ravi Gupta

INTRODUCTION

Sleep is a state of altered consciousness which is reversible, characterized by absence of interaction to and from the environment—both internal as well as external but, not a state of passivity as many changes take place in the body during sleep. Sleep has been found to influence emotions, cognition, behavior, tissue repair, and brain plasticity across many studies and hence plays a vital role in functioning.[1-4] Exercise is defined as "regular use of bodily organ" in an attempt to maintain "physical fitness" in dictionary.[5]

Sleep as well as exercise plays an important role in maintaining state of good health and in recuperating from the state of illness. These facts suggest that "mental health" is essentially a part of "physical health" where both are interdependent, rather than independent. They both interact and a plethora of literature suggests that brain interacts with body through multiple axes—brain–gut axis,[6] brain–heart axis,[7] psychoneuroendocrinal axis, and psychoneuroimmunlogical axis. Though research in this area is limited, preliminary evidence favor that sleep and exercise are important domains in the management of psychiatric disorders. Available literature related to the role of sleep and exercise in management of important psychiatric disorders shall be examined in this review.

SLEEP AND HEALTH

As already mentioned, sleep plays an important role in management of healthy state of body. Sleep deprivation, voluntary as well as arising out of sleep disorders, has been found to induce emotional changes, cognitive impairment, obesity, and metabolism.[4,8]

Sleep, Obesity, Metabolism, and Psychiatric Disorders

Sleep restriction has been found to reduce the amount of circulating high-density lipoprotein (HDL).[9] These effects were probably mediated through alteration of expression of genes involved in metabolic pathways, such as reduction in the expression of genes encoding for the cholesterol transporters with an increase in expression of genes encoding for inflammatory markers like interleukin 1β (IL-1β) and toll-like receptor 4 (TLR4).[9] A 4-year follow-up study that assessed incidental metabolic syndrome in adults aging between 40 years and 70 years with normal metabolic profile reported that sleeping less than 6 hours a day was associated with development of metabolic syndrome.[10] Not only the sleep deprivation, but also the longer sleep duration increases chances of metabolic syndrome suggesting that sleep and metabolic syndrome have a U-shaped relationship.[11] In other words, sleeping shorter than 6 hours or more than 8 hours increases chances of metabolic syndrome.[11] However, sleep requirement varies across all ages and sleep deprivation should be seen relative to the sleep requirement relative to the age. For example, among adolescents, sleep duration shorter than 8 hours was found to increase central deposition of fat and reduce the insulin sensitivity.[12]

However, in addition to sleep duration, sleep fragmentation, altered sleep timing, and altered sleep architecture have been found to be associated with development of diabetes.[13] While a number of studies suggest that metabolic syndrome in subjects with short sleep duration is associated with alteration in gherlin and leptin, a recent systematic review failed to identify role of these factors.[14] Instead, this review suggested that relationship between sleep duration and insulin resistance is mediated through sedentary habits and unhealthy lifestyle.[14] Another meta-analysis suggested that short sleep duration leads to change in dietary habits and physical activity, thus leading to development of obesity. Moreover, it also suggested a reverse causation where obesity leads to sleep apnea resulting in sleep disruption and consequent metabolic syndrome.[15] A study conducted among middle-aged females reported this reversed association. It suggested that obesity was associated with hypertension, diabetes, poor sleep, depression, and anxiety.[16] Thus, while association between altered quantity or quality of sleep and development of metabolic syndrome/obesity is clear, underlying mechanisms are not clear. Moreover, further research is required if correction of sleep problems improves metabolic profile and obesity.[17]

Sleep and Cognition

Sleep disturbances and sleep disorders have been linked to cognitive impairment across a number of studies. For example, a community-based study reported that poor attention, concentration, and memory lapses were common in younger subjects with insomnia; however, these symptoms were more common among subjects having a diagnosis of depression and were taking psychotropics.[18] Not only insomnia, but also other sleep disorders may pave way for cognitive impairment. One of the common sleep disorders is obstructive sleep apnea (OSA) that is characterized by recurrent apneas during sleep, which are often associated with micro-arousals and consequently sleep disturbance. Depending upon the severity, OSA is treated using mandibular advancement devices or continuous positive airway pressure (CPAP) therapy. CPAP therapy has been found to improve working memory and attention among patients with OSA.[19] Interestingly, improvement in attention and vigilance can be seen after only one night of CPAP therapy; however, effects on memory consolidation perhaps require long-term CPAP therapy.[20] Episodic memory, short-term memory, and executive functioning have been reported to improve after 3 months of CPAP therapy.[21] Improvements in cognitive functions among patients with OSA are possibly associated with improving neurogenesis or reducing neurodegeneration as CPAP has been found to increase connectivity in right middle frontal gyrus and serum level of insulin-like growth factor-1 (IGF-1).[21,22] Further, CPAP therapy has been found to not only improve cognitive functions, but also to slow down cognitive decline in a longitudinal study among patients with mild-to-moderate Alzheimer's disease having comorbid OSA.[23]

Sleep and Mood

A significant advancement has been observed in our understanding between sleep and depression. Earlier, sleep disturbance was considered as an essential part of depression and thus they were not considered as target symptoms of the management plan.[24] However, sleep disturbance has been found to vary with severity of depression, with increasing prevalence with greater severity of depression.[25] Further advancement in understanding suggested a bidirectional relationship between insomnia and depression where both have been considered to work in feed forward manner to aggravate each other.[26] Interestingly, worsening of mood has been reported even after one night of complete sleep deprivation among adolescents.[27] However, recent trials have shown that daytime symptoms of insomnia may masquerade depression and treatment of insomnia may actually reduce the symptoms of depression.

Disturbed sleep have negative impact on daytime mood and these subjects often become irritable and are likely to qualify for the diagnosis of depression.[18] However, there is a possibility that daytime symptoms of insomnia and poor sleep overlap that of depression and may be mistaken for that or augment the severity of symptoms. This issue was made clearer in the studies assessing role of therapeutic techniques for various sleep disorders on daytime mood. In patients with comorbid depression and insomnia, addition of cognitive behavior therapy for insomnia (CBT-I) to the pharmacotherapy for depression led to greater symptoms resolution.[28] CBT-I is an effective technique to treat insomnia. However, delivery of behavior therapies has multiple challenges, especially availability of trained therapists, time consumed in delivery of therapy, cost of treatment, to name a few. CBT-I has been delivered in various formats to overcome these limitations, e.g. delivery in a group and development of internet modules. Whether all of them are equally effective in reducing symptoms of depression has been a challenge.

A meta-analysis has shown significant effect of face-to-face delivered CBT-I on depressive symptoms among adults; however, other modes of CBT-I delivery were not found as effective.[29] Similar results have been reported in older adults where improvement in insomnia, but not sleep quality has been found to correlate with reduction in depressive symptomatology.[30] CBT-I has also been found to be effective in improving the daytime functioning, reducing stress, and anxiety in addition to depressive symptoms, an effect that was not observed with the pharmacotherapy alone.[31] Further, improvement in depressive symptoms was found to be mediated through improvement in insomnia, further suggesting that daytime symptoms of insomnia are often mistaken for depression.[32]

Considering the advancement of our understanding that insomnia may either pave way for depression or symptoms may be mistaken for depression, further research was carried out to understand the underlying mechanism. It was found that insomnia increases the development of negative cognition by increasing the period of arousal.[33]

Among patients with OSA, CPAP has been found to correlate with improvement in depressive scores.[34] Additionally, subjects having residual OSA even after CPAP therapy had lesser improvement in depressive symptoms.[34] More than half of the patients with OSA report depressive symptoms which improve after CPAP therapy to a significant extent.[35] Apparently, depressive symptomatology in patients with OSA is not related to physical activity as improvement in depressive symptoms was found to be independent of it after CPAP therapy.[36] However, results of available meta-analysis and systematic reviews on this subject are mixed. While one meta-analysis showed that CPAP and mandibular advancement devices improve depressive symptoms, others did not find any difference between standard CPAP and sham CPAP.[37,38] Latter meta-analysis argued that improvement in depressive symptoms could be related to the patient's expectations and meeting with healthcare provider. In view of contradictory evidences, this is an area for further exploration.

Sleep and Addiction

Restless legs syndrome (RLS) is a sleep disorder that is characterized by an urge to move legs, especially at night with worsening of symptoms at rest and an improvement by movement.[39] This disorder has been linked to the dopamine abnormalities in brain, which in turn have been found to be regulated by opioid receptors.[40,41] Furthermore, opioid has been found a place in the management of RLS in selected cases.[42]

Opioid withdrawal presents with muscle aches and pains, often along with the restlessness.[43] These features often overlap with the symptoms of RLS and considering the neurobiological underpinnings, it may be possible that some of the patients develop RLS during opioid withdrawal. Case reports and case series suggested that RLS is seen in the patients during opioid withdrawal, including dextropropxyphene and tramadol.[44,45] However, large studies in this area are limited and to the best of our knowledge, only one study is available that suggested the prevalence of RLS as 13% among patients with opiate withdrawal.[46] Recognition of RLS and its distinction from myalgia that occurs during opioid/opiate withdrawal is important for a number of reasons. First, RLS may induce sleep disturbance in these patients, which is completely amenable to treatment.[44,45] Addressing the RLS may, thus, facilitate the detoxification process. Second, in contrast to myalgia, which generally lasts for only initial 3–5 days after opiate/opioid withdrawal, symptoms of RLS may persist for a longer duration, thus, requiring treatment to be continued during post-detoxification process.[44,45] A recent study from India suggested that RLS is seen in around 50% subjects during opioid withdrawal.[47] Moreover, there are evidences that concurrent cannabis use or cannabis itself may prevent or ameliorate symptoms of RLS.[47,48] Similarly, tobacco, in particular smoking, is considered as a risk factor for development of RLS.[49] However, contradictory data is also available suggesting improvement in RLS following tobacco chewing and absence of effect of smoking over RLS.[50-53] However, still gaps exist in literature and further research is required in this area.

EXERCISE AND HEALTH

Exercise and Neuronal Changes

Exercise is thought to induce a host of neuronal changes including synaptogenesis, neurogenesis, and increase in neurotrophic factors. Exercise has been found to partially reverse apoptosis, cell proliferation, demyelination, and increase brain-derived neurotrophic factor (BDNF) in a mouse model.[54] Exercise has been found to increase neurogenesis in hippocampal region, an area that has been found to lose neurons in depressed as well as demented patients.[55] It not only influences the neurogenesis, but also alters the cerebrovascular structures to improve angiogenesis, which in turn improved blood supply to neurons, an effect considered to be mediated through IGF-1.[56] In short, exercise mediates positive effect on brain that is mediated through specific cellular mechanisms.

Exercise and Depression

Exercise in addition to CBT has been found to improve depression and suicidal ideation to a greater extent compared to therapy alone in subjects with moderate depression.[57] Exercise has also been found to improve depression as an adjunct therapy to antidepressants.[58] Preliminary evidence suggest that exercise improves mood and depression during pregnancy irrespective of type of exercise—aerobic versus nonaerobic.[59] There is some controversy whether exercise alone has any effect on depressive symptoms.

One meta-analysis reported that exercise is not useful as standalone therapy for depression due to small effect size and short-lasting effect.[58] However, another paper reported that physical exercise alone is beneficial in management of mild-to-moderate depression and is as effective as standard treatments, i.e. pharmacotherapy or psychotherapy.[60]

Exercise imparts positive effect in depression through various mechanisms. One of the proposed mechanisms involved improving BDNF and consequently increasing neurogenesis.[61] Another view postulates that this effect could be mediated through exercise-induced alteration in gut microbiota, which, in turn, is known to influence neuronal functioning.[62]

Exercise and Schizophrenia

Patients with schizophrenia have lower exercise capacity and cognitive decline among them is also known. Regular exercise training improves not only the exercise capacity but also the symptoms in patients with schizophrenia.[63] Both aerobic exercise as well as yoga have been reported to improve attention and memory in long-term when used along with usual pharmacotherapy for schizophrenia.[64] However, mechanisms underlying the cognitive improvement secondary to exercise are still dubious and more research is required. Controversial data exists that reports that this effect could be mediated through increasing the neurogenesis, preventing neurodegeneration in hippocampal area and lastly, increasing BDNF.[65] Interestingly, proinflammatory markers have not been found to have any role in cognitive decline or improvement in schizophrenia, though results of these studies are confounded by obesity, smoking, and measurement of serum levels of inflammatory markers that may not truly represent brain levels of the same.[65] Additionally, exercise has been found to have beneficial effect on both positive and negative symptoms of schizophrenia. However, limited data exists regarding type of exercise, its dosing, frequency, intensity, duration, and method of execution among patients with schizophrenia; all these variables can influence the results of the studies.[66]

Exercise and Addiction

Human studies have shown that physically active individuals have lesser chances of initiating the drug use; however, contradictory data also exists. This finding varies with the type of sports the teens are involved in, intensity and duration of exercise that they are involved in during the exercise.[67] Animal studies also reported similar results where modest exercise has been found to be protective effect while chronic high level exercise predisposed to addiction.[67] From initiation to addiction, exercise has been found to have mixed effect in both human and animal studies, and at present no conclusive evidence is available regarding protective effect of exercise against addiction.[67]

Exercise has been found to reduce craving of the smoking but data related to other substances is limited.[67] Preliminary evidences suggest that exercise can be an important adjunctive therapy to prevent relapse.[67] This has also been found that gender may be a determinant factor in relation between exercise and addiction since neurobiological mechanisms of addiction differ, i.e. synaptogenesis, neurogenesis, second messenger systems, and receptor modulation differ between genders.[68]

CONCLUSION

There are sufficient evidences to conclude that management of disturbed sleep and sleep problems can alter the management of psychiatric disorders and improve the outcome. Hence, adequate knowledge of sleep disorders is necessary for psychiatry practice. However, data related to the effect of exercise in management of psychiatric disorders is preliminary but promising. Further research is required in this area to explore potential mechanisms of exercise on brain, especially in perspective of psychiatric disorders.

REFERENCES

1. Perogamvros L, Schwartz S. Sleep and emotional functions. Curr Top Behav Neurosci. 2015;25:411-31.
2. Basner M, Rao H, Goel N, et al. Sleep deprivation and neurobehavioral dynamics. Curr Opin Neurobiol. 2013;23(5):854-63.
3. Killgore WD. Effects of sleep deprivation on cognition. Prog Brain Res. 2010;185:105-29.
4. Cassé-Perrot C, Lanteaume L, Deguil J, et al. Neurobehavioral and cognitive changes induced by sleep deprivation in healthy volunteers. CNS Neurol Disord Drug Targets. 2016;15(7):777-801.
5. Exercise/Definition of Exercise by Merriam-Webster n.d. [online] Available from https://www.merriam-webster.com/dictionary/ exercise [Last accessed December, 2019].
6. Kelly JR, Kennedy PJ, Cryan JF, et al. Breaking down the barriers: The gut microbiome, intestinal permeability and stress-related psychiatric disorders. Front Cell Neurosci. 2015;9:392.
7. Bazo-Alvarez JC, Quispe R, Pillay TD, et al. Glycated haemoglobin (HbA1c) and fasting plasma glucose relationships in sea-level and high-altitude settings. Diabet Med. 2017;34(6):804-12.
8. Kohyama J. Neural basis of brain dysfunction produced by early sleep problems. Brain Sci. 2016;6(1):E5.
9. Aho V, Ollila HM, Kronholm E, et al. Prolonged sleep restriction induces changes in pathways involved in cholesterol metabolism and inflammatory responses. Sci Rep. 2016;6:24828.
10. Kim JY, Yadav D, Ahn SV, et al. A prospective study of total sleep duration and incident metabolic syndrome: The ARIRANG study. Sleep Med. 2015;16(12):1511-5.

11. Li X, Lin L, Lv L, et al. U-shaped relationships between sleep duration and metabolic syndrome and metabolic syndrome components in males: a prospective cohort study. Sleep Med. 2015;16(8):949-54.
12. De Bernardi Rodrigues AM, da Silva C de C, Vasques AC, et al. Association of sleep deprivation with reduction in insulin sensitivity as assessed by the hyperglycemic clamp technique in adolescents. JAMA Pediatr. 2016;170(5):487-94.
13. Koren D, O'Sullivan KL, Mokhlesi B. Metabolic and glycemic sequelae of sleep disturbances in children and adults. Curr Diab Rep. 2015;15(1):562.
14. Felső R, Lohner S, Hollódy K, et al. Relationship between sleep duration and childhood obesity: systematic review including the potential underlying mechanisms. Nutr Metab Cardiovasc Dis. 2017;27(9):751-61.
15. Ogilvie RP, Patel SR. The epidemiology of sleep and obesity. Sleep Health. 2017;3(5):383-8.
16. Blümel JE, Chedraui P, Aedo S, et al. Obesity and its relation to depressive symptoms and sedentary lifestyle in middle-aged women. Maturitas. 2015;80(1):100-5.
17. Coughlin JW, Smith MT. Sleep, obesity, and weight loss in adults: is there a rationale for providing sleep interventions in the treatment of obesity? Int Rev Psychiatry. 2014;26(2):177-88.
18. Ohayon MM, Lemoine P. Daytime consequences of insomnia complaints in the French general population. Encephale. 2004;30(30):222-7.
19. Hobzova M, Hubackova L, Vanek J, et al. Cognitive function and depressivity before and after CPAP treatment in obstructive sleep apnea patients. Neuro Endocrinol Lett. 2017;38(3):145-53.
20. Djonlagic I, Guo M, Matteis P, et al. First night of CPAP: impact on memory consolidation attention and subjective experience. Sleep Med. 2015;16(6):697-702.
21. Dalmases M, Solé-Padullés C, Torres M, et al. Effect of CPAP on cognition, brain function, and structure among elderly patients with OSA: A randomized pilot study. Chest. 2015;148(5):1214-23.
22. Kanbay A, Demir NC, Tutar N, et al. The effect of CPAP therapy on insulin-like growth factor and cognitive functions in obstructive sleep apnea patients. Clin Respir J. 2017;11(4):506-13.
23. Cooke JR, Ayalon L, Palmer BW, et al. Sustained use of CPAP slows deterioration of cognition, sleep, and mood in patients with Alzheimer's disease and obstructive sleep apnea: a preliminary study. J Clin Sleep Med. 2009;5(4):305-9.
24. Mendlewicz J. Sleep disturbances: core symptoms of major depressive disorder rather than associated or comorbid disorders. World J Biol Psychiatry. 2009;10(4):269-75.
25. Gupta R, Dahiya S, Bhatia MS. Effect of depression on sleep: qualitative or quantitative? Indian J Psychiatry. 2009;51(2):117-21.
26. Sivertsen B, Salo P, Mykletun A, et al. The bidirectional association between depression and insomnia: the HUNT study. Psychosom Med. 2012;74(7):758-65.
27. Short MA, Louca M. Sleep deprivation leads to mood deficits in healthy adolescents. Sleep Med. 2015;16(8):987-93.
28. Manber R, Edinger JD, Gress JL, et al. Cognitive behavioral therapy for insomnia enhances depression outcome in patients with comorbid major depressive disorder and insomnia. Sleep. 2008;31(4):489-95.

29. Ballesio A, Aquino MRJV, Feige B, et al. The effectiveness of behavioural and cognitive behavioural therapies for insomnia on depressive and fatigue symptoms: a systematic review and network meta-analysis. Sleep Med Rev. 2018;37:114-29.
30. Li MJ, Kechter A, Olmstead RE, et al. Sleep and mood in older adults: Coinciding changes in insomnia and depression symptoms. Int Psychogeriatr. 2018;30(3):431-5.
31. Morin CM, Beaulieu-Bonneau S, Bélanger L, et al. Cognitive-behavior therapy singly and combined with medication for persistent insomnia: impact on psychological and daytime functioning. Behav Res Ther. 2016;87:109-16.
32. Manber R, Buysse DJ, Edinger J, et al. Efficacy of cognitive-behavioral therapy for insomnia combined with antidepressant pharmacotherapy in patients with comorbid depression and insomnia: a randomized controlled trial. J Clin Psychiatry. 2016;77(10):e1316-23.
33. Kalmbach DA, Pillai V, Drake CL. Nocturnal insomnia symptoms and stress-induced cognitive intrusions in risk for depression: a 2-year prospective study. PLoS One. 2018;13(2):e0192088.
34. Wells RD, Freedland KE, Carney RM, et al. Adherence, reports of benefits, and depression among patients treated with continuous positive airway pressure. Psychosom Med. 2007;69(5):449-54.
35. El-Sherbini AM, Bediwy AS, El-Mitwalli A. Association between obstructive sleep apnea (OSA) and depression and the effect of continuous positive airway pressure (CPAP) treatment. Neuropsychiatr Dis Treat. 2011;7:715-21.
36. Diamanti C, Manali E, Ginieri-Coccossis M, et al. Depression, physical activity, energy consumption, and quality of life in OSA patients before and after CPAP treatment. Sleep Breath. 2013;17(4):1159-68.
37. Povitz M, Bolo CE, Heitman SJ, et al. Effect of treatment of obstructive sleep apnea on depressive symptoms: systematic review and meta-analysis. PLoS Med. 2014;11(11):e1001762.
38. Gupta MA, Simpson FC, Lyons DC. The effect of treating obstructive sleep apnea with positive airway pressure on depression and other subjective symptoms: A systematic review and meta-analysis. Sleep Med Rev. 2016;28:55-68.
39. Allen RP, Picchietti DL, Garcia-Borreguero D, et al.; International Restless Legs Syndrome Study Group. Restless legs syndrome/Willis-Ekbom disease diagnostic criteria: Updated International Restless Legs Syndrome Study Group (IRLSSG) consensus criteria—history, rationale, description, and significance. Sleep Med. 2014;15(8):860-73.
40. Sun YM, Hoang T, Neubauer JA, et al. Opioids protect against substantia nigra cell degeneration under conditions of iron deprivation: a mechanism of possible relevance to the Restless Legs Syndrome (RLS) and Parkinson's disease. J Neurol Sci. 2011;304(1-2):93-101.
41. Fulda S, Wetter TC. Where dopamine meets opioids: A meta-analysis of the placebo effect in restless legs syndrome treatment studies. Brain. 2008;131(Pt 4):902-17.
42. Aurora RN, Kristo DA, Bista SR, et al. The treatment of restless legs syndrome and periodic limb movement disorder in adults—an update for 2012: Practice parameters with an evidence-based systematic review and meta-analyses: an American Academy of Sleep Medicine Clinical Practice Guideline. Sleep. 2012;35(8):1039-62.

43. American Psychiatric Association. Diagnostic and Statistical Manual of Mental Disorders, 5th edition. Arlington: American Psychiatric Association; 2013.
44. Ghosh A, Basu D. Restless legs syndrome in opioid dependent patients. Indian J Psychol Med. 2014;36(1):85-7.
45. Park YM, Park HK, Kim L, et al. Acute-withdrawal restless legs syndrome following abrupt cessation of short-term tramadol. Psychiatry Investig. 2014;11(2):204-6.
46. Scherbaum N, Stüper B, Bonnet U, et al. Transient restless legs-like syndrome as a complication of opiate withdrawal. Pharmacopsychiatry. 2003;36(2):70-2.
47. Gupta R, Ali R, Ray R. Willis-Ekbom disease/restless legs syndrome in patients with opioid withdrawal. Sleep Med. 2018;45:39-43.
48. Megelin T, Ghorayeb I. Cannabis for restless legs syndrome: a report of six patients. Sleep Med. 2017;36:182-3.
49. Benediktsdottir B, Janson C, Lindberg E, et al. Prevalence of restless legs syndrome among adults in Iceland and Sweden: lung function, comorbidity, ferritin, biomarkers and quality of life. Sleep Med. 2010;11(10):1043-8.
50. Lahan V, Ahmad S, Gupta R. RLS relieved by tobacco chewing: paradoxical role of nicotine. Neurol Sci. 2012;33(5):1209-10.
51. Vizcarra-Escobar D, Mendiola-Yamasato A, Risco-Rocca J, et al. Is restless legs syndrome associated with chronic mountain sickness? Sleep Med. 2015;16(8): 976-80.
52. Budhiraja P, Budhiraja R, Goodwin JL, et al. Incidence of restless legs syndrome and its correlates. J Clin Sleep Med. 2012;8(2):119-24.
53. Gupta R, Ulfberg J, Allen RP, et al. High prevalence of restless legs syndrome/ Willis Ekbom Disease (RLS/WED) among people living at high altitude in the Indian Himalaya. Sleep Med. 2017;35:7-11.
54. Kim TW, Sung YH. Regular exercise promotes memory function and enhances hippocampal neuroplasticity in experimental autoimmune encephalomyelitis mice. Neuroscience. 2017;346:173-81.
55. Ma CL, Ma XT, Wang JJ, et al. Physical exercise induces hippocampal neurogenesis and prevents cognitive decline. Behav Brain Res. 2017;317:332-9.
56. Nishijima T, Torres-Aleman I, Soya H. Exercise and cerebrovascular plasticity. Prog Brain Res. 2016;225:243-68.
57. Abdollahi A, LeBouthillier DM, Najafi M, et al. Effect of exercise augmentation of cognitive behavioural therapy for the treatment of suicidal ideation and depression. J Affect Disord. 2017;219:58-63.
58. Kvam S, Kleppe CL, Nordhus IH, et al. Exercise as a treatment for depression: a meta-analysis. J Affect Disord. 2016;202:67-86.
59. Daley AJ, Foster L, Long G, et al. The effectiveness of exercise for the prevention and treatment of antenatal depression: systematic review with meta-analysis. BJOG. 2015;122(1):57-62.
60. Andersson E, Hovland A, Kjellman B, et al. Physical activity is just as good as CBT or drugs for depression. Lakartidningen. 2015;112. pii: DP4E.
61. Phillips C. Brain-derived neurotrophic factor, depression, and physical activity: Making the neuroplastic connection. Neural Plast. 2017;2017:7260130.
62. Yuan TF, Ferreira Rocha NB, Paes F, et al. Neural mechanisms of exercise: effects on gut microbiota and depression. CNS Neurol Disord Drug Targets. 2015;14(10):1312-4.

63. Curcic D, Stojmenovic T, Djukic-Dejanovic S, et al. Positive impact of prescribed physical activity on symptoms of schizophrenia: Randomized clinical trial. Psychiatr Danub. 2017;29(4):459-65.
64. Bhatia T, Mazumdar S, Wood J, et al. A randomised controlled trial of adjunctive yoga and adjunctive physical exercise training for cognitive dysfunction in schizophrenia. Acta Neuropsychiatr. 2017;29(2):102-14.
65. Firth J, Cotter J, Carney R, et al. The pro-cognitive mechanisms of physical exercise in people with schizophrenia. Br J Pharmacol. 2017;174(19):3161-72.
66. Rimes RR, de Souza Moura AM, Lamego MK, et al. Effects of exercise on physical and mental health, and cognitive and brain functions in schizophrenia: Clinical and experimental evidence. CNS Neurol Disord Drug Targets. 2015;14(10):1244-54.
67. Lynch WJ, Peterson AB, Sanchez V, et al. Exercise as a novel treatment for drug addiction: a neurobiological and stage-dependent hypothesis. Neurosci Biobehav Rev. 2013;37(8):1622-44.
68. Zhou Y, Zhao M, Zhou C, et al. Sex differences in drug addiction and response to exercise intervention: from human to animal studies. Front Neuroendocrinol. 2016;40:24-41.

CHAPTER 15

Recent Advances in Drug Treatment of Chronic Depression

Kaustav Chakraborty

INTRODUCTION

Depression is a disorder of major public health importance, in terms of its prevalence and the suffering, dysfunction, morbidity, and economic burden. The report on Global Burden of Disease estimates the point prevalence of unipolar depressive episodes to be 1.9% for men and 3.2% for women, and the 1-year prevalence has been estimated to be 5.8% for men and 9.5% for women. Global Burden of Diseases report also shows that unipolar depressive disorders place an enormous burden on society and are ranked as the fourth leading cause of burden among all diseases, accounting for 4.4% of the total disability adjusted life years (DALYs) and are the leading cause of years lived with disability (YLD), accounting for 11.9% of total YLD. It is estimated that, by the year 2020, if current trends for demographic and epidemiological transition continue, the burden of depression will increase to 5.7% of the total burden of disease and it would be the second leading cause of DALYs, second only to ischemic heart disease.[1]

Chronic major depression has been subsumed under persistent depressive disorder in Diagnostic and Statistical Manual of Mental Disorders, fifth edition (DSM-5)[2] which also includes dysthymic disorder hitherto described in DSM, 4th edition, Text Revision (DSM-IV-TR). The criteria for chronic major depression requires a depressed mood for most of the day, for more days than not, as indicated by either subjective account or observation by others, for at least 2 years. During this 2-year period (1 year for children or adolescents) of the disturbance, the individual has never been without the symptoms for more than 2 months at a time. It also requires the presence of, while depressed, of two (or more) of the following: poor appetite or overeating; insomnia or hypersomnia; low energy or fatigue; low self-esteem; poor concentration or difficulty making decisions; and feelings of hopelessness.

Antidepressants are the first-line treatments for a major depressive episode (moderate-to-severe depressive episode) in the context of major depressive disorder (MDD). While choosing an antidepressant certain factors should be taken into account, e.g. patient's prior experience with the drug (response, tolerability, adverse effects), coexisting medical conditions and use of medicines other than psychotropics, a particular drug's short- and long-term side effects, safety in overdose, physician's own comfortability to the medicine, history of patient's adherence to medication, history of response to medicine in a first-degree relative, patient preferences, affordability, availability of specific antidepressants, and whether the antidepressant has been approved by the appropriate drug controlling authority. No single class of antidepressant has been proved to be more efficacious or have faster onset of action compared to others, although some tricyclic antidepressants (TCAs) (amitriptyline and clomipramine), and venlafaxine are slightly more effective than selective serotonin reuptake inhibitors (SSRIs) in severely depressed hospitalized patients. Different classes of antidepressants have different side-effect profile, potential for drug–drug interaction and safety issues when taken in overdose. Second (e.g. bupropion, maprotiline, mianserin, trazodone) and third [e.g. SSRI, serotonin-noradrenaline reuptake inhibitors (SNRIs), mirtazapine] generation antidepressants are generally well tolerated than the first-generation TCAs, and therefore, patients are less likely to discontinue them. This may have a significant impact on "real-life" efficacy. It has now been established that, in at least one-third of the cases, patients do not respond to first-line treatment with any chosen antidepressant. In this scenario, a careful review of the diagnosis, comorbid axis II pathology, compliance to the medication should be performed. Thereafter, clinician can do the following things: (1) increase the dose of the initial antidepressant to its maximum dose; (2) switching to another antidepressant from a different pharmacological class (e.g. from a SSRI to a TCA or a dual-acting antidepressant); (3) switching to another antidepressant within the same pharmacological class (e.g. from a SSRI to another SSRI); (4) combining two antidepressants from different classes (e.g. an SSRI or a dual-acting AD with e.g. mirtazapine); (5) augmenting the antidepressant with other agents (e.g. lithium, thyroid hormone or atypical antipsychotics) to enhance antidepressant efficacy; (6) combining the antidepressant with a psychotherapeutic intervention; and (7) combining the antidepressant with nonpharmacological biological therapies [e.g. wake therapy, light therapy, electroconvulsive therapy (ECT)]. Augmentation with lithium, quetiapine, and aripiprazole are the best-documented strategies at present.[3]

With this brief introduction, in subsequent sections, the author will review the evidences available for existing antidepressants and will also explore the recent advances in drug treatment of chronic major depression.

DATA SEARCH METHODOLOGY

The data search strategies used included electronic databases as well as hand-search of relevant publications or cross-references. The electronic search included PUBMED, Google Scholar, PsycINFO, etc. Cross-searches of electronic and hand-search key references yielded other relevant material. Besides this, American Psychiatric Association (APA) guidelines, British

Association of Psychopharmacology (BAP) guidelines, World Federation of Societies of Biological Psychiatry (WFSBP) guidelines, Canadian Network for Mood and Anxiety Treatment (CANMAT) guidelines, Royal Australian and New Zealand College of Psychiatrists (RANZCP) clinical practice guidelines for mood disorders, and Maudsley guidelines were very much useful[3-8] **(Table 1)**. The search terms used, in various combinations, were unipolar major depression, chronic depression, management, treatment, novel, molecules, drugs, antidepressants, clinical, and trials.

ANTIDEPRESSANTS: GENERAL OVERVIEW

The severity of depression at which antidepressants show consistent benefits over placebo is poorly defined. Although it is generally accepted that the more severe the symptoms, the greater the benefit from antidepressant treatment, there is some evidence to support the view that response may be independent of symptom severity.[9] Antidepressants are normally recommended as first-line treatment in patients whose depression is of at least moderate severity. Of this patient group, approximately 20% will recover with no treatment at all, 30% will respond to placebo and 50% will respond to antidepressant drug treatment.[10] This gives a number needed to treat (NNT) of 3 for antidepressant over true no-treatment control and an NNT of 5 for antidepressant over placebo. Drug–placebo differences have diminished over time largely because of methodological changes.[11] Recent studies have reappraised drug–placebo differences. Hieronymus et al. did patient-level post hoc analyses of 18 industry-sponsored placebo-controlled trials of sertraline, paroxetine, fluoxetine, or citalopram which included 6,669 adults with major depression, with the aim to assess the outcome with single-item depressed mood (rated 0–4) being used as the measure of efficacy.[12] In total, 32 drug–placebo comparisons were reassessed. While 18 out of 32 comparisons (56%) failed to separate active drug from placebo at week 6 with respect to reduction in Hamilton Depression Rating Scale (HDRS/HAM-D)-17 score, only 3 out of 32 comparisons (9%) were negative when depressed mood was used as an effect parameter ($p \leq 0.001$). Even when whole depression scales are used, a recent network meta-analysis showed robust superiority for antidepressants over placebo, with amitriptyline being the most efficacious.[13] In patients with subsyndromal depression, it is difficult to separate antidepressant response rate from that of placebo. In such cases, antidepressant treatment is not indicated unless the patient has a definite history of moderate-to-severe depression or symptoms persist. Patients with dysthymia also benefit from antidepressant treatment; however, the minimum duration of symptoms associated with benefit is not known. In other patients, the adverse effects associated with antidepressant treatment may not justify their use compared to the small benefit seen.

Table 1: Comparison between different guidelines regarding pharmacological treatment of major depressive disorder (MDD).	
Guidelines	Summary of recommendations
APA guideline, 2002[4]	If preferred by the patient, antidepressant medications may be provided as an initial primary treatment modality for mild MDD. Antidepressant medications should be provided for moderate-to-severe MDD unless electroconvulsive therapy (ECT) is planned. A combination of antipsychotic and antidepressant medications or ECT should be used for psychotic depression.
WFSBP guidelines, 2013[3]	Antidepressants are the first-line treatments for a major depressive episode (moderate–to-severe depressive episode) in the context of MDD. No single class of antidepressants has proven to be more effective or have a more rapid onset than any other, although some tricyclic antidepressants (TCAs) (amitriptyline and clomipramine), and venlafaxine are slightly more effective than selective serotonin reuptake inhibitor (SSRI) in severely depressed hospitalized patients.
BAP guidelines, 2015[5]	Antidepressants are a first-line treatment for moderate and severe major depression in adults irrespective of environmental factors and depression symptom profile; and depression of any severity that has persisted for 2 years or more. In more severely ill patients, and in other situations where maximizing efficacy is of overriding importance, consider clomipramine, venlafaxine (150 mg), escitalopram (20 mg), sertraline, amitriptyline, or mirtazapine in preference to other antidepressants.
RANZCP guidelines, 2015[7]	In mild-to-moderate episodes of MDD, psychological management alone may be adequate, especially early in the course of illness. However, episodes of greater severity, and those that run a chronic course, are likely to require the addition of antidepressant medication. In severe episodes of MDD pharmacotherapy is typically needed and, where there is a high risk of suicide or when the patient's welfare is threatened by a lack of nutrition or fluid intake, urgent intervention is sometimes necessary and may include ECT.
CANMAT guidelines, 2016[6]	Most second-generation antidepressants are recommended as first-line treatments for patients with a major depressive episode of moderate or greater severity (as determined by symptom scales and/or functional impairment). The SSRIs, serotonin norepinephrine reuptake inhibitors (SNRIs), agomelatine, bupropion, and mirtazapine remain first-line recommendations for pharmacotherapy for MDD. Vortioxetine is also a first-line recommendation. Recommended second-line agents include TCAs, quetiapine and trazodone (owing to higher side-effect burden), moclobemide and selegiline (potential serious drug interactions), levomilnacipran (lack of comparative and relapse prevention data), and vilazodone (lack of comparative and relapse prevention data and the need to titrate and take with food). Third-line recommendations include monoamine oxidase inhibitors (owing to higher side-effect burden and potential serious drug and dietary interactions) and reboxetine (lower efficacy).
Maudsley guidelines, 2018[8]	Antidepressants are recommended for the treatment of moderate-to-severe depression and subthreshold depressive symptoms that persist for more than 2 years. When an antidepressant is prescribed, a generic SSRI is recommended.

(APA: American Psychological Association; BAP: British Association for Psychopharmacology; CANMAT: Canadian Network for Mood and Anxiety Treatment; RANZCP: Royal Australian and New Zealand College of Psychiatrists; WFSBP: The World Federation of Societies of Biological Psychiatry)

Selective serotonin reuptake inhibitors (SSRIs) are well-tolerated compared with the older TCAs and monoamine oxidase inhibitors (MAOIs), and are generally recommended as first-line pharmacological treatment for depression.[14] There is a suggestion from network meta-analyses that some antidepressants may be more effective overall than others but this has not been consistently demonstrated in head-to-head studies and should therefore be treated with caution.[13,15] Adverse-effect profiles of antidepressants do differ. For example, paroxetine has been associated with weight gain and sexual dysfunction, and sertraline with diarrhea compared to other SSRIs. Dual reuptake inhibitors such as venlafaxine and duloxetine are better tolerated than TCAs but less well-tolerated than SSRIs. A flexible approach is usually required to find the right drug for a particular patient. SSRIs as a class are associated with a range of other adverse effects including sexual dysfunction, hyponatremia and gastrointestinal (GI) bleeds. TCAs have adverse cardiovascular side effects, e.g. hypotension, tachycardia and QTc prolongation, and can be life threatening in cases of overdose. MAOIs, which are rarely used nowadays, have the propensity to interact with tyramine-containing foods to cause hypertensive crisis. All antidepressant drugs can cause discontinuation symptoms, the problem being more evident with drugs having short half-life.

Antidepressants do not treat the underlying cause of depression, but they just relieve the symptoms. Therefore, they should be taken for 6–9 months after recovery from a single episode. In patients having multiple episodes, there is evidence of benefit from maintenance treatment for at least 2 years; although in selected cases treatment may have to be continued for lifelong. However, research data is lacking on the duration of augmentation strategies.[8]

Approximately one-third of patients do not respond to the first antidepressant. Options in this group include increasing the dose, switching to a different drug of same or different class and augment with different agents. The Sequenced Treatment Alternatives to Relieve Depression (STAR*D) has shown that a small proportion of nonresponders will respond with each treatment change, but that effect sizes are modest and there is no advantage of one strategy over the other.[16]

MANAGEMENT OF PERSISTENT AND CHRONIC DEPRESSION

A systematic review and network meta-analysis examined the efficacy and acceptability of treatments for persistent depressive disorder (PDD) which included 45 randomized controlled trials (RCTs) (N = 5,804) involving 28 drugs.[17] Most of the studied drugs were more effective compared to placebo, including fluoxetine, paroxetine, sertraline, moclobemide, and imipramine, with no differences in acceptability compared to placebo. Among the active comparators, sertraline had higher efficacy over imipramine and fluoxetine had superior acceptability over moclobemide.[17] These results were similar to a meta-analysis (20 trials, N = 2,918) of chronic depression showing that SSRIs were similar in efficacy but superior in tolerability compared with TCAs.[18] The network meta-analysis also identified differences in effects between combined psychotherapy + medication and medication-only studies in dysthymia compared to studies of chronic MDD, suggesting that the new diagnosis of PDD may not have homogeneous treatment response.[17] Although antidepressants showed some positive results in treating chronic depression and PDD, experts have argued that patients with chronic course of depression and recurrent treatment failure should have a chronic management approach, i.e. less reliance on drug management, lesser emphasis on remission and cure, more emphasis on psychotherapeutic and nonmedication management, and more focus on improving the quality of life and functioning.[19]

NEWER ANTIDEPRESSANT MOLECULES

Vortioxetine

Vortioxetine probably acts through enhancement of serotonergic activity via reuptake inhibition; other potential mechanisms include agonism and/or antagonism of various serotonin receptors (e.g. 5-HT1A, 5-HT1B, 5-HT3, 5-HT1D, and 5-HT7).[20] Vortioxetine is usually taken orally with or without food; the recommended starting dose is 10 mg/day in a single dose, which can be increased to 20 mg/day.[20] In patients having tolerability issues, dosage can be lowered to 5 mg/day. Because of its relatively long elimination half-life, vortioxetine is associated with a low level of discontinuation symptoms and abrupt discontinuation can be attempted.[21] In Canada, approval of vortioxetine for the acute treatment of MDD was based on a review of 11 short-term (6 or 8 weeks) Phase III studies, which included 6 positive studies of vortioxetine 5–20 mg/day in adults, vortioxetine 20 mg/day in adults, and vortioxetine 5 mg/day in older adults (>65 years).[22-24] In non-US trials, all the 4 doses (5 mg, 10 mg, 15 mg, and 20 mg) showed efficacy against placebo. In US trials, only the 20 mg/day dose was significantly efficacious than placebo, which led the US Food and Drug Administration to recommend a starting dose of 10 mg/day, with an increase to 20 mg/day as tolerated.[20] In a meta-analysis of vortioxetine studies, significantly greater decreases in Montgomery–Åsberg Depression Rating Scale (MADRS) total score were shown for vortioxetine (5, 10, and 20 mg/day) versus placebo.[25] Treatment effects appeared to be dose-related, which is consistent with the dose-related pharmacokinetics of vortioxetine.[20] Placebo-controlled studies have shown improvement in cognitive functioning with vortioxetine irrespective of its effect on depressive symptoms.[26-27] This procognitive effects of vortioxetine involve a combination of monoaminergic and glutamatergic effects.[26] Vortioxetine has also been effective in preventing relapse and was well-tolerated as maintenance agent.[28] Nausea was the only adverse event (AE) reported in >10% of all vortioxetine-treated patients during placebo-controlled trials.[20] Vortioxetine has demonstrated placebo-level sexual dysfunction at initiation doses of 10 mg/day.[21] Although rates of sexual dysfunction are higher at doses of 15-20 mg/day compared with 10 mg/day (lower than SSRI treatment), switching to vortioxetine has been shown to be beneficial for patients experiencing sexual dysfunction during antidepressant therapy with SSRIs.[21]

Levomilnacipran

Levomilnacipran ER, the more active enantiomer of the racemic drug milnacipran, is an SNRI with preferential inhibition of norepinephrine reuptake *in vitro*.[29,30] Levomilnacipran exhibits higher affinity for norepinephrine and serotonin transporters compared to milnacipran.[30] The recommended dose is 40-120 mg once daily, with or without food; levomilnacipran ER is started at 20 mg/day for 2 days and then increased to 40 mg/day. Based on response and side effects, the dose can be increased in 40 mg/day increments every 2 or more days until the highest recommended dose of 120 mg/day is reached.[29] To prevent emergence of discontinuation symptoms, gradual dose reduction is recommended for levomilnacipran ER whenever possible.[29] In the Health Canada review, four short-term (8 or 10 weeks) placebo-controlled trials of levomilnacipran ER were included, including three positive studies (2 fixed dose and 1 flexible dose).[31-33] In these studies, levomilnacipran ER showed significant changes from baseline in MADRS total score (primary endpoint) and Sheehan Disability Scale (SDS; secondary endpoint) compared to placebo, indicating greater improvement in depressive symptoms and functional impairment. At the time of the Health Canada review, a levomilnacipran ER relapse prevention study had not been completed (NCT02288325); however, subsequently reported results showed that continued treatment with levomilnacipran ER (40-120 mg/day) significantly reduced risk of relapse compared to placebo over a 26 weeks' period.[34]

Post hoc analyses of clinical study data indicated that levomilnacipran ER can improve motivation and energy, which is consistent with its noradrenergic effects.[35,36] A meta-analysis of five randomized placebo-controlled studies showed that levomilnacipran ER improved range of symptoms and symptom domains of depression, including anhedonia and retardation.[37] In placebo-controlled trials, nausea was the only AE reported in 10% of all levomilnacipran ER-treated patients.[29] No untoward safety concerns were found during a 48-week open-label extension study in which patients received levomilnacipran ER (40, 80, or 120 mg/day) or during the relapse prevention trial.[34,38]

Vilazodone

Vilazodone is a serotonin reuptake inhibitor and partial serotonergic 5-HT1A receptor agonist.[39] The recommended dose is 20–40 mg/day taken once daily with food. The initial 10-mg/day dose is taken for 7 days, followed by an increase to 20 mg/day then to 40 mg/day at an interval of 7 days or more to avoid acute GI side effects.[39,40] Additionally, gradual dosage reduction is recommended to avoid reactions associated with serotonin discontinuation syndrome.[39] In the four short-term (8 or 10 weeks) phase III trials, significantly greater improvements in depression scores were seen with vilazodone (20–40 mg/day) compared to placebo.[41] In a post hoc pooled analysis of data from two clinical trials, statistically significant differences were seen for vilazodone on rating scales measuring depression, anxiety and global illness severity compared to placebo. Vilazodone showed significant improvement on individual items of MADRS, suggesting efficacy across a myriad of depressive symptoms compared to placebo. Vilazodone might be well suited for patients with depression and high levels of anxiety, as suggested by post hoc analyses of MDD trials' data and results from studies in patients with generalized anxiety disorder.[42,43] Diarrhea, nausea, and headache were the adverse effects reported in >10% of all vilazodone-treated patients in placebo-controlled trials.[39] Weight gain in the long-term MDD study was small (mean increase +1.7 kg), in contrast to mean weight gains seen in long-term studies of other SSRI drugs (up to ~10 kg).[44,45] Vilazodone was relatively safe in sexually active male depressed patients compared to placebo.[46]

Ketamine

Ketamine, which is known to affect descending glutamatergic systems represent a novel approach for managing treatment-resistant depression (TRD).[47] Many well-controlled clinical trials indicate that a single ketamine infusion (0.5 mg/kg) induces a rapid but generally transient, antidepressant effect in addition to small, but significant, increases in psychotomimetic and dissociative symptoms.[48] The ketamine-induced antidepressant effect occurs within 1–2 hours following its intravenous administration and may sustain for up to 2 weeks.[49] This rapid onset of action has encouraged studies to explore the role of ketamine as a potential life-saving drug for treatment-resistant depression (TRD) patient with high suicidality.[50] Twice- and thrice-weekly administration of ketamine at 0.5 mg/kg provides antidepressant efficacy for over 2 weeks with no signs of tolerance.[51] It is hypothesized that by blocking N-methyl-D-aspartate (NMDA) receptors on GABAergic interneurons, ketamine causes a rapid, but transient, increase in extracellular glutamate in the prefrontal cortex. At the molecular level, the ketamine-induced blockade of NMDA receptors results in inhibition of elongation factor 2 (eF2) kinase, dephosphorylation of eF2, and a consequent increase in brain-derived neurotrophic factor (BDNF) synthesis.[47] Recent studies suggest that pharmacological profile of ketamine is more complex and goes beyond NMDA receptor blockade because it also shows significant affinity for dopamine D2 receptor (D2R) and opioid receptors as well as for monoamine transporters.

NOVEL DRUGS IN THE PIPELINE

The link between glutamate system and rapid antidepressant effect of ketamine has enthused the researchers to explore for related molecules, including esketamine (the S-enantiomer of ketamine, delivered intranasally), lanicemine, and memantine.[52,53] Other molecules which hold promise include GluN2B antagonists (e.g. CERC-301); GLYX13, which targets the glycine coagonist site on the NMDA receptor; and basimglurant, which targets the metabotropic glutamate (mGlu) receptors.[54] Other target molecules with antidepressant actions are those which target the endocannabinoid systems and drugs affecting the cerebral neuroplasticity, which is thought to have sustained antidepressant effects. Nonsteroidal anti-inflammatory drugs (NSAIDs) have also been researched. In a meta-analysis (4 studies, N = 150), higher response and remission rates were reported with adjunctive celecoxib compared to placebo.[55] Preliminary studies of pramipexole, a dopaminergic D2, D3, and D4 receptor agonist that has efficacy in bipolar depression, was shown to have some benefit in TRD.[56] Other investigational drugs for MDD include cariprazine, a novel atypical antipsychotic.[57]

EVIDENCE FROM RECENT META-ANALYSIS

A meta-analysis by Cipriani et al. included 522 trials of antidepressants comprising 116,477 participants.[15] It found that all antidepressants were more effective than placebo, with odds ratios (ORs) ranging between 2.13 [95% credible interval (CrI) 1.89–2.41] for amitriptyline and 1.37 (1.16–1.63) for reboxetine. Regarding acceptability, only agomelatine (OR 0.84, 95% CrI 0.72–0.97) and fluoxetine (0.88, 0.80–0.96) were associated with fewer dropouts than placebo, whereas clomipramine performed worse than placebo (1.30, 1.01–1.68). When all trials were considered, differences in ORs between antidepressants ranged from 1.15 to 1.55 for efficacy and from 0.64 to 0.83 for acceptability.[15] In head-to-head comparison, escitalopram, mirtazapine, paroxetine, agomelatine, venlafaxine, amitriptyline, and vortioxetine were more effective than other antidepressants (range of ORs 1.19–1.96), whereas reboxetine, fluoxetine, fluvoxamine, and trazodone underperformed (0.51–0.84). Agomelatine, fluoxetine, sertraline, citalopram, escitalopram, and vortioxetine were more tolerable than other antidepressants (range of ORs 0.43–0.77), whereas clomipramine, duloxetine, amitriptyline, fluvoxamine, trazodone, reboxetine, and venlafaxine had the highest dropout rates (1.30–2.32).[15] 46 (9%) of 522 trials were rated as having high risk of bias, 380 (73%) trials as moderate, and 96 (18%) as low; and the certainty of evidence was moderate to very low. The meta-analysis concluded that all antidepressants were more efficacious compared to placebo for treatment of MDD in adults. There was more variability in efficacy and acceptability among the antidepressants in head-to-head trials.

CONCLUSION

Antidepressants remain the mainstay of treatment of moderate-to-severe depressive episode and chronic depression persisting for more than 2 years. Antidepressants have been proven to be efficacious compared to placebo in treating the abovementioned conditions. However, there was no difference between antidepressants in terms of efficacy. A recent meta-analysis by Cipriani et al. suggested that few of them might be superior to the rest in terms of efficacy and tolerability. Newer molecules such as vortioxetine, levomilnacipran, and agomelatine have come up with the promises of dual action of blocking serotonin transporter (SERT) and agonist/partial agonist/antagonistic action on certain subtypes of 5-HT receptors, but they need to withstand the test of time and real world experiences to become comparable to established agents, e.g. the SNRIs and SSRIs. Nevertheless, the available guidelines guide the clinicians in choosing antidepressants based upon the evidence for/against a particular molecule and at the same time empower them to exercise their own expertise in choosing a particular molecule depending upon its side effects, patient preference, affordability, treatment response in index/prior episodes, family history of treatment response, and presence of medical comorbidities. With the advent of newer neuroimaging modalities and more insight into the neurochemical pathways of brain, newer/novel antidepressants molecules which are in the pipeline are expected to aid in the treatment of MDD.

REFERENCES

1. Lopez AD, Mathers CD, Ezzati M, et al. Global Burden of Disease and Risk Factors. Washington: The World Bank; 2006.
2. American Psychiatric Association. Diagnostic and Statistical Manual of Mental Disorders, 5th edition. Washington, DC: American Psychiatric Association; 2013.
3. Bauer M, Pfennig A, Severus E, et al. World Federation of Societies of Biological Psychiatry (WFSBP) guidelines for biological treatment of unipolar depressive disorders, part 1: update 2013 on the acute and continuation treatment of unipolar depressive disorders. World J Biol Psychiatry. 2013;14(5):334-85.
4. Work Group on Major Depressive Disorder. Practice guideline for the treatment of patients with major depressive disorder, 2nd edition. Washington, DC: American Psychiatric Association; 2002.

5. Cleare A, Pariante CM, Young AH, et al. Evidence-based guidelines for treating depressive disorders with antidepressants: a revision of the 2008 British Association for Psychopharmacology guidelines. J Psychopharmacol. 2015;29(5): 459-525.
6. Kennedy SH, Lam RW, McIntyre RS, et al. Canadian Network for Mood and Anxiety Treatments (CANMAT) 2016 Clinical Guidelines for the Management of Adults with Major Depressive Disorder: Section 3. Pharmacological Treatments. Can J Psychiatry. 2016;61(9):540-60.
7. Malhi GS, Bassett D, Boyce P, et al. Royal Australian and New Zealand College of Psychiatrists clinical practice guidelines for mood disorders. Aust NZJ Psychiatry 2015;49(12):1-185.
8. Taylor D, Barnes TRE, Young AH. The Maudsley. Prescribing Guidelines in Psychiatry, 13th edition. West Sussex, UK: Wiley Blackwell; 2018.
9. Kirsch I, Deacon BJ, Huedo-Medina TB, et al. Initial severity and antidepressant benefits: a meta-analysis of data submitted to the Food and Drug Administration. PLoS Med. 2008;5:e45.
10. Anderson IM, IN Ferrier, RC Baldwin, et al. Evidence-based guidelines for treating depressive disorders with antidepressants: a revision of the 2000 British Association for Psychopharmacology guidelines. J Psychopharmacol. 2008;22: 343-96.
11. Khan A, Bhat A, Kolts R, et al. Why has the antidepressant-placebo difference in antidepressant clinical trials diminished over the past three decades? CNS Neurosci Ther. 2010;16:217-26.
12. Hieronymus F, Emilsson JF, Nilsson S, et al. Consistent superiority of selective serotonin reuptake inhibitors over placebo in reducing depressed mood in patients with major depression. Mol Psychiatry. 2016;21:523-30.
13. Cipriani A, Furukawa TA, Salanti G, et al. Comparative efficacy and acceptability of 21 antidepressant drugs for the acute treatment of adults with major depressive disorder: a systematic review and network meta-analysis. Lancet. 2018;391: 1357-66.
14. National Institute for Health and Care Excellence (2009). Depression in adults: recognition and management. Clinical guideline 90. [online] Available from https://www.nice.org.uk/guidance/cg90 [Last accessed January, 2020].
15. Cipriani A, Furukawa TA, Salanti G, et al. Comparative efficacy and acceptability of 12 new-generation antidepressants: a multiple-treatments meta-analysis. Lancet. 2009;373:746-58.
16. Rush AJ, Warden D, Wisniewski SR, et al. STAR*D: revising conventional wisdom. CNS Drugs. 2009;23:627-47.
17. Kriston L, von Wolff A, Westphal A, et al. Efficacy and acceptability of acute treatments for persistent depressive disorder: a network meta-analysis. Depress Anxiety. 2014;31:621-30.
18. von Wolff A, Hölzel LP, Westphal A, et al. Selective serotonin reuptake inhibitors and tricyclic antidepressants in the acute treatment of chronic depression and dysthymia: a systematic review and meta-analysis. J Affect Disord. 2013;144:7-15.
19. Keitner GI, Mansfield AK. Management of treatment resistant depression. Psychiatr Clin North Am. 2012;35:249-65.

20. Trintellix (vortioxetine). US prescribing information. Deerfield (IL): Takeda Pharmaceuticals America, Inc; 2016.
21. Baldwin DS, Chrones L, Florea I, et al. The safety and tolerability of vortioxetine: analysis of data from randomized placebo-controlled trials and open-label extension studies. J Psychopharmacol. 2016;30(3):242-52.
22. Boulenger JP, Loft H, Olsen CK. Efficacy and safety of vortioxetine (Lu AA21004), 15 and 20 mg/day: a randomized, double-blind, placebocontrolled, duloxetine-referenced study in the acute treatment of adult patients with major depressive disorder. Int Clin Psychopharmacol. 2014;29(3):138-49.
23. Mahableshwarkar AR, Jacobsen PL, Chen Y, et al. A randomized, double-blind, duloxetine-referenced study comparing efficacy and tolerability of 2 fixed doses of vortioxetine in the acute treatment of adults with MDD. Psychopharmacology (Berl). 2015;232(12):2061-70.
24. Jacobsen PL, Mahableshwarkar AR, Serenko M, et al. A randomized, double-blind, placebo-controlled study of the efficacy and safety of vortioxetine 10 mg and 20 mg in adults with major depressive disorder. J Clin Psychiatry. 2015;76(5):575-82.
25. Thase ME, Mahableshwarkar AR, Dragheim M, et al. A meta-analysis of randomized, placebo-controlled trials of vortioxetine for the treatment of major depressive disorder in adults. Eur Neuropsychopharmacol. 2016;26(6):979-93.
26. McIntyre RS, Harrison J, Loft H, et al. The effects of vortioxetine on cognitive function in patients with major depressive disorder: a meta-analysis of three randomized controlled trials. Int J Neuropsychopharmacol. 2016. pii: pyw055.
27. Rosenblat JD, Kakar R, McIntyre RS. The cognitive effects of antidepressants in major depressive disorder: a systematic review and metaanalysis of randomized clinical trials. Int J Neuropsychopharmacol. 2015;19(2):1-13.
28. Boulenger JP, Loft H, Florea I. A randomized clinical study of Lu AA21,004 in the prevention of relapse in patients with major depressive disorder. J Psychopharmacol. 2012;26:1408-16.
29. Fetzima (levomilnacipran extended release). US prescribing information. Irvine, CA: Allergan USA, Inc; 2017.
30. Auclair AL, Martel JC, Assie MB, et al. Levomilnacipran (F2695), a norepinephrine-preferring SNRI: profile in vitro and in models of depression and anxiety. Neuropharmacology. 2013;70:338-47.
31. Asnis GM, Bose A, Gommoll CP, et al. Efficacy and safety of levomilnacipran sustained release 40 mg, 80 mg, or 120 mg in major depressive disorder: a phase 3, randomized, double-blind, placebo-controlled study. J Clin Psychiatry. 2013;74(3):242-8.
32. Bakish D, Bose A, Gommoll C, et al. Levomilnacipran ER 40 mg and 80 mg in patients with major depressive disorder: a phase III, randomized, double-blind, fixed-dose, placebo- controlled study. J Psychiatry Neurosci. 2014;39(1):40-9.
33. Sambunaris A, Bose A, Gommoll CP, et al. A phase III, doubleblind, placebo-controlled, flexible-dose study of levomilnacipran extended-release in patients with major depressive disorder. J Clin Psychopharmacol. 2014;34(1):47-56.
34. Durgam S, Chen C, Migliore R, et al. Relapse prevention with levomilnacipran ER in adults with major depressive disorder: a multicenter, randomized, double-blind, placebo-controlled study [abstract]. American Psychiatric Association Annual Meeting. San Diego, CA; 2017.

35. Thase ME, Gommoll C, Chen C, et al. Effects of levomilnacipran extended-release on motivation/energy and functioning in adults with major depressive disorder. Int Clin Psychopharmacol. 2016;31(6):332-40.
36. Bruno A, Morabito P, Spina E, et al. The role of levomilnacipran in the management of major depressive disorder: a comprehensive review. Curr Neuropharmacol. 2016;14(2):191-9.
37. McIntyre RS, Gommoll C, Chen C, et al. The efficacy of levomilnacipran ER across symptoms of major depressive disorder: a post hoc analysis of 5 randomized, double-blind, placebo-controlled trials. CNS Spectr. 2016;21(5):385-92.
38. Mago R, Forero G, Greenberg WM, et al. Safety and tolerability of levomilnacipran ER in major depressive disorder: results from an open-label, 48-week extension study. Clin Drug Investig. 2013;33(10):761-71.
39. Viibryd (vilazodone). US prescribing information. Irvine, CA: Allergan USA, Inc; 2017.
40. Singh M, Schwartz TL. Clinical utility of vilazodone for the treatment of adults with major depressive disorder and theoretical implications for future clinical use. Neuropsychiatr Dis Treat. 2012;8:123-30.
41. Mathews M, Gommoll C, Chen D, et al. Efficacy and safety of vilazodone 20 and 40 mg in major depressive disorder: a randomized, double-blind, placebo-controlled trial. Int Clin Psychopharmacol. 2015;30(2):67-74.
42. Gommoll C, Forero G, Mathews M, et al. Vilazodone in patients with generalized anxiety disorder: a double-blind, randomized, placebocontrolled, flexible-dose study. Int Clin Psychopharmacol. 2015;30(6):297-306.
43. Durgam S, Gommoll C, Forero G, et al. Efficacy and safety of vilazodone in patients with generalized anxiety disorder: a randomized, double-blind, placebo-controlled, flexible-dose trial. J Clin Psychiatry. 2016;77(12):1687-94.
44. Robinson DS, Kajdasz DK, Gallipoli S, et al. A 1-year, open-label study assessing the safety and tolerability of vilazodone in patients with major depressive disorder. J Clin Psychopharmacol. 2011;31(5):643-6.
45. Ferguson JM. SSRI Antidepressant medications: adverse effects and tolerability. Prim Care Companion J Clin Psychiatry. 2001;3(1):22-7.
46. Clayton AH, Kennedy SH, Edwards JB, et al. The effect of vilazodone on sexual function during the treatment of major depressive disorder. J Sex Med. 2013;10(10):2465-76.
47. Duman RS. Neurobiological advances identify novel antidepressant targets. World Psychiatry. 2013;12(3):207-9.
48. Rasmussen KG. Has psychiatry tamed the "ketamine tiger?" Considerations on its use for depression and anxiety. Prog Neuropsychopharmacol Biol Psychiatry. 2016;64:218-24.
49. Sanacora G, Schatzberg AF. Ketamine: promising path or false prophecy in the development of novel therapeutics for mood disorders? Neuropsychopharmacology. 2015;40(2):259-67.
50. Bobo WV, Voort JL, Croarkin PE, et al. Ketamine for treatment-resistant unipolar and bipolar major depression: critical review and implications for clinical practice. Depress Anxiety. 2016;33(8):698-710.
51. Singh JB, Fedgchin M, Daly EJ, et al. A Double-Blind, Randomized, Placebo Controlled, Dose-Frequency Study of Intravenous Ketamine in Patients with Treatment-Resistant Depression. Am J Psychiatry. 2016;173(8):816-26.

52. Segmiller F, Rüther T, Linhardt A, et al. Repeated S-ketamine infusions in therapy resistant depression: a case series. J Clin Pharmacol. 2013;53:996-8.
53. Dale E, Bang-Andersen B, Sa´nchez C. Emerging mechanisms and treatments for depression beyond SSRIs and SNRIs. Biochem Pharmacol. 2015;95:81-97.
54. Quiroz JA, Tamburri P, Deptula D, et al. The efficacy and safety of basimglurant as adjunctive therapy in major depression: a randomised, double-blind, placebo controlled study. Eur Neuropsychopharmacol. 2014;24(Suppl 2):S468.
55. Na KS, Lee KJ, Lee JS, et al. Efficacy of adjunctive celecoxib treatment for patients with major depressive disorder: a meta-analysis. Prog Neuropsychopharmacol Biol Psychiatry. 2014;48:79-85.
56. Dell'Osso B, Ketter TA. Assessing efficacy/effectiveness and safety/tolerability profiles of adjunctive pramipexole in bipolar depression: acute versus long-term data. Int Clin Psychopharmacol. 2013;28:297-304.
57. Veselinovic´ T, Paulzen M, Grunder G. Cariprazine, a new, orally active dopamine D2/3 receptor partial agonist for the treatment of schizophrenia, bipolar mania and depression. Expert Rev Neurother. 2013;13:1141-59.

16

CHAPTER

Current Status of Cognitive Enhancers

AQ Jilani, Santosh Kumar

INTRODUCTION

In rapidly changing demography of world, due to improved health and longer life expectancy, there is increased risk for the development of neurocognitive disorders, especially Alzheimer's disease (AD) and related dementias, where cognition is the first casualty. Cognition is an important aspect of an individual's daily functioning. This is the faculty of brain, which is advanced in humans in comparison to all living creatures on the earth. Highly developed cognitive abilities such as critical and creative thinking, learning to learn, innovative and creative abilities differentiate humans from others.

Cognitive enhancement is not a new concept. The quest for a healthy mind is gaining much importance with the advent of alternative and complementary medicine, which not only appears safer but may also promise good results. Since times, unknown people have used various strategies to increase their ability to learn and improve performance. Our ancestors used various plant extracts to improve memory, attention, and concentration. The use of cognitive-enhancing drugs appears to be common among people under pressure to perform, where they are usually taken to fight fatigue and improve their performance on the work front.

Also, whenever there is an insult to the brain, cognitive abilities usually suffer, which may produce substantial medical and functional impairment. Therefore, cognitive enhancement is not only reserved for people with decline in cognitive functioning but is also used by healthy people. There are so many cognitive enhancers, although, majority of which are not evidence, but experience based. The authors have tried to classify the available cognitive enhancers for remedial purpose and briefed about their current status and their future course.

CLASSIFICATION

At present, cognitive enhancers may be classified under following broad categories, some of which are indicated for the use in the disease state of primary neurocognitive disorders such as dementias, and secondary cognitive decline associated with chronic psychiatric disorders, e.g. depression, schizophrenia, etc. Others categories are usually promoted for

uses by healthy people as supplements or as add on in the diseases affecting cognitive abilities.
- Acetylcholinesterase inhibitors (AChE I)
- N-methyl-D-aspartate (NMDA) receptors antagonists
- Disease-modifying agents
- *Others*: Antioxidant drugs/natural nootropics.

Among the above classes of drugs, the first two categories namely cholinesterase inhibitors and NMDA receptor antagonist are currently approved by regulatory agencies such as the US Food and Drug Administration (FDA) and the European Medicines Agency (EMA) to treat the cognitive symptoms of AD with aim to improve quality of life of the patients and to reduce the burden of care of the caregivers. These are donepezil, rivastigmine, and galantamine as reversible AChE inhibitors, and Memantine as an NMDA receptor antagonist.[1-3] Although, the molecule tacrine was the first to get approval for AD treatment in 1993, but was withdrawn due to high incidence of side effects including hepatotoxicity.[4] At present, the other classes of drugs are not evidence based, and most are being tested by clinical trials.

Acetylcholinesterase Inhibitors

Acetylcholinesterase inhibitors are currently the mainstay of cognitive enhancement in clinical practice for the management of neurodegenerative disorders, e.g. AD and related dementia. These classes of drugs are first to be approved by FDA. These drugs have been shown to slow down the progression of dementia and improve alertness, but have negligible impact on underlying disease process. In this way, AChEs inhibitors provide symptomatic benefits.

The enzyme acetylcholinesterase (AChE) is responsible for termination of impulses transmission by acetylcholine in the cholinergic pathway of central and peripheral nervous system. Thus, the inactivation of AChE enzyme by inhibitors leads to increased availability of acetylcholine and its accumulation leading to hyperstimulation of nicotinic and muscarinic receptors and improvement in the disrupted neurotransmission. This way, AChE inhibitors are used as relevant drugs and toxins for various purposes.

There are two types of AChE inhibitors—reversible and irreversible. The reversible agents are either commonly used in the treatment of neurodegenerative disorders, e.g. Alzheimer disease (donepezil, rivastigmine, and galantamine), or as pesticides, e.g. toxic carbamates. The irreversible inhibitors are generally toxics and are used as pesticides, e.g. organophosphorus compounds.

Since, the cholinergic projection from nucleus basalis of Meynert in the basal forebrain to the forebrain neocortex and associated limbic areas are the first structures, where the neuropathology of AD starts leading to deficit of acetylcholine neurotransmitter with consequent symptomatology.[5] Hence, the aim of management is to increase the synthesis and availability of acetylcholine by preventing its breakdown by acetylcholinesterase enzyme. This way, the AChE inhibitors play their therapeutic role by making the availability of acetylcholine for neurotransmission and compensate for the loss of functioning cholinergic and other neurons. There are many AChE inhibitors, of which some are approved for clinical uses and others are being researched for their efficacy and safety profiles.

These are followings:
- Approved AChE inhibitors—donepezil, rivastigmine, and galantamine
- Other AChE inhibitors

Approved AChE Inhibitors

Donepezil: It is a selective and reversible inhibitor of AChE enzyme and is indicated for mild-to-moderate stages of AD. Studies indicate that beside symptomatic effects, donepezil also delays deposition of amyloid plaques.[6,7]

The usual dose is 5–10 mg per day and is available as disintegrating tablet and oral solution. The oral bioavailability is 100% with ease to cross the blood–brain barrier and slow excretion. The maximum daily dose is 23 mg once daily.[8]

Although it is used in other cognitive disorders such as Lewy body dementia, vascular dementia, frontotemporal dementia, and cognitive decline of schizophrenia and Autism, but is not approved by regulatory agencies.[9–11]

Rivastigmine: It is a powerful and slow reversible carbamates inhibitor. This is approved for the treatment of mild-to-moderate stage of AD.[12] Rivastigmine is given orally as capsules or liquid formulations. The starting dose is 1.5 mg twice daily, and is increased gradually over weeks to 6 mg twice daily. Recently, transdermal patches, in the strength of 9.5–13.5 mg/day, are approved to reduce the gastrointestinal adverse effects.[13]

Furthermore, among AChEs, rivastigmine is also recommended for the treatment of Lewy body and Parkinson's disease dementia.[12,14]

Galantamine: It is an alkaloid derivative, indicated for the treatment of mild-to-moderate stages of AD. It is a selective, competitive, and rapidly reversible AChE inhibitor. Unlike other agents, galantamine is an allosteric modulating ligand at nicotinic cholinergic receptors. It acts specifically to enhance the activity (sensitize) of nicotinic receptors in the presence of acetylcholine.[15] Since, the severity of cognitive impairment in AD is correlated with loss of nicotinic receptors; this effect appears to be beneficial.[16] Due to allosteric potentiating effects at nicotinic receptors, galantamine also has effects on the other neurotransmitter systems such as monoamines, glutamate, and γ-aminobutyric acid (GABA). Thus, it could also be considered to improve cognitive dysfunction in other psychiatric illnesses such as schizophrenia, major depression, bipolar disorder, and alcohol abuse.[17]

The oral bioavailability of galantamine is 80–100% after oral administration with the half-life of about 7 hours. The starting dose is 4 mg twice daily and could be increased gradually up to 12 mg twice daily.[18]

The above three mentioned AChE inhibitors do not differ in term of efficacy. However, donepezil is better tolerated than rivastigmine and galantamine.[18]

Other AChE Inhibitors

There are many other AChE inhibitors, which have been shown to be effective but still not approved by regularizing bodies like FDA for clinical uses. For example, 7-methoxytacrine, a derivative of hepatotoxic tacrine, has been tested both *in vivo* and *in vitro* and has been found to be having less toxic effect and stronger inactivating action against acetylcholinesterase enzyme.[19]

Similarly, a natural alkaloid, known as Huperzine-A, is potent acetylcholinesterase enzyme inhibitor, and like donepezil, it has also potential to prevent deposition of amyloid plaque.[20]

Furthermore, in search of potent and selective AChE inhibitors, drugs are combined for having dual mode of action. For example, *donepezil-tacrine* and *oxoisoaporphine-tacrine* derivatives, and *coumarin-huperzine* derivatives have shown greater acetylcholinesterase inhibitory activity with ability to bind on both peripheral and catalytic site of acetylcholinesterase enzyme. These are considered to be promising compounds for development as disease-modifying agents in future.[21-24]

The main disadvantages of AChE inhibitors are that their effect is modest, temporary, and short lasting for a maximum of 12–24 months, as these drug do not decrease the rate of cognitive and functional decline over long term.[25,26] But still they provide significant symptomatic relief, hence at present, they are mainstay of pharmacotherapy in AD.[18]

NMDA Receptors Antagonists

N-methyl-D-aspartate receptor antagonists is a class of drug (Memantine), which is approved by FDA and EMA for the treatment of moderate-to-severe stage of AD. The excitatory state of glutaminergic system along with overactivation of NMDA receptors is one mechanism responsible for degeneration of neurons. Memantine acts by blocking the NMDA glutamate receptors and normalizes the glutaminergic overactivity and thus may ameliorate cognitive and memory deficits in AD.

Memantine is uncompetitive partial blocker of NMDA receptor with low affinity and rapid take-off kinetics. This helps in preservation of normal physiological function of NMDA receptors and makes it tolerable.[27]

The starting dose of Memantine is 5 mg/day and can be titrated up to 20 mg/day over weeks. Memantine has also been found to be effective in mild-to-moderate vascular dementia.[27]

Randomized controlled trials (RCTs) favor the combination of Donepezil and Memantine in cases of AD with moderate-to-severe stages with consequent benefit in cognitive function, language, ADL (activities of daily living), behaviors, and global state,[28,29] but such benefits are not demonstrable among cases with mild-to-moderate severity.[30]

Disease-modifying Agents

Like AChE inhibitors, Memantine has also shown only a moderate decrease in clinical deterioration in AD and VD. Hence, efforts must be taken to design newer drugs with novel mechanism of actions, which would be disease-modifying drugs and hopefully provide greater efficacy.

Briefing the pathogenesis of AD, the cascade of neurodegeneration is supposed to start from excessive formation of Aβ fibrils, which gets deposited to form Aβ amyloid plaques. This concomitantly also initiates the hyperphosphorylation of tau proteins in the mitochondria resulting in the mitochondrial dysfunction with consequent synaptic disconnections and neuronal death. The significant synaptic loss and neuronal death manifest the symptoms of AD.[31]

Considering the various underlying steps of neurodegenerative process, drugs could be developed in future, which could halt the disease progression by action on one or other underlying steps leading to neurodegeneration. Thus, the primary target could be Aβ and tau for disease-modifying therapies. In this way, the neuropathological cascade leading to AD either could be prevented or effectively treated by inhibiting the production of Aβ and tau, preventing aggregation or misfolding of these proteins, enhancing the removal of the toxic aggregate or misfolded forms of these proteins, or a combination of these modalities. These various future targets for antidementia drugs could be following:
- Modulation of amyloid (Aβ) deposition
- Modulation of tau deposition.

Modulation of Amyloid Deposition

Table 1 summarizes various ongoing trials with aim to target various substeps in the amyloid deposition.[32]

At present, the results of various ongoing trials are at primitive levels, and these will be matter of time, only after that any conclusion about the safety and potency of these agents could be made with certainty.

Modulation of Tau Deposition

Various molecules have been identified as tau aggregation agents and are currently being evaluated in humans as AD trials. A Phase II trial testing for 6 month of methylene blue (MB) has shown significant improvement in cognitive functions and may be considered as a potential therapy for AD.[33]

Table 1: Various ongoing trials with aim to target various substeps in the amyloid deposition.

Interference with Aβ aggregation	Selective Aβ42-lowering agents	Immunotherapy
Anti-amyloid aggregation agents: • Tramiprosate—Phase III trial (–) • Colostrinin—Phase II trial (±) • Scyllo-inositol—Phase II trial (±)	Inhibition of β-secretase: • Nonpeptidic inhibitors—trial in animal models (+) • CTS-21166—Phase I trial (+)	Active immunization (vaccination): • AN-1792—Phase II trial (–) • CAD-106, V950, ACC-001—Phase II trials • MABT5102A, PF-04360365, R1450—Phase I trials (+) • DNA epitope vaccine antibodies against the β-secretase cleavage site mucosal vaccination—trials in animal models (+)
Drugs interfering with metal: PBT2—Phase IIa trial (+)	Inhibition of γ-secretase: • Semagacestat—Phase III trial (–) • Tarenflurbil—Phase III trial (–) • Avagacestat—Phase II trial	
	Activation of α-secretase: Etazolate—Phase IIa trial (+)	Passive immunization (monoclonal antibodies): • Bapineuzumab—Phase II trial (+) • Solanezumab—Phase II trial • IVIg—Phase III trial

[(+): encouraging results; (–): negative results; (±): mixed results]

Kinases, which induce hyperphosphorylation of tau, are also considered as target for tau kinase inhibitors and could be potential therapeutic in future.[34] The main target is glycogen synthase kinase 3 (GSK3β), which is inhibited by lithium and other compounds, e.g. *pyrazolopyridines*, the *aminothiazole* AR-A014418, and sodium *valproate*.[35] Although the result of GSK3 inhibition trail is negative, but recently, a RCT has shown promising effect on cognition in patient with amnestic mild cognitive impairment (MCI).[36] Since, tau proteins are intracellular, hence development of vaccination therapy targeting tau is complicated at present.[37]

Others: Antioxidant Drugs/Natural Nootropics

In addition to Aβ and tau-related pathogenesis, other overlapping pathogenic causations have also been described, and these could also be an approach to treat/prevent AD in coming future. The examples are neuroinflammation, oxidative damage to neurons, iron deregulation, and cholesterol metabolism.[32] Various antioxidants and nootropics, although frequently used as supplement for cognitive enhancement and remedies, lack clinical trials and are yet to be approved by regulatory body like FDA. These are Ginkgo biloba, ginseng, Ashwagandha, brahmi, vitamins (A, B_6, B_9, B_{12}, and C), and cerebrolysin.

CONCLUSION

Since currently there is no approved medication, which could either halt the neurodegeneration or revoke the regenerative process of neurons, therefore the current treatments of neurodegenerative dementias are only symptomatic based on AChE inhibitors (donepezil, rivastigmine, and galantamine) and NMDA antagonists (Memantine).[38] However, these drugs do demonstrate modest, but consistent benefit for cognition, global status, and functional ability.[39]

The need of the time is to have disease-modifying interventions, which could interfere with Aβ and tau pathways. At present, drugs targeting this pathway, such as tarenflurbil, tramiprosate, and semagacestat, have been found inefficacious in the final clinical stages of testing.[40,41]

There is also need to explore the role of other possible neuronal mechanisms such as neuroinflammation, iron deregulation, and oxidative stress, so that promising therapeutic targets could be researched. Till now, vitamin E and omega-3 fatty acids, used as antioxidants, have not shown positive effects in patients with AD.[42]

REFERENCES

1. Birks J. Cholinesterase inhibitors for Alzheimer's disease. Cochrane Database Syst Rev. 2006;(1):CD005593.
2. Hyde C, Peters J, Bond M, et al. Evolution of the evidence on the effectiveness and cost-effectiveness of acetylcholinesterase inhibitors and memantine for Alzheimer's disease: systematic review and economic model. Age Ageing. 2013;42(1):14-20.
3. Bond M, Rogers G, Peters J, et al. The effectiveness and cost-effectiveness of donepezil, galantamine, rivastigmine, and memantine for the treatment of Alzheimer's disease (review of Technology Appraisal No. 111): a systematic review and economic model. Health Technol Assess. 2012;16(21):1-470.
4. Birks J, Grimley Evans J, Iakovidou V, et al. Rivastigmine for Alzheimer's disease. Cochrane Database Syst Rev. 2009;(2):CD001191.
5. Perry E, Walker M, Grace J, et al. Acetylcholine in mind: a neurotransmitter correlate of consciousness? Trends Neurosci. 1999;22(6):273-80.
6. Arce MP, Rodríguez-Franco MI, González-Muñoz GC, et al. Neuroprotective and cholinergic properties of multifunctional glutamic acid derivatives for the treatment of Alzheimer's disease. J Med Chem. 2009;52(22):7249-57.
7. Castro A, Martinez A. Targeting beta-amyloid pathogenesis through acetylcholinesterase inhibitors. Curr Pharm Des. 2006;12(33):4377-87.
8. Farlow MR, Alva G, Meng X, et al. A 25-week, open-label trial investigating rivastigmine transdermal patches with concomitant memantine in mild-to-moderate Alzheimer's disease: a post hoc analysis. Curr Med Res Opin. 2010;26(2): 263-9.
9. Rojas-Fernandez CH. Successful use of donepezil for the treatment of dementia with Lewy bodies. Ann Pharmacother. 2001;35(2):202-5.

10. Malouf R, Birks J. Donepezil for vascular cognitive impairment. Cochrane Database Syst Rev. 2004;(1):CD004395.
11. Thakurathi N, Vincenzi B, Henderson DC. Assessing the prospect of donepezil in improving cognitive impairment in patients with schizophrenia. Expert Opin Investig Drugs. 2013;22(2):259-65.
12. Desai AK, Grossberg GT. Rivastigmine for Alzheimer's disease. Expert Rev Neurother. 2005;5(5):563-80.
13. Winblad B, Grossberg G, Frölich L, et al. IDEAL: a 6-month, double-blind, placebo-controlled study of the first skin patch for Alzheimer disease. Neurology. 2007;69(4 Suppl 1):S14-22.
14. Chitnis S, Rao J. Rivastigmine in Parkinson's disease dementia. Expert Opin Drug Metab Toxicol. 2009;5(8):941-55.
15. Pohanka M. Cholinesterases, a target of pharmacology and toxicology. Biomed Pap Med Fac Univ Palacky Olomouc Czech Repub. 2011;155(3):219-29.
16. Bajgar J. Organophosphates/nerve agent poisoning: Mechanism of action, diagnosis, prophylaxis, and treatment. Adv Clin Chem. 2004;38:151-216.
17. Ago Y, Koda K, Takuma K, et al. Pharmacological aspects of the acetylcholinesterase inhibitor galantamine. J Pharmacol Sci. 2011;116(1):6-17.
18. Tayeb HO, Yang HD, Price BH, et al. Pharmacotherapies for Alzheimer's disease: beyond cholinesterase inhibitors. Pharmacol Ther. 2012;134(1):8-25.
19. Pohanka M, Kuca K, Kassa J. New performance of biosensor technology for Alzheimer's disease drugs: in vitro comparison of tacrine and 7-methoxytacrine. Neuro Endocrinol Lett. 2008;29(5):755-8.
20. Gao X, Zheng CY, Yang L, et al. Huperzine A protects isolated rat brain mitochondria against beta-amyloid peptide. Free Radic Biol Med. 2009;46(11):1454-62.
21. Alonso D, Dorronsoro I, Rubio L, et al. Donepezil-tacrine hybrid related derivatives as new dual binding site inhibitors of AChE. Bioorgan Med Chem. 2005;13(24):6588-97.
22. Tang H, Zhao LZ, Zhao HT, et al. Hybrids of oxoisoaporphine-tacrine congeners: Novel acetylcholinesterase and acetylcholinesterase-induced β-amyloid aggregation inhibitors. Eur J Med Chem. 2011;46(10):4970-9.
23. Catto M, Pisani L, Leonetti F, et al. Design synthesis and biological evaluation of coumarin alkylamines as potent and selective dual binding site inhibitors of acetylcholinesterase. Bioorgan Med Chem. 2013;21(1):146-52.
24. Yan J, Sun L, Wua G, et al. Rational design and synthesis of highly potent anti-acetylcholinesterase activity huperzine A derivatives. Bioorgan Med Chem. 2009;17(19):6937-41.
25. Courtney C, Farrell D, Gray R, et al. Long-term donepezil treatment in 565 patients with Alzheimer's disease (AD2000): randomised double-blind trial. Lancet. 2004;363(9427):2105-15.
26. Giacobini E. Cholinesterase inhibitors stabilize Alzheimer's disease. Ann N Y Acad Sci. 2000;920:321-7.
27. Olivares D, Deshpande VK, Shi Y, et al. N-methyl D-aspartate (NMDA) receptor antagonists and memantine treatment for Alzheimer's disease, vascular dementia and Parkinson's disease. Curr Alzheimer Res. 2012;9(6):746-58.

28. Feldman HH, Schmitt FA, Olin JT, et al. Activities of daily living in moderate-to-severe Alzheimer disease: an analysis of the treatment effects of memantine in patients receiving stable donepezil treatment. Alzheimer Dis Assoc Disord. 2006;20(4):263-8.
29. Howard R, McShane R, Lindesay J, et al. Donepezil and memantine for moderate-to-severe Alzheimer's disease. N Engl J Med. 2012;366(10):893-903.
30. Farlow MR, Salloway S, Tariot PN, et al. Effectiveness and tolerability of high-dose (23 mg/d) versus standard-dose (10 mg/d) donepezil in moderate to severe Alzheimer's disease: A 24-week, randomized, double-blind study. Clin Ther. 2010;32(7):1234-51.
31. Wang R, Reddy PH. Role of glutamate and NMDA receptors in Alzheimer's disease. J Alzheimers Dis. 2017;57(4):1041-8.
32. Konstantina GY, Sokratis GP. Current and future treatments for Alzheimer's disease. Ther Adv Neurol Disord. 2013;6(1):19-33.
33. Gura T. Hope in Alzheimer's fight emerges from unexpected places. Nat Med. 2008;14(9):894.
34. Yiannopoulou K, Karydakis K, Sakka P. Therapeutic targets in Alzheimer's disease. Prim Psychiatry. 2009;16:29-36.
35. Martinez A, Perez DI. GSK-3 inhibitors: a ray of hope for the treatment of Alzheimer's disease? J Alzheimers Dis. 2008;15(2):181-91.
36. Forlenza OV, Diniz BS, Radanovic M, et al. Disease-modifying properties of long-term lithium treatment for amnestic mild cognitive impairment: randomised controlled trial. Br J Psychiatry. 2011;198(5):351-6.
37. Galimberti D, Scarpini E. Disease-modifying treatments for Alzheimer's disease. Ther Adv Neurol Disord. 2011;4(4):203-16.
38. Stahl SM. The new cholinesterase inhibitors for Alzheimer's disease, Part 2: illustrating their mechanisms of action. J Clin Psychiatry. 2000;61(11):813-4.
39. Herrmann N, Chau SA, Kircanski I, et al. Current and emerging drug treatment options for Alzheimer's disease: a systematic review. Drugs. 2011;71(15):2031-65.
40. Gauthier S, Aisen PS, Ferris SH, et al. Effect of tramiprosate in patients with mild-to-moderate Alzheimer's disease: exploratory analyses of the MRI sub-group of the Alphase study. J Nutr Health Aging. 2009;13(6):550-7.
41. Imbimbo BP, Giardina GA. γ-secretase inhibitors and modulators for the treatment of Alzheimer's disease: disappointments and hopes. Curr Top Med Chem. 2011;11(12):1555-70.
42. Barten DM, Albright CF. Therapeutic strategies for Alzheimer's disease. Mol Neurobiol. 2008;37:171-86.

CHAPTER 17

Pharmacogenomics in Psychiatry

Anil Kakunje, Manoj Shettar

INTRODUCTION

In psychiatry, there was an era of treating patients by keeping them in captivity to protect general public from being harmed. During captivity, many nonscientific methods were used as a treatment modality. Psychiatric treatment has moved from pharmacological methods of treatment by serendipitous discovery to introduction of psychotropic medications for treating patients, to development of various drugs for treating disorders which has revolutionized the treatment strategy where drug selection is based on patient's symptom profile, medical comorbidities, tolerability of the drug, and the side effects and the improvement achieved with drugs.

A new era started in 1953, when double helix model of deoxyribonucleic acid (DNA) was discovered by Watson and Crick. Motulsky in 1957 proposed that inheritance might explain individual differences in the occurrence of adverse drug reactions and efficacy of drugs. In 1959, Friedrich Vogel used the term "Pharmacogenetics".[1]

During early days of pharmacogenomics, the studies revolved around the genes involved in drug metabolisms where inherited variations in a single gene caused abnormal response to the drug. For example, association of prolonged muscle paralysis leading to apnea by muscle relaxant succinylcholine was due to pseudocholinesterase.[2,3] A major breakthrough in the field of pharmacogenomics happened with the successful completion of the human genome project in 2003 which led to drug therapy through personalized medicine approaches, where genotype-guided medication prescription could be done. Pharmacogenomic markers are used for inter-individual drug response (safety and efficacy) and also for pretreatment genetic testing.[4]

It is seen that patients who seek treatment for depression, treatment remission is seen in one-third of individuals.[5] Predicting clinical response of an individual to a specific antidepressant drug is not yet possible as treatment choice is based on doctor's discretion and experience. An important factor that guides in choosing a specific antidepressant drug is the occurrence of adverse effects among which some are desired, such as sleep; while others are not, such as weight gain. Another limitation of antidepressants is that there is a considerable lag between the onset of treatment and full remission of depressive symptoms which can last several weeks.[6]

There is a vast variation in medication response ranging from 20% to 95% which can be attributed to patient's genetic profile.[7] Lack of benefit from medication can lead to multiple failed medication trials and as a result the patients are considered treatment-resistant.[8]

With the advancement in pharmacogenomics, one can give personalized treatments to every patient using genetic markers. It helps to identify drugs which may work better than other drugs with improved efficacy and lesser side effect profile.[9]

Pharmacogenomics utilizes the genetic information to predict responses to medications at a personalized level using gene-drug interactions for pharmacokinetic and pharmacodynamic genes. Pharmacokinetic response is controlled by cytochrome P450 enzymes which metabolize these drugs in the body and in turn determine their levels. Pharmacodynamic genes predict the medication response at the site of its action.[10]

DEFINITIONS
Pharmacogenetics
It is study of genetic basis for variation in drug response. Pharmacogenetics looks at how variation in a single gene brings about differences in individual drug response **(Fig. 1)**.

Pharmacogenomics
Pharmacogenomics is the study of the role of the genome in drug response. Pharmacogenomics analyzes how the genetics of an individual affects his/her response to drugs. The name (pharmaco + genomics) reflects its combining of pharmacology and genomics together.

It is identification of genome variants which influence drug effects, by altering drug's pharmacokinetics (absorption, distribution, metabolism, and excretion) or by drug's pharmacodynamics (e.g. modifying a drug's target that alters sensitivity to the drug's pharmacological effects).[11]

Pharmacogenomics looks at whole of the genome how it influences variation in drug response. Therefore, pharmacogenomics is a broader term. Pharmacogenomics includes pharmacogenetics **(Fig. 1)**.

Epigenetics
Conrad Waddington defined epigenetics as "the branch of biology which studies the causal interactions between genes and their products which bring the phenotype into being."[12]

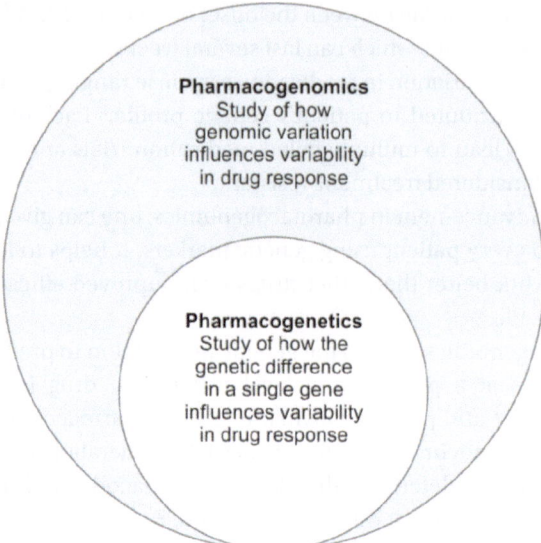

Fig. 1: Pharmacogenomics and pharmacogenetics.

INDICATIONS[13-15]

- Identification of responders and nonresponders to medications
- To avoid side effects
- For dosing of medications based on individual's metabolizing capacity
- Identification of drug exposure and clinical response variability
- To unleash mechanisms of drug action
- To identify trial design features
- It increases the efficiency in drug discovery process by screening the targets for variation.

It also helps in reducing the costs and duration of clinical trials either by including or excluding particular patients by genotype who are prone to develop side effects from drug treatment.

ADVANTAGES

For treating a person who suffers from infectious disease antibiotics are used and antibiotic selection is based on antibiotic sensitivity test which gives an idea about the antibiotic, the microorganism is sensitive, and to which it is resistant. In the same way, pharmacogenomics helps the clinician to identify which one of the many psychotropics works out in better way compared to other in cost-effective manner with least possible side effects.[15]

It reduces the trial and error method of finding an appropriate medication that suits the particular patient. Using this, one can readily identify who will respond to a particular drug and have better tolerability to that medication. When a drug is prescribed to a patient in the beginning of treatment that is most effective to him and which he can tolerate without experiencing much of the side effects, this reduces the time spent in choosing a medication by trial and error method. Dose optimization for psychotropic medications can take several weeks.[16]

Pharmacogenetic usage in psychiatric intervention will lead to improved adherence and cost savings.[17]

Individuals according to the inherited CYP2D6 alleles can be grouped as poor metabolizer (PM), intermediate metabolizer (IM), extensive metabolizer (EM), and ultrarapid metabolizers (UM). An increased risk of toxic reactions has been reported in PM while certain drugs may get eliminated early and may not reach therapeutic plasma concentrations in UM.[18] Pharmacogenomics helps to identify these types of variations and helps in providing an individualized approach.

SINGLE/INDIVIDUAL GENE TESTING VERSUS COMBINATORIAL GENE TESTING

Pharmacogenomics testing can be done either by using individual gene testing (IGT) or combinatorial gene testing (CPGx).

Individual gene testing is testing pharmacogenomic markers ad hoc and revealing each gene's results to a clinician in an attempt to positively intervene in the medication management of the patient.[9]

Individual clinical pharmacogenomic testing began in 2004 with Food and Drug Administration (FDA) approval of Roche's AmpliChip testing for CYP2D6 and CYP2C19.[19]

AmpliChip gives information about two genes—it can be conceptualized as an IGT because each gene's resultant phenotypes are reported individually. Newly found alleles could not be added to AmpliChip as it was FDA approved test.[20]

In IGT, individual genes are selected for their potential to illuminate clinically relevant information. As our understanding of genes and alleles is expanding, the clinical utility of individual pharmacogenomic testing is reducing;[9] predictably, with IGT, the clinical relevance has been only validated in medications that are metabolized by one, or may be two, enzymes (e.g. tricyclic antidepressants, paroxetine, aripiprazole, etc.).

Earlier, pharmacogenomic testing had limited ability to predict patient's response to medications based upon single gene.[21]

Combinatorial gene testing is the approach of combining genetic markers into sophisticated risk categories as an attempt to collect more relevant information to improve the clinical utility of pharmacogenomic testing.[9]

Recent use of combinatorial pharmacogenomic testing has better success rates in identifying patients taking genetically incompatible medications, who are less likely to respond, compared with patients taking more genetically compatible medications.[22]

WHETHER TO OPT FOR SINGLE-GENE TESTING OR MULTIPLE-GENE TESTING

Single-gene testing guides treatment for a particular drug. In multiple-gene testing, multiple genes are tested. When single gene is tested, it does not give any idea of other genetic mechanisms involved in drug pharmacokinetics and pharmacodynamics. For multiple-gene testing, selecting multiple genes is more complex as one should consider interaction between multiple genes, drug and clinical area targeted for implementation. Gene panel of multigene testing may cover only few genes or it may cover hundreds of genes comprehensively. Thus, one should select the required gene panel based on available resources considering the genetic variants for that ethnic mix of population.[23]

Factors to be considered for pharmacogenomic testing are the evidence threshold for drug–gene pair, single versus multigene testing, patient's comorbidities, allele frequency, and technical aspects of genotyping.[23]

Study by Hall-Flavin et al. showed that patients whose treatment was guided by using the combinatorial pharmacogenomic test result had 70% greater improvement in symptoms when compared with patients whose treatment was not guided by such results.[24]

ADVANTAGES AND DISADVANTAGES OF INDIVIDUAL- AND MULTIPLE-GENE TESTING

Individual gene testing has clinical validity with only a limited number of antidepressant and antipsychotic medications;[25] but single-gene pharmacogenomic testing has been significantly studied, particularly for pharmacokinetic genes.[26]

Multiple genes on a pharmacogenomic panel create more complexity and increase the requirement for analysis on the part of the clinician who would have very little experience with pharmacogenomics.[27] When multiple enzymes are tested for, the burden falls on the clinician to "reverse engineer" the effects of several genes on medications.[9]

The clinician is wholly interested in the fate of the medication in the body, not the enzyme. Examining pharmacogenomics information from the perspective of each medication's unique metabolic profile, as opposed to each enzyme's profile, reveals the most useful clinical information. CPGx is the process of simultaneously assessing the combined effects of multiple pharmacokinetic and pharmacodynamic genes for a given medication so that the information from each relevant gene is conveyed in a way that gives integrated information about the pharmacology of the medication for an individual.[9]

Neuropsychiatric medications are metabolized by multiple enzymes and interact with multiple neuronal pathways to provide clinical response. The genes that inform this response often do so in piecemeal fashion. As an example, a physician might order pharmacogenomic testing to inform their choice and dosing of escitalopram. Escitalopram is metabolized by three different P450 enzymes—CYP2D6, CYP2C19, and CYP3A4. In a scenario if patient is CYP2D6 UM, CYP2C19 PM, and a CYP3A4 EM, the clinical information provided to the physician would be conveyed from the perspective of each of the genes tested. For CYP2D6, the clinical inference might be to increase the dose due to the patient's ultrarapid metabolic capacity. However, for CYP2C19, the suggestion might be to lower the dose due to the patient's poor metabolizing status. In such situation, the clinical path forward is unclear. Such situations can lead to conflicting treatments and likely to contribute to the dilution of the clinical effect of pharmacogenomics in psychiatry.[9]

The combinatorial categorical approach showed that side effects were most accurately predicted when both enzymes were considered. The highest side effect burden was noted when an individual had deficiencies in CYP2D6 but overactivity in CYP2C19.

The GeneSight test includes pharmacokinetic and pharmacodynamic genes; it addresses both the safety and efficacy of psychiatric medications. This combinatorial approach accounts for both single and multiple metabolic pathways for each medication synergistically combined with genetic changes to brain pathways affecting the mechanism of drug action. Additional information is given to the treating clinician through the use of drug-specific footnotes for those medications in the yellow and red advisory categories, which supply the details of the gene–drug interactions. Genotype and phenotype result with interpretive comments for each of the genes with more elaborate details. This layering process allows for complex genomic and pharmacologic data to be presented in discrete, increasingly informative layers that provide useful clinical insight.[9]

The GeneSight psychotropic test provides clinicians with a list of preselected psychiatric genes yielding a composite phenotype that integrates the known pharmacology of 38 medications compromising the large majority of psychotropic medication prescriptions in the United States.[9]

DISADVANTAGES OF PHARMACOGENOMICS[28]

- Very expensive and are time-consuming
- Educating healthcare professional who are unaware of this
- Ethical issues that can arise out of testing.

COST-EFFECTIVENESS

For including a pharmacogenetic test in routine clinical practice, the test should be valid and should have clinical utility. The test should be cost-effective so that the test can be applied to vast majority of population.

Clinical validity is the accuracy of a genetic test to predict the clinical outcome such as the chances of response to treatment. Two open-label prospective clinical trials have shown the clinical validity of treatment guided by combinatorial pharmacogenomics in major depressive disorders.[24,29,30]

Clinical utility is the improved outcome when pharmacogenomics is used for individuals compared to standard care.[31]

When Herbild investigated a population which consisted extreme phenotypes of both CYP2D6 and CYP2C19 separating them into treatment as usual and pharmacogenomic-informed treatment group, it was observed that costs for the extreme metabolizers in pharmacogenomically tested group were comparatively less.[14]

Individual gene testing was associated with an increase in pharmacy costs and decrease in healthcare utilization.[32]

The clinical validity of the GeneSight CPGx information is shown by its predictive capacity to reveal that patients who are placed on red category medications have higher chances of poorer outcomes.[32]

Teresa et al.[23] gave the reference laboratory parameters for pharmacogenomic implementation broadly divided into four domains:
1. Pharmacogene and variant selection
2. Logistics
3. Reporting of results
4. Test costs along with reimbursement.

Selection of pharmacogene and its variants is dependent on single-gene testing or multiple-gene testing. When single gene is tested, it does not give any idea of other genetic mechanisms involved in drug metabolism. For multiple-gene testing, one should select the required gene panel based on relevant genetic variants for that ethnic mix of population. The evidence threshold for drug–gene pair, single-versus multiple-gene testing, patient's comorbidities, allele frequency, and technical aspects of genotyping are the factors to be considered for pharmacogenomic testing. For laboratory logistics, the factors to be considered are sample type, time to result reporting, consent processes, and sample storage. Testing requires samples such as blood, saliva or buccal swabs. Results reported vary from single-gene information to multigene information which can be comprehensive based on single-gene analysis to multigene analysis at a time. Result can also be in terms of single or multiple medication specific or disease specific medications.[23] The gene–drug interactions can be reported in terms of three color codes—little or no gene–

drug interaction (green "use as directed"), moderate gene-drug interaction (yellow "use with caution"), and severe gene-drug interaction (red "use with caution and with more frequent monitoring").[9] The cost of the test differs from laboratory to laboratory. If the test has insurance coverage, then it has a significant impact on implementation of pharmacogenomics.[23]

Bousman et al. systematically evaluated CYP2D6 and CY2C19 star (*) allele contents of 20 pharmacogenetic testing panels and concluded that a consensus should be reached on which star alleles should be included in pharmacogenetic testing panel and also pharmacogenetic testing report should improve considerably.[33]

The costs related to developing, manufacturing, and obtaining approval for genetic tests, in addition to defining the role of ethnic genetic differences, may force poor and middle income countries and communities to miss the benefits of personalized medicine advances. To overcome this, there should be further advances in genomic technologies so that there is a reduction in costs of implementing them.

After a thorough evaluation, Center for Medicare Services looked at clinical validity, clinical utility, and economic data following which it released its decision for the combinatorial GeneSight psychotropic test (Center for Medicare and Medicaid Services, 2014), thus increasing the affordability and access to combinatorial testing for patients.[10]

WEBSITES THAT HELP CLINICIANS ON PHARMACOGENOMICS

The Clinical Pharmacogenetics Implementation Consortium (CPIC®) is an international consortium of individual volunteers and few staffs who are interested to promote the use of pharmacogenetic tests for patient care. They provide specific guidance to clinicians and laboratories so that pharmacogenetic tests can be better utilized.[34]

United States FDA lists over 100 medications with applicable pharmacogenomics biomarkers which are given in the website in drug labeling and 33 of these are psychotropic medications.[13]

To collect, encode, and help disseminate knowledge about the impact of human genetic variations on drug response, pharmacogenomics knowledgebase (*www.PharmGKB.org*) initiated a program.[35]

GeneSight psychotropic testing gives information on multiple prospective clinical trials supporting its clinical validity and utility over the usual treatment as it is powered by combinatorial pharmacogenomic testing.[36]

International HapMap project provides data resource to investigate the association of variants across the human genome with a wide range of clinical phenotypes.[37]

CONCLUSION

A challenge for pharmacogenomics is application of genetic markers when there is a variable drug response while prescribing psychotropics.[28] Routine use of phamrcogenomic testing is not recommended as a usual practice for prescribing psychotropic medications. Clinicians should utilize the pharmacogenomic principles to reduce stigma associated with psychiatric illness. For implementation of pharmacogenomics, clinicians should be ready to accept and apply it, and wherever necessary, convince patients; finally insurance companies should be willing to provide insurance coverage for the same. Pharmacogenomics provides opportunity to practice personalized medicine in the field of mental health.

REFERENCES

1. Vogel F. Moderne Probleme der Humangenetik. In: Heilmeyer L, Schoen R, de Rudder B (Eds). Ergebnisse der Inneren Medizin und Kinderheilkunde. Germany: Springer Berlin Heidelberg; 1959. pp. 52-125.
2. Charlab R, Zhang L. Pharmacogenomics: historical perspective and current status. Methods Mol Biol. 2013;1015:3-22.
3. Lehmann H, Ryan E. Familial incidence of low pseudocholinesterase level. Lancet. 1956;271(6934):124.
4. Carr D, Alfirevic A, Pirmohamed M. Pharmacogenomics: current state-of-the-art. Genes (Basel). 2014;5(2):430-43.
5. Warden D, Rush AJ, Trivedi MH, et al. The STAR*D Project results: a comprehensive review of findings. Curr Psychiatry Rep. 2007;9(6):449-59.
6. Reynolds GP, McGowan OO, Dalton CF. Pharmacogenomics in psychiatry: the relevance of receptor and transporter polymorphisms. Br J Clin Pharmacol. 2014;77(4):654-72.
7. Evans WE, McLeod HL. Pharmacogenomics—drug disposition, drug targets, and side effects. N Engl J Med. 2003;348(6):538-49.
8. Mrazek DA, Hornberger JC, Altar CA, et al. A review of the clinical, economic, and societal burden of treatment-resistant depression: 1996-2013. Psychiatr Serv. 2014;65(8):977-87.
9. Winner JG, Dechairo B. Combinatorial versus individual gene pharmacogenomic testing in mental health: A perspective on context and implications on clinical utility. Yale J Biol Med. 2015;88(4):375-82.
10. Benitez J, Jablonski MR, Allen JD, et al. The clinical validity and utility of combinatorial pharmacogenomics: enhancing patient outcomes. Appl Transl Genom. 2015;5:47-9.
11. Relling MV, Evans WE. Pharmacogenomics in the clinic. Nature. 2015;526(7573):343-50.
12. Waddington CH. Towards a theoretical biology. Nature. 1968;218(5141):525-7.
13. Research C for DE and. Science & Research (Drugs)—Table of Pharmacogenomic Biomarkers in Drug Labeling. [online] Available from https://www.fda.gov/drugs/scienceresearch/ ucm572698.htm [Last accessed December, 2019].

14. Moore TR, Hill AM, Panguluri SK. Pharmacogenomics in psychiatry: implications for practice. Recent Pat Biotechnol. 2014;8(2):152-9.
15. Kleyn PW, Vesell ES. Genetic variation as a guide to drug development. Science. 1998;281(5384):1820-1.
16. Leckband SG, Bishop JR, Ellingrod VL. Pharmacogenomics in psychiatry. J Pharm Pract. 2007;20(3):252-64.
17. Fagerness J, Fonseca E, Hess GP, et al. Pharmacogenetic-guided psychiatric intervention associated with increased adherence and cost savings. Am J Manag Care. 2014;20(5):e146-56.
18. De Luca V, Mueller DJ, de Bartolomeis A, et al. Association of the HTR2C gene and antipsychotic induced weight gain: a meta-analysis. Int J Neuropsychopharmacol. 2007;10(5):697-704.
19. Phillips KA, Van Bebber SL. Measuring the value of pharmacogenomics. Nat Rev Drug Discov. 2005;4(6):500-9.
20. Raimundo S, Toscano C, Klein K, et al. A novel intronic mutation, 2988G>A, with high predictivity for impaired function of cytochrome P450 2D6 in white subjects. Clin Pharmacol Ther. 2004;76(2):128-38.
21. Teutsch SM, Bradley LA, Palomaki GE, et al. The Evaluation of Genomic Applications in Practice and Prevention (EGAPP) initiative: methods of the EGAPP Working Group. Genet Med. 2009;11(1):3-14.
22. Altar CA, Carhart JM, Allen JD, et al. Clinical validity: combinatorial pharmacogenomics predicts antidepressant responses and healthcare utilizations better than single gene phenotypes. Pharmacogenomics J. 2015;15(5):443-51.
23. Vo TT, Bell GC, Owusu Obeng A, et al. Pharmacogenomics implementation: considerations for selecting a reference laboratory. Pharmacotherapy. 2017;37(9):1014-22.
24. Hall-Flavin DK, Winner JG, Allen JD, et al. Utility of integrated pharmacogenomic testing to support the treatment of major depressive disorder in a psychiatric outpatient setting. Pharmacogenet Genomics. 2013;23(10):535-48.
25. Relling MV, McDonagh EM, Chang T, et al. Clinical Pharmacogenetics Implementation Consortium (CPIC) guidelines for rasburicase therapy in the context of G6PD deficiency genotype. Clin Pharmacol Ther. 2014;96(2):169-74.
26. Gordon AS, Tabor HK, Johnson AD, et al.; NHLBI GO Exome Sequencing Project. Quantifying rare, deleterious variation in 12 human cytochrome P450 drug-metabolism genes in a large-scale exome dataset. Hum Mol Genet. 2013;23(8):1957-63.
27. Winner JG, Goebert D, Matsu C, et al. Training in psychiatric genomics during residency: A new challenge. Acad Psychiatry. 2010;34(2):115-8.
28. Poste G. Bring on the biomarkers. Nature. 2011;469(7329):156-7.
29. Hall-Flavin DK, Winner JG, Allen JD, et al. Using a pharmacogenomic algorithm to guide the treatment of depression. Transl Psychiatry. 2012;2:e172.
30. Winner JG, Carhart JM, Altar CA, et al. A prospective, randomized, double-blind study assessing the clinical impact of integrated pharmacogenomic testing for major depressive disorder. Discov Med. 2013;16(89):219-27.
31. Becquemont L, Alfirevic A, Amstutz U, et al. Practical recommendations for pharmacogenomics-based prescription: 2010 ESF-UB Conference on Pharmacogenetics and Pharmacogenomics. Pharmacogenomics. 2011;12(1):113-24.

32. Kitzmiller JP, Groen DK, Phelps MA, et al. Pharmacogenomic testing: relevance in medical practice: Why drugs work in some patients but not in others. Cleve Clin J Med. 2011;78(4):243-57.
33. Bousman CA, Jaksa P, Pantelis C. Systematic evaluation of commercial pharmacogenetic testing in psychiatry: a focus on CYP2D6 and CYP2C19 allele coverage and results reporting. Pharmacogenet Genomics. 2017;27(11):387-93.
34. Relling MV, Klein TE. CPIC: Clinical Pharmacogenetics Implementation Consortium of the Pharmacogenomics Research Network. Clin Pharmacol Ther. 2011;89(3):464-7.
35. Klein TE, Chang JT, Cho MK, et al. Integrating Genotype and Phenotype Information: An overview of the PharmGKB project. Pharmacogenetics Research Network and Knowledge Base. Pharmacogenomics J. 2001;1(3):167.
36. GeneSight Psychotropic-Tests-GTR–NCBI. [online] Available from https:// www.ncbi.nlm.nih.gov/gtr/tests/508961/ [Last accessed December, 2019].
37. International HapMap Consortium. The International HapMap Project. Nature. 2003;426(6968):789-96.

CHAPTER 18

Stem Cell Therapy for Psychiatric Disorders

Naresh Nebhinani, Pooja Patnaik Kuppili

INTRODUCTION AND RELEVANCE

Psychiatric illnesses are associated with significant global morbidity. Despite this, the neurobiological basis of many of the psychiatric illnesses is not clear.[1] There are no consistently proven biomarkers as well as objective markers of prognostication in psychiatry.[2] Further, limitations of pharmacological management exist. There are limited means for prediction of treatment response in psychiatric illness and hence, often the treatment progresses on "trial and error basis", exposing patient to the undesirable adverse effects of psychotropic medication.[3] Hence, there is increasing focus on personalized medicine or precision-based medicine. Newer modalities such as stem cell research are a step forward in this direction.[4]

Stem cells are those cells which are capable of renewing self, unlimited number of times as well as engaging in asymmetrical cell division, i.e. producing one stem cell and one committed somatic cell.[5] Induced pluripotent stem cell (iPSC) and adult as well as fetal stem cells have been used in stem cell research in psychiatry. iPSCs are derived from reprogramming of adult somatic cells such as fibroblasts, hair follicles, keratinocytes *in vivo* by the means of some transcription factors such as Oct4, Klf4, Nnaog, Sox2, and c-Myc. The derived iPSCs can differentiate into cells belonging to any of the germ layers (ectoderm/endoderm/mesoderm).[6] iPSCs confer advantage over embryonic stem cells in terms of ethical concerns associated with origin of embryonic stem cells as well as the spontaneous differentiation of embryonic stem cells into unwanted cells,[7] whereas adult stem cells can be directly obtained from bone marrow, fat cells, dental pulp tissue, and skin.[8]

The evidence for use of adult and fetal stem cells in psychiatry is largely limited to autism spectrum disorders (ASD). They are purported to act through the mechanisms of improving plasticity, enhancing production of survival-promoting factors, viability of neurons as well as anti-inflammatory molecules, increasing neurogenesis, and promoting neuronal homeostasis.[8,9] The relevance of iPSC to psychiatric illnesses is based on the findings of abnormal neurogenesis noted in patients with depression, schizophrenia, bipolar disorder, and anxiety disorders.[10] The correction of the reduced neurogenesis by the iPSC could thereby lead to promising results.

For example, functional midbrain dopaminergic neurons, GABAergic interneurons, and serotonergic neurons have been produced from iPSCs subsequently over the last decade.[11] This could lead to pathbreaking results as role of dopamine, GABA, and serotonin in the pathophysiology of psychiatric illness is well-known. The iPSCs can be used primarily for developing models for psychiatric illnesses and thereby understanding the neurobiology and developing high-throughput screening for drugs.[11] iPSCs described in this chapter are restricted to human-derived iPSCs, and preclinical models are beyond the scope of this chapter.

PROCEDURE AND IMPLICATIONS OF INDUCED PLURIPOTENT STEM CELL IN PSYCHIATRIC ILLNESSES

Procedure of Generation of iPSCs

Induced pluripotent stem cells generation can be broadly divided into two steps. In the first step of induction, iPSCs are derived from somatic cells of humans such as fibroblasts, blood cells by integrating methods using viruses (retrovirus, lentivirus) or by nonintegrating methods such as chemical induction with the aid of stem cell reprogramming factors. Further in the next step of differentiation, the patient-derived iPSCs can differentiate into various types of neuronal cells.[12]

Modeling of Psychiatric Illnesses

Compared to other models of psychiatric illnesses such as animal models, genome wide association studies or neuroimaging, iPSC confers advantages in terms of generation of subtypes of neurons, preserving genetics as well as helps in conducting disease pertinent assays.[13] Studies on human iPSC are almost exclusively limited to schizophrenia and bipolar disorder. Studies on iPSCs derived from patients with schizophrenia primarily demonstrated deficits in synapse, mitochondria, and microRNAs,[14] whereas, studies on bipolar disorder demonstrated deficits in expression of genes of cell cycle and signaling pathways.[14] iPSC models of psychiatric illnesses are described here under.

Schizophrenia

Schizophrenia was the first psychiatric illness for generation of iPSC from patients in 2011.[15] Subsequently in the same year, neural progenitor cells (NPC) and neurons were generated which demonstrated deficits of several structures and pathways such as number of neurites, connectivity, AMP, signaling of Wnt as well as PSD95 throwing light on the neurobiology of the illness.[16]

Further adding to the neurobiological understanding of the illness, the model of chromosome 22q11 studied in glutaminergic neurons derived from patients was also published in 2011.[17] Studies on 22q11 mutation subsequently revealed higher copy number variants of L1, underexpression of genes involved in apoptosis and cell cycle, varied expression of miRNA as well as decrease in neural differentiation, and reduced neuron to glia ratio.[18-21]

In 2013, generation of NPC, dopaminergic and glutaminergic neurons aided in demonstrating the deficits in the process of neurogenesis in terms of differentiation and maturation as well as mitochondrial defects.[22] Further, increased production of catecholamines was noted.[23] DISC1 (disrupted-in-schizophrenia 1) mutation such as frameshift and translocation studied in neurons of the forebrain neurons demonstrated decreased release of synaptic vesicles and delay in mitosis through modulation of attachment of kinetochores during mitosis.[24,25]

In 2015, miR-137 pathway was studied in neurons directly produced from fibroblasts. It was found that overexpression of miR-137 led to reduced synaptic plasticity as well as downregulation of genes in the presynaptic region in the hippocampus. Further, these changes were found to be reversible with sequestration of miR-137.[26] NPCs generated from mutation of DISC1 cells aided in understanding the Wnt signaling pathways. This model showed that increased Wnt signaling was associated with alteration in expression of Foxg1 and Tbr2 which was reversible by sequestering the Wnt signaling.[27] These studies could have important clinical implications as these molecular changes could lead to reversal of disease phenotype.

Bipolar Disorder and Depression

In 2014, glutaminergic and GABAergic neurons were derived from patients for the first time which showed overexpression of ion channels as well as membrane-bound receptors.[28] In 2015, neurons derived from the patients showed overexpression of miR-34a and it was interesting to note that reduced expression of miR-34a was associated with increased dendrite connectivity.[29] Neural progenitor cells demonstrated deficits in neurogenesis, WNT/GSK3 signaling pathways as well as ion channels. Further, the deficits in proliferation were found to be reversible with inhibition of GSK3 pathways.[30] Deficits in Wnt/GSK3 signaling pathway were also demonstrated in iPSCs derived from patients of the Amish pedigree.[31] Hippocampal dentate gyrus like neurons were generated in 2015 which showed altered expression of mitochondrial genes as well as decreased mitochondrial size with hyperexcitability of neurons.[32]

DISC1 gene mutation has been studied in glutaminergic cortical neurons derived from patients with major depression and deficits in release of presynaptic vesicles were noted.[23]

Autism Spectrum Disorder and Syndromes Associated with Autism Spectrum Disorder

Induced pluripotent stem cells have been produced in patients with ASD as well as various syndromes associated with ASD such as Phelan McDermid syndrome, Timothy syndrome, Fragile X syndrome, and Angelman syndrome.[12,33,34] Deficits in neuronal as well as synaptic maturation with altered expression of GABRA4, ROBO, SLITRK5, and HTR7 have been noted in iPSCs generated from hair follicle obtained from patients with ASD.[33]

Induced pluripotent stem cells generated from patients of ASD who were carriers of duplication or deletion of 16p chromosome demonstrated greater size of soma as well as length of dendrites length in neurons obtained from carriers of 16p deletion and decreased size of neurons as well as dendrites length in neurons obtained from carriers of 16p duplication.[34] Glutamatergic and GABAergic iPSCs were derived from patients with Rett syndrome which showed decreased dendritic branching, size of cyton as well as spinal density.[12]

Psychotropic Drug Modeling

Induced pluripotent stem cells can also be used to understand the mechanism of action of psychotropic medication as well as assess the efficacy.[35] Loxapine was found to reverse deficits in connectivity of neurons as well as upregulating the glutamate receptors.[16] Clozapine was found to improve cell adhesion.

Atypical antipsychotics such as clozapine, aripiprazole, risperidone, etc. were more potent in inducing differentiating iPSC compared to typical antipsychotics such as chlorpromazine and haloperidol.[36] Valproate was found to revert zinc and potassium levels, increase oxygen supply extramitochondrially as well as reduce reactive oxygen species in iPSCs.[37,38]

Responsiveness to lithium was to be associated with better cell adhesion in iPSCs derived from fibroblasts of patients with bipolar disorder.[39] Lithium was also found to reverse the hyperexcitability of the iPSCs.[32] A recently published study in 2018 also highlighted the role of chronic lithium consumption in reducing hyperexcitability in patients of bipolar disorder responsive to lithium compared to nonresponders.[40] Lithium was found to affect the phosphorylation of collapsin response mediator protein-2 (CRMP2). Another interesting point to note is that pCRMP2:CRMP2 is higher in iPSCs generated from lithium responsive patients of bipolar disorder.[41] Hence, the iPSCs could aid in understanding the specific pathways responsible for responsiveness to lithium and thereby help in identifying subset of subjects of bipolar disorder who would be responsive to lithium.

PROCEDURE AND EVIDENCE BASE OF ADULT/FETAL STEM CELLS IN AUTISM SPECTRUM DISORDERS

Procedure

As a part of autologous stem cell transplantation, patients are administered granulocyte-colony stimulating factor (GCSF) prior to the harvest and transplantation. About 80–100 mL of bone marrow aspirate is collected from anterior superior iliac spine and mononuclear cells are separated from the aspirate and transplanted intrathecally between L4 and L5 lumbar vertebrae. This is followed by injection of prednisolone in ringer lactate solution,[42] whereas, in fetal stem cell transplantation, cells from liver and brain are collected from aborted fetuses and stem cells are cultured and transplanted into recipient tissue such as adipocytes.[43]

Evidence Base

The first clinical study of adult stem cell therapy in ASD dates back to 2013. This was an open labeled study of intrathecal transplantation of autologous bone marrow mononuclear cells in 32 patients with age ranging from 3 years to 33 years. All these patients were receiving multidisciplinary therapies such as occupational therapy, training of activities of daily living behavioral therapy and speech therapy in addition to dietary modification following the stem cell transplantation. At the end of 26 months, significant improvement was noted with 91% patients having better total Indian Scale for Assessment of Autism (ISAA) scores and 96% subjects showing improvement on Clinical Global Impression (CGI-II) scale. Most common adverse effect was nausea and vomiting, and seizures were noted in three patients.[42] Similar findings in improvement of ISAA scores were noted following autologous bone marrow mononuclear cell transplantation in a 25-year-old male with ASD at the end of 6 months.[44]

Allogeneic fetal stem cell transplantation was done from fetal cells derived from liver and brain and were followed up for 1 year in a recent study by Bradstreet et al. 2014. Significant improvement was noted in eye-to-eye contact as well as socialization with increase of $CD3^+$ T-lymphocytes and $CD4^+$ T helper cells with decrease in $CD19^+$ B-cells. No major adverse effects were noted.[43] Autologous stem cell transplantation using intravenous infusion of umbilical cord blood has been carried out in two recent studies in children with ASD with conflicting results.[45,46] One phase 1 open labeled study by Dawson et al., 2017 on 25 children demonstrated significant improvement in parent-rated as well as clinician-rated measures in eye tracking, social communication, vocabulary as well as overall symptoms of autism at the end of 12 months.[45] Another study was a randomized placebo-controlled, cross-over study with follow-up period of 24 weeks. The study did not find any significant improvement in symptoms of autism.[46] No major adverse events were noted in both the studies.[45,46]

An interesting finding of better therapeutic efficacy of combined transplantation of mononuclear cells derived from human cord blood and mesenchymal cells was noted in an open labeled non-randomized Phase I/II trial. The study demonstrated significant improvement in the Childhood Autism Rating Scale scores in children receiving combined transplantation compared to children who received transplantation of mononuclear cells derived from human cord blood and rehabilitation groups at the end of 24 weeks.[47]

LIMITATIONS

Induced pluripotent stem cell model, however, has certain limitations. Firstly, there is loss of epigenetic modifications in the iPSC. This might be important in psychiatric illnesses where genetic environment interaction is implicated in pathogenesis. Further, the iPSC cell lines are found to be immature. Heterogeneity in the patient genetics is another drawback which could result from the somatic mosaicism demonstrated by the cells of the donor.[14] Apart from patient-related variability, variation in neuronal differentiation as well as differences among the type of iPSCs generated also can lead to varied outcomes.[48,49]

It is important to interpret the findings of the studies in the light of variations in study methodology such as protocols used to induce differentiation globally, limited sample size, etc. Also, some of the studies had used family members as controls in comparison to some studies which used nonrelated controls which could have influenced the study findings.[14] Nevertheless, the differences in *in vivo* and *in vitro* conditions need to be acknowledged.[32]

Studies on adult stem cell therapies are also limited by small sample size, lack of randomization, the confounding effect of patients receiving multidisciplinary therapies, and shorter duration of follow-up.[42,43,45,46]

CONCLUSION AND FUTURE DIRECTION

Stem cell research aids in understanding neurobiology of psychiatric illnesses as well as identifying the mechanism of action of psychotropic medication. There is need for future studies to compare iPSC derived from various disease phenotypes. For example, it would be interesting to note differences in neurobiology as well as study mechanism of action of psychotropic medication among patients with predominant negative symptoms compared to those with predominant disorganization.[50]

There is definitely need for studies which are adequately powered as well as studies on patients at risk for psychiatric illnesses which will help in better understanding of the neurobiology and possible prevention.[51] There is need for studies with homogeneous sample of cases and controls in terms of disease characteristics, response to treatment, family history, neuroimaging, and neurocognitive functioning to decrease the heterogeneity.[48,52] Studies assessing the varying effect of adult stem cell transplant as per age and route of transplantation are warranted to gain further insights regarding efficacy and tolerability.[42]

Variability in differentiation of neurons among the subjects is a challenge which needs to be addressed in the further research.[48,49,52] Further, heterogeneity among the iPSC neurons can be overcome by newer methods such as quantitative trait loci (eQLTs).[48]

Future studies employing gene editing techniques such as CRISPR (clustered regularly interspaced short palindromic repeats) are warranted for better matching and decreasing genetic variations between cases and controls.[53] Newer genetic techniques for faster generation of neurons which are homogenous from iPSCs can be incorporated.[52] There is need for more studies on iPSCs from patients with depression and anxiety disorders as well as ASD as the majority of literature on iPSC research on these disorders is limited to animal models.[11]

Currently, the research on stem cell therapy in various psychiatric illnesses is still in infantile stage with increasing research being done only over the last 5 years. Considering the encouraging results being reported in the background of several limitations discussed above, it could take several decades for effective translation of research from bench to bedside practice. Advancements of stem cell research could thereby pave way forward toward precision medicine by early identification of disease phenotypes and further targeted treatments.

REFERENCES

1. Insel TR, Quirion R. Psychiatry as a clinical neuroscience discipline. JAMA. 2005;294(17):2221-4.
2. Dave KP. Field of psychiatry: Current trends and future directions: an Indian perspective. Mens Sana Monogr. 2016;14(1):108-17.
3. McMahon FJ. Prediction of treatment outcomes in psychiatry—where do we stand? Dialogues Clin Neurosci. 2014;16(4):455-64.
4. Fernandes BS, Williams LM, Steiner J, et al. The new field of "precision psychiatry". BMC Med. 2017;15(1):80.
5. Potten CS, Loeffler M. Stem cells: attributes, cycles, spirals, pitfalls and uncertainties. Lessons for and from the crypt. Development. 1990;110(4):1001-20.
6. Ratajczak M, Kucharska-Mazur J, Samochowiec J. Stem cell research and its growing impact on contemporary psychiatry. Psychiatr Pol. 2014;48(6):1073-85.
7. Benninghoff J. Stem cell approaches in psychiatry—challenges and opportunities. Dialogues Clin Neurosci. 2009;11(4):397-404.
8. Siniscalco D, Kannan S, Semprún-Hernández N, et al. Stem cell therapy in autism: becent insights. Stem Cells Cloning. 2018;11:55-67.

9. Siniscalco D, Bradstreet JJ, Sych N, et al. Perspectives on the use of stem cells for autism treatment. Stem Cells Int. 2013;2013:262438.
10. Cocks G, Carta MG, Arias-Carrión O, et al. Neural plasticity and neurogenesis in mental disorders. Neural Plast. 2016;2016;3738015.
11. Soliman MA, Aboharb F, Zeltner N, et al. Pluripotent stem cells in neuropsychiatric disorders. Mol Psychiatry. 2017;22(9):1241-9.
12. Lim CS, Yang JE, Lee YK, et al. Understanding the molecular basis of autism in a dish using hiPSCs-derived neurons from ASD patients. Mol Brain. 2015;8(1):57.
13. Vadodaria KC, Amatya DN, Marchetto MC, et al. Modeling psychiatric disorders using patient stem cell-derived neurons: a way forward. Genome Med. 2018;10(1):1.
14. Liu YN, Lu SY, Yao J. Application of induced pluripotent stem cells to understand neurobiological basis of bipolar disorder and schizophrenia. Psychiatry Clin Neurosci. 2017;71(9):579-99.
15. Chiang CH, Su Y, Wen Z, et al. Integration-free induced pluripotent stem cells derived from schizophrenia patients with a DISC1 mutation. Mol Psychiatry. 2011;16:358-60.
16. Brennand KJ, Simone A, Jou J, et al. Modelling schizophrenia using human induced pluripotent stem cells. Nature. 2011;473(7346):221-5.
17. Pedrosa E, Sandler V, Shah A, et al. Development of patient-specific neurons in schizophrenia using induced pluripotent stem cells. J Neurogenet. 2011;25(3):88-103.
18. Lin M, Pedrosa E, Hrabovsky A, et al. Integrative transcriptome network analysis of iPSC-derived neurons from schizophrenia and schizoaffective disorder patients with 22q11.2 deletion. BMC Syst Biol. 2016;10(1):105.
19. Zhao D, Lin M, Chen J, et al. MicroRNA profiling of neurons generated using induced pluripotent stem cells derived from patients with schizophrenia and schizoaffective disorder, and 22q11.2 Del. PLoS One. 2015;10(7):e0132387.
20. Toyoshima M, Akamatsu W, Okada Y, et al. Analysis of induced pluripotent stem cells carrying 22q11.2 deletion. Transl Psychiatry. 2016;6(11):e934.
21. Bundo M, Toyoshima M, Okada Y, et al. Increased l1 retrotransposition in the neuronal genome in schizophrenia. Neuron. 2014;81(2):306-13.
22. Robicsek O, Karry R, Petit I, et al. Abnormal neuronal differentiation and mitochondrial dysfunction in hair follicle-derived induced pluripotent stem cells of schizophrenia patients. Mol Psychiatry. 2013;18(10):1067-76.
23. Wen Z, Nguyen HN, Guo Z, et al. Synaptic dysregulation in a human iPS cell model of mental disorders. Nature. 2014;515(7527):414-8.
24. Ye F, Kang E, Yu C, et al. DISC1 regulates neurogenesis via modulating kinetochore attachment of Ndel1/Nde1 during mitosis. Neuron. 2017;96(5):1041-54.e5.
25. Hook V, Brennand KJ, Kim Y, et al. Human iPSC neurons display activity-dependent neurotransmitter secretion: aberrant catecholamine levels in schizophrenia neurons. Stem Cell Reports. 2014;3(4):531-8.
26. Siegert S, Seo J, Kwon EJ, et al. The schizophrenia risk gene product miR-137 alters presynaptic plasticity. Nat Neurosci. 2015;18(7)1008-16.
27. Srikanth P, Han K, Callahan DG, et al. Genomic DISC1 disruption in hiPSCs alters Wnt signaling and neural cell fate. Cell Rep. 2015;12(9):1414-29.

28. Chen HM, DeLong CJ, Bame M, et al. Transcripts involved in calcium signaling and telencephalic neuronal fate are altered in induced pluripotent stem cells from bipolar disorder patients. Transl Psychiatry. 2014;4:e375.
29. Bavamian S, Mellios N, Lalonde J, et al. Dysregulation of miR-34a links neuronal development to genetic risk factors for bipolar disorder. Mol Psychiatry. 2015; 20(5):573-84.
30. Madison JM, Zhou F, Nigam A, et al. Characterization of bipolar disorder patient-specific induced pluripotent stem cells from a family reveals neurodevelopmental and mRNA expression abnormalities. Mol Psychiatry. 2015;20(6):703-17.
31. Kim KH, Liu J, Sells Galvin RJ, et al. Transcriptomic analysis of induced pluripotent stem cells derived from patients with bipolar disorder from an old order Amish pedigree. PLoS One. 2015;10(11):e0142693.
32. Mertens J, Wang QW, Kim Y, et al. Differential responses to lithium in hyperexcitable neurons from patients with bipolar disorder. Nature. 2015;527(7576):95-9.
33. Adhya D, Swarup V, Nowosaid P, et al. Shared gene co-expression networks in autism from induced pluripotent stem cell (iPSC) neurons. bioRxiv. 2018:349415.
34. Deshpande A, Yadav S, Dao DQ, et al. Cellular phenotypes in human iPSC-derived neurons from a genetic model of autism spectrum disorder. Cell Rep. 2017;21(10):2678-87.
35. LaMarca EA, Powell SK, Akbarian S, et al. Modeling neuropsychiatric and neurodegenerative diseases with induced pluripotent stem cells. Front Pediatr. 2018;6:82.
36. Asada M, Mizutani S, Takagi M, et al. Antipsychotics promote neural differentiation of human iPS cell-derived neural stem cells. Biochem Biophys Res Commun. 2016;480(4):615-21.
37. Paulsen Bda S, de Moraes Maciel R, Galina A, et al. Altered oxygen metabolism associated to neurogenesis of induced pluripotent stem cells derived from a schizophrenic patient. Cell Transplant. 2012;21:1547-59.
38. Paulsen Bda S, Cardoso SC, Stelling MP, et al. Valproate reverts zinc and potassium imbalance in schizophrenia-derived reprogrammed cells. Schizophr Res. 2014;154(1-3):30-5.
39. Wang JL, Shamah SM, Sun AX, et al. Label-free, live optical imaging of reprogrammed bipolar disorder patient-derived cells reveals a functional correlate of lithium responsiveness. Transl Psychiatry. 2014;4:e428.
40. Stern S, Santos R, Marchetto MC, et al. Neurons derived from patients with bipolar disorder divide into intrinsically different sub-populations of neurons, predicting the patients' responsiveness to lithium. Mol Psychiatry. 2018;23(6):1453-65.
41. Pernia CD, Nathan NH, Tobe BTD, et al. Modeling complex neurological diseases with stem cells: a study of bipolar disorder. Results Probl Cell Differ. 2018;66: 265-82.
42. Sharma A, Gokulchandran N, Sane H, et al. Autologous bone marrow mononuclear cell therapy for autism: an open label proof of concept study. Stem Cells Int. 2013;2013:623875.
43. Bradstreet JJ, Sych N, Antonucci N, et al. Efficacy of fetal stem cell transplantation in autism spectrum disorders: An open-labeled pilot study. Cell Transplant. 2014;23(Suppl 1):S105-12.

44. Sharma A, Gokulchandran N, Sane H, et al. Therapeutic effects of cellular therapy in a case of adult autism spectrum of disorder. Int Biol Biomed J. 2018;4(2):98-103.
45. Dawson G, Sun JM, Davlantis KS, et al. Autologous cord blood infusions are safe and feasible in young children with autism spectrum disorder: Results of a single-center phase I open-label trial. Stem Cells Transl Med. 2017;6(5):1332-9.
46. Chez M, Lepage C, Parise C, et al. Safety and observations from a placebo-controlled, crossover study to assess use of autologous umbilical cord blood stem cells to improve symptoms in children with autism. Stem Cells Transl Med. 2018;7(4):333-41.
47. Lv YT, Zhang Y, Liu M, et al. Transplantation of human cord blood mononuclear cells and umbilical cord-derived mesenchymal stem cells in autism. J Transl Med. 2013;11:196.
48. Brennand KJ, Gage FH. Concise review: the promise of human induced pluripotent stem cell-based studies of schizophrenia. Stem Cells. 2011;29(12):1915-22.
49. Hoffmann A, Sportelli V, Ziller M, et al. From the psychiatrist's couch to induced pluripotent stem cells: Bipolar disease in a dish. Int J Mol Sci. 2018;19(3). pii: E770.
50. Wright R, Réthelyi JM, Gage FH. Enhancing induced pluripotent stem cell models of schizophrenia. JAMA Psychiatry. 2014;7(3):334-45.
51. Miller ND, Kelsoe JR. Unraveling the biology of bipolar disorder using induced pluripotent stem-derived neurons. Bipolar Disord. 2017;19(7):544-51.
52. Kim S, Kim MK, Oh D, et al. Induced pluripotent stem cells as a novel tool in psychiatric research. Psychiatry Investig. 2016;13(1):8-17.
53. O'Shea KS, McInnis MG. Neurodevelopmental origins of bipolar disorder: iPSC models. Mol Cell Neurosci. 2016;73:63-83.

CHAPTER 19

Psychobiotic Therapy

Aswin Krishnan Ajit, Shahul Ameen

INTRODUCTION

The term "Probiotics" is used to refer to "live microorganisms which when ingested in adequate amounts, confer a health benefit on the host". Though their existence had been identified for more than a hundred years, scientific evidence based on research data had been published only in the recent period. Initially studied extensively by Ilya Metchnikoff who was a Russian Biologist and Nobel laureate, in 1907, there is a significantly overwhelming interest in the beneficial aspects of probiotics toward the central nervous system (CNS) via various hypothetical neural and neurochemical mediated mechanisms involving the endocrinological, immunological, and humoral systems.[1,2]

The term "Psychobiotic" was coined in 2013 by Dinan TG, as "a live microorganism that when ingested in adequate amounts, confers mental health benefits through interactions with commensal gut bacteria".[3] Though initially this term referred to only the neuromodulatory effects of probiotics, later prebiotics, which are essentially compounds which nurture the growth of these bacteria, were also included.

WHY IS THE MICROBIOME IMPORTANT?

The microbial colonization of mammals was considered to be one of the most important evolutionary events. It is postulated that each one of us has a microbiome composition as unique as our finger prints and no two people can have the same flora profile. Whatever experiences and environmental influences we have from birth, makes a contribution which leads to the formation of a unique and diversified flora profile. It is so dynamic that a lot of factors modulate the composition of the flora such as our age, gender, lifestyle habits, geographical location, dietary patterns, psychological and physiological stress, and effect of treatment with antibiotics for other illnesses.[4] The microbiome also exerts certain influences and may affect the way we think, behave and also how we react to stress. It may also modulate our predisposition to certain neurological and psychological disorders.[5] Researchers have even hypothesized that our gut flora can play a role in shaping our personality. This is supported by animal studies using germ-free mice (mice with no gut bacteria) where they have demonstrated that when a germ-free mouse comes in contact with the bacterial flora of a regular mouse, there is a change in the behavioral characteristics of the germ-free mouse as if it has adopted it from the new donor mouse.[6]

The influence of the microbiome is most significantly elaborated in the gastrointestinal (GI) system, where 95% of the entire human microbiota is present. The microbiome mainly comprises of commensal (symbiotic) microbial organisms and serves an adjunctive role in a multitude of physiological functions. The physiological functions in which the microbiome exerts a mediatory influence include digestion, growth, nutrition, neurotropism, immunity, inflammation, and growth, and also in the synthesis of B-Vitamins and Vitamin K.[7] It is proposed that a healthy gut should ideally contain "good" or friendly bacteria and "bad" bacteria in a ratio of 85:15. When this balance is not maintained, it is termed as "dysbiosis".[8] Dysbiosis can present in a variety of symptoms **(Table 1)**.

It is hypothesized that nearly 1,000 species of bacteria are present in the gut, which accounts to a total number of about 100 trillion organisms.[7] Such a sophisticated microbiome is thought to play an important role in the regulation of multiple neurochemical and neurometabolic pathways. They may do that with the help of a complicated mechanism which involves highly interactive and symbiotic host–microbiome signaling systems.[9] The presence of the small noncoding ribonucleic acid (RNA) and microRNA of microbial origin in the signaling cascades in the GI tract and in the systemic and lymphatic circulation in the CNS has been of evidence.[10-12] The studies with germ-free mice have elaborated and identified the role of the microbiome in the conventional development of the physiological functioning of the enteric nervous system (ENS).[9]

Table 1: Symptoms of dysbiosis.	
Fatigue	Skin rash
Poor memory	Palpitations
Insomnia and hypersomnia	Gas or bloating
Anxiety or depression	Diarrhea or constipation
Mood swings	Candida
Muscle and joint aches and pains	Body odors and bad breath
Alcohol intolerance	Eczema
Itching	Psoriasis
Frequent urination	Frequent colds

HUMAN BIOCHEMICAL AND GENETIC INDIVIDUALITY: POTENTIAL ROLE OF THE MICROBIOME

The Human Genome Project had reported that the human genome is composed of about 26,600 protein encoding transcripts, which results in a very complex phenotypic expression. Ironically, *Oryza sativa* (rice) genome, with about 46,000 functional genes, has a very noncomplex phenotypic expression.[13,14] What could explain such a varied diversity? It has been postulated that the 1,000 species of bacteria contribute about 4,000,000 genetic transcripts which, when come in association with the host genome, add up to more than 4,026,000 genes and such great numbers can possibly explain the conundrum of genome complexity.[13,15,16]

HOW DO PSYCHOBIOTICS WORK: THE BRAIN-GUT CONNECTION

In order to understand how psychobiotics work, it is essential to have an insight about the brain-gut connection and the field of psychoneurogastroenterology which is fast emerging.

The field of research involving the ENS had been neglected till recently. It was the remarkable observation by Michael Gershon that 90% of the body's serotonin is stored within the walls of the GI tract, that reignited the curiosity of various neuroscientists and psychiatrists, about the GI nervous system.[17]

According to Dr David Wingate, a developmental biologist, the earlier tubular organisms which stuck to rock surfaces to allow food to pass through them, had only an abdominal neuronal system. As living organisms evolved and the challenges for sustaining life increased, the "reptile brain" or limbic system evolved and catered to those higher needs. It is understood beyond doubt that, like the CNS neuron, the ENS too originates from neural crest cells. Gershon had hypothesized that the body maintained the GI or enteric brain as a distinct entity in higher animals, and this local mini brain got connected to the higher brain via the vagus nerve later in the evolutionary process.[18] The ENS is considered as a single entity which comprises of a network of neuronal plexuses namely the Meissner's and Auerbach's plexus, and surrounded by a pool of more than 30 neurotransmitters such as dopamine, serotonin, glutamate, nitric oxide, norepinephrine, and other chemical mediators like enkephalins and neuropeptides. It also contains glia-like supportive cells, and when combined together contain nearly 100 million neurons which is similar to as that in the spinal cord.[19,20] Though the ENS is considered to have independent activity, it is influenced significantly by the CNS. Though initially it was considered that the higher brain (CNS) had complete and unidirectional influence over the ENS, current research evidence propose that the gut brain may also influence the higher brain, hence making it a bidirectional interaction.[20]

MECHANISMS BY WHICH PSYCHOBIOTICS EXERT THEIR INFLUENCE IN THE CENTRAL NERVOUS SYSTEM

Most of the studies examining the psychophysiological effects of probiotics and prebiotics have been done in rodents and surprisingly the rodents to human translation have been robust. However, a lot more human research is required to concretely verify the claims made.

Synthesis of Neurotransmitters

As described earlier, the ENS uses and produces more than 30 types of neurotransmitters and hence acts as a local mini brain.[21] It is reported that 90% of the body's serotonin and 50% of dopamine are present in the ENS.[17] The major neurotransmitters such as dopamine, gamma-aminobutyric acid (GABA), serotonin, norepinephrine, and acetylcholine have all been demonstrated to be synthesized by the gut microbiome as well **(Table 2)**.[22,23]

Reduction of Level of Stress Hormones

A pivotal study done with germ-free mice had demonstrated exaggerated physiological responses to stress in comparison to normal controls. These abnormal responses were reversible by means of probiotic-induced bacterial recolonization. This observation revealed that the microbiome may have a causative influence in the normal physiological development of the hypothalamo-pituitary-adrenal (HPA) axis.[24]

Stress has also been demonstrated to bring about changes in the overall constitution of the GI microbiome and in turn may potentially lead to an elevation in the levels of neurotoxins which may lead to cognitive dysfunction.[16,25-27] Chronically elevated levels of the stress hormone cortisol are observed in many chronic stressful conditions (physiological and psychological). Similar findings are seen in a variety of psychiatric illnesses as evidenced by dexamethasone nonsuppression and exaggerated waking cortisol, which is a biomarker of depression.[28] Certain strains of psychobiotics

Table 2: Neurotransmitters produced by gut microbiome.	
Bacteria	Neurotransmitters
Bacillus	Dopamine, norepinephrine
Bifidobacterium	Gamma-aminobutyric acid (GABA)
Enterococcus	Serotonin
Escherichia	Norepinephrine, serotonin
Lactobacillus	Acetylcholine, GABA
Streptococcus	Serotonin

Source: Dinan TG, Stilling R, Stanton C, et al. Collective unconscious: How gut microbes shape human behavior. J Psychiatr Res. 2015;63:1-9.

have been demonstrated to significantly lead to a reduction in the levels of cortisol.[29] In one of the studies, the participants who took a combination of *Bifidobacterium longum* and *Lactobacillus helveticus* for a 1-month period, experienced a significant reduction in the levels of cortisol and associated improvement of mood.[30] One of the first human studies which examined the psychophysiological effects of prebiotics in which healthy female and male participants consumed either fructo-oligosaccharides or galacto-oligosaccharides or a placebo, the participants who consumed galacto-oligosaccharides demonstrated a significantly attenuated waking-cortisol response, compared to the other two groups.[31]

Reduce Inflammation

Chronic inflammation may be attributed as a cause for depression according to the neuroinflammatory hypothesis.[32] High levels of circulating proinflammatory cytokines have been linked to depression, anxiety, dementia, and other major and minor cognitive disorders.[33] The proinflammatory cytokines have also been demonstrated to be capable of increasing the permeability of the blood–brain barrier and lead to various adverse consequences.[34] Cytokines have been demonstrated to alter the concentrations of various neurotransmitters that modulate communication in the brain, mainly dopamine, serotonin, and glutamate.[35] A recent meta-analysis had demonstrated that injection of interferon-α which is a proinflammatory cytokine, leads to the induction of depression, which could be reversed with the use of antidepressants.[36] The good bacteria may have a protective effect on the brain by modulating the levels of proinflammatory cytokines and keeping them under control. Few studies have shown that some strains and species of psychobiotic bacteria reduce inflammation which leads to a reduction in depressive and anxiety symptoms.[37,38]

Promote Neurotrophic Growth

Brain derived neurotrophic factor (BDNF), which is one of the most important neurotrophic factors, is observed to have a reduced expression in the brains of patients with depressive illness, schizophrenia, and anxiety disorders.[39] Similar deficiency of BDNF has also been demonstrated in the hippocampus and cortex of germ-free mice.[40-42] Whether the microbiome has a role in the expression of BDNF may be an important area of research on the origin of psychological morbidity and may have a promising role to play in the quest for the etiology of various psychiatric illnesses and their treatment.

Protect the Brain from Free Radical Damage

Certain strains of bifidobacteria and lactobacilli have antioxidant effects and protect the neuronal cells from free radical damage.[43] They also lack proinflammatory lipopolysaccharides and may help to sensitize the immune system to differentiate between anti- and pro-inflammatory agents and help develop appropriate immunogenic responses.

Good bacteria play a positive role in preventing the growth of bad bacteria which are responsible for the production of lipopolysaccharides (present in their cytoskeleton) which are toxic to the brain cells.[44] Lipopolysaccharides may have the following deleterious effects as follows:

- Lower the levels of dopamine and serotonin
- Cause damage to the hippocampus and impair memory processing
- Increase levels of stress hormone cortisol
- Produce neuroinflammation
- Increase production of free radicals.

Neuromodulation

Neuroimaging studies using functional MRI (fMRI) have demonstrated the effects of probiotics as having an effect in the modulation of vigilance and attention to negative emotional stimuli. One study employed healthy female subjects who consumed either a placebo or a mixture of probiotics (*Streptococcus thermophiles*, *Bifidobacterium animalis*, *Lactococcus lactis*, and *Lactobacillus bulgaricus*), or did not consume anything as part of a passive control. During image acquisition in fMRI, the study subjects were shown different emotional faces that are identified to capture attention and increase brain activation. In relation to placebo-treated subjects, probiotic-treated subjects showed a reduction in the activity in the functional network associated with somatosensory, emotional and interoceptive processing, which included the insula, somatosensory cortex, and periaqueductal gray. Placebo subjects showed an increase in the activity in these regions in response to emotional faces. This may be interpreted as a probiotic-induced reduction in network-level neural reactivity to emotional information.[45]

Communication via the Vagus Nerve

The vagus nerve is known to play a very essential and important role in coordinating the parasympathetic activity, which includes the regulation of gut motility and heart rate. Vagal stimulation has been shown to exert anti-inflammatory effects and has also been used as a therapeutic modality for refractory pain, depression, and epilepsy.[46-50] There is also significant evidence about anxiolytics and antidepressants exerting actions via the vagus, suggesting that vagal modulation may be a common pathway for the effects of anxiolytics, antidepressants, and psychobiotics.[51-53] Ted Dinan and his colleagues demonstrated that the probiotics exerted their influence via the vagus nerve. They observed that the mice which were inoculated with the probiotic *Lactobacillus rhamnosus* had shown fewer signs of anxiety, stress, and depression while the mice with a severed vagus did not elicit a similar response.[4,54]

The human microbiome is found to have a potential role to play in the etiopathogenesis of various neuropsychiatric disorders. These are based on certain observations by researchers as follows:

- The bacterial species *Bifidobacterium* and *Lactobacillus* are demonstrated to have the capability to metabolize glutamate to GABA, which is one of the key mediators in anxiety disorders.[40,55,56] One randomized-controlled trial had even demonstrated the anxiolytic properties of the probiotics *B. longum* and *L. helveticus* in humans with anxiety disorders.[57]

- β-N-methylamino-L-alanine (BMAA), which is an amino acid present in certain bacteria, which has a role to play in the formation of structural compounds and mediating resistance to host immunity, is observed to be elevated in the brains of patients suffering from Parkinson-dementia complex of Guam, amyotrophic lateral sclerosis, or Alzheimer's dementia. BMAA is understood to be a neurotoxic amino acid, as it has been observed to have deleterious effects in the functioning of the N-methyl D-aspartate (NMDA) glutamate receptors mainly by means of its propensity to cause glutathione depletion and oxidative stress induction. BMAA is thought to originate from cyanobacterium, which is a constituent of the human microbiome.[58]

- Schizophrenia, depression, obsessive compulsive disorder, and autistic spectrum disorders have all been proposed to have autoimmune and infective theories as an etiopathogenetic mechanism. Molecular mimicry induced by exposure to some strains of streptococci in the GI tract and the cross reactivity with the mitochondria has been hypothesized to be a plausible phenomenon supporting this theory. Mitochondria are believed to have a bacterial origin via endosymbiotic relationships in the evolutionary history of eukaryotes and this relation has been hypothesized to lead to the potential for molecular mimicry due to similar immunological profiles. It is suggested that differences in exposure and genetic vulnerability toward human microbiota-mediated autoimmunity may be significant determinants in the etiopathogenesis.[56,59-61] Obsessive compulsive disorder and pediatric autoimmune neuropsychiatric disorders associated with streptococcal infections (PANDAS) are two conditions which are hypothesized to emerge as a result of an infective etiology.

- The comorbidity of GI disorders with autism spectrum disorders (ASD) is very common. Studies have even shown that the number of GI symptoms may be directly proportional to the severity of the ASD.[62] Studies have demonstrated that the bacterial flora in autistic patients had a predominance of *Bacteroidetes* species as compared to *Firmicutes* which were found to be predominant in normal healthy controls.[63] It has also been speculated that certain bacterial neurotoxins, especially those produced by *Clostridia* species, may lead to a worsening of the behavioral symptoms in patients suffering from ASD.[64] Researchers have demonstrated how treatment with antibiotics for a short period can ameliorate the behavioral symptoms in some cases of ASD.[65] Because of such findings, probiotics are currently under research for their potential efficacy in treating some of the behavioral symptoms in ASD.

- A 38-study review found that probiotics effectively reduced the symptoms of depression, anxiety, obsessive-compulsive disorder, and autism and also had a positive effect in improving cognitive deficits.[66]
- One study demonstrated the serotonin altering effects of *Bifidobacterium infantis*, which was comparable to the action of the antidepressant fluoxetine.[54] Similar effects have been shown with other bacterial species such as *Mycobacterium vaccae* as well. *Mycobacterium vaccae* is found in soil and their inhalation can improve mood by elevating serotonin levels.[67] Is that the reason for the "feel good" effect of gardening?

HOW TO OPTIMIZE THE BENEFICIAL EFFECTS OF PSYCHOBIOTICS?

Bifidobacteria and lactobacilli are two of the most ubiquitous groups of bacteria in our GI tract. They are also the major constituents in most of the probiotic supplements and are found abundantly in probiotic foods. Though they are commercially available in various combinations and in use in other specialties like in the management of irritable bowel syndrome (IBS), researchers are of the opinion that clinically tested psychobiotics with mental health benefits would not be commercially available for the next 5–10 years.

Dr Dinan categorically states in his book "The Psychobiotic Revolution: Mood, Food, and the New Science of the Gut-Brain Connection" that "Eating the right kinds of foods has always been and still is the best way to achieve and maintain a healthy gut."

Eating probiotic foods, which contain beneficial microbes in adequate quantities, is the most sensible and sustainable way to increase the good gut flora. Eating traditionally prepared fermented foods such as yogurt, pickles, kimchi, etc. forms a major source of probiotic bacteria. Foods rich in fat and less sugar are ideal for the growth and preservation of probiotics.

Eat prebiotic foods which aid in the growth of probiotics. Some examples of foods rich in prebiotic properties are black pepper, asparagus, bananas, bamboo shoots, barley, broccoli, beets, chicory, dark chocolate, coffee, fennel root, ginger, garlic, leeks, legumes (especially lentils and lima beans), mustard greens, tomatoes, onions, etc.

And most importantly, stop killing the good bacteria by the indiscriminate and rampant use of broad-spectrum antibiotics. Other factors which lead to destruction/deficiency of good bacteria are stress, poor diet, alcohol, prescription medications, sugar, food emulsifiers, chlorinated tap water, artificial sweeteners, and the rampant use of hand sanitizers and antibacterial soaps. So, use them wisely.

CONCLUSION

Several conceptual and knowledge gaps exist even now regarding the development of psychobiotics as shown in **Table 3**.[68]

Psychobiotics are definitely at the frontier of advancement in the field of mental healthcare. They can positively influence our mental health and neurological functions in an amazing variety of ways. The definition of psychobiotics should ideally be expanded to "any exogenous influence whose effect on the brain is bacterially mediated". They are definitely going to have a significant role to play in the treatment of various psychiatric disorders in the future.

Table 3: Knowledge gaps.	
Ecosystem and structural change	Do psychobiotics alter the architecture of the microbiome? Do probiotics and prebiotics differ in this regard?
Age	Do psychobiotics exert age-specific effects, given impaired-homeostatic integrity of the microbiome in aging individuals?
Dose-response functions	Are psychobiotic effects dose-sensitive?
Time-course of emergence of effects	How long after the beginning of ingestion do psychobiotic effects emerge?
Long-term effects	Do psychobiotics produce long-term changes in the central nervous system?
Zero-sum effects	Are changes in one brain region broadly offset by changes in the opposing direction elsewhere?
Cognitive enhancement	Can psychobiotics confer cognitive benefits?
Detrimental effects	Are psychobiotic benefits accompanied by undetected costs?
Joint effects of probiotics and prebiotics	What are the independent and interactive effects of prebiotics and probiotics?
Strain specificity	Why do some strains of probiotic or prebiotic produce effects but not others?
Role of moderators	What factors moderate psychobiotic effects?
Drug interactions	How do psychobiotics interact with other psychotropic substances?

REFERENCES

1. Buryachkovskaya L, Sumarokov A, Lomakin N. Historical overview of studies on inflammation in Russia. Inflamm Res. 2013;62(5):441-50.
2. Saulnier DM, Ringel Y, Heyman MB, et al. The intestinal microbiome, probiotics and prebiotics in neurogastroenterology. Gut Microbes. 2013;4(1):17-27.
3. Dinan TG, Stanton C, Cryan JF. Psychobiotics: A novel class of psychotropic. Biol Psychiatry. 2013;74(10):720-6.
4. Zhou L, Foster JA. Psychobiotics and the gut-brain axis: In the pursuit of happiness. Neuropsychiatr Dis Treat. 2015;11:715-23.
5. Foster JA. Gut feelings: bacteria and the brain. Cerebrum. 2013;2013:9.
6. Schmidt C (2015). [online] Available from https://www.scientificamerican.com/article/mental-health-may-depend-on-creatures-in-the-gut/ [Last accessed December, 2019].
7. Hill JM, Bhattacharjee S, Pogue AI, et al. The gastrointestinal tract microbiome and potential link to Alzheimer's disease. Front Neurol. 2014;5:43.
8. American Nutrition Association. [online] Available from http://americannutritionassociation.org/newsletter/science-probiotics [Last accessed December, 2019].
9. Bhattacharjee S, Lukiw WJ. Alzheimer's disease and the microbiome. Front Cell Neurosci. 2013;7:153.
10. Zhao Y, Cui JG, Lukiw WJ. Natural secretory products of human neural and microvessel endothelial cells: implications in pathogenic "spreading" and Alzheimer's disease. Mol Neurobiol. 2006;34(3):181-92.
11. Alexandrov PN, Dua P, Hill JM, et al. microRNA (miRNA) speciation in Alzheimer's disease (AD) cerebrospinal fluid (CSF) and extracellular fluid (ECF). Int J Biochem Mol Biol. 2012;3(4):365-73.
12. Sarkies P, Miska EA. Molecular biology. Is there social RNA? Science. 2013;341(6145):467-8.
13. Lukiw WJ. Variability in micro RNA (miRNA) abundance, speciation and complexity amongst different human populations and potential relevance to Alzheimer's disease (AD). Front Cell Neurosci. 2013;7:133.
14. Yu J, Hu S, Wang J, et al. A draft sequence of the rice genome (Oryza sativa L. ssp. indica). Science. 2002;296(5565):79-92.
15. Venter JC, Adams MD, Myers EW, et al. The sequence of the human genome. Science. 2001;291(5507):1304-51.
16. Foster JA, McVey Neufeld KA. Gut-brain axis: How the microbiome influences anxiety and depression. Trends Neurosci. 2013;36(5):305-12.
17. Gershon M. The second brain: a groundbreaking new understanding of nervous disorders of the stomach and intestine. New York, NY: HarperCollins Publishers; 1999. pp. 1-336
18. A Contemporary View of Selected Subjects from the Pages of The New York Times, January 23, 1996. Printed in Themes of the Times: General Psychology, Fall 1996. Distributed Exclusively by Prentice-Hall Publishing Company.
19. McMillin DL, Richards DG, Mein EA, et al. The abdominal brain and enteric nervous system. J Altern Complement Med. 1999;5(6):575-86.

20. Wood JD, Alpers DH, Andrews PL. Fundamentals of neurogastroenterology. Gut. 1999;45(Suppl 2):II6-II16.
21. Hurley D (2011). Your backup brain. [online] Available from https://www.psychologytoday.com/us/articles/201111/your-backup-brain [Last accessed December, 2019].
22. Wall R, Cryan JF, Ross RP, et al. Bacterial neuroactive compounds produced by psychobiotics. Adv Exp Med Biol. 2014;817:221-39.
23. ScienceNews. Microbes can play games with the mind. [online] Available from https://www.sciencenews.org/article/microbes-can-play-games-mind [Last accessed December, 2019].
24. Sudo N, Chida Y, Aiba Y, et al. Postnatal microbial colonization programs the hypothalamic-pituitary-adrenal system for stress response in mice. J Physiol. 2004;558(Pt 1):263-75.
25. Henckens MJ, Hermans EJ, Pu Z, et al. Stressed memories: How acute stress affects memory formation in humans. J Neurosci. 2009;29(32):10111-9.
26. [online] Available from https://news.yale.edu/2012/08/12/yale-team-discovers-how-stress-and-depression-can-shrink-brain. [Last accessed December, 2019].
27. Issa G, Wilson C, Terry AV Jr, et al. An inverse relationship between cortisol and BDNF levels in schizophrenia: Data from human postmortem and animal studies. Neurobiol Dis. 2010;39(3):327-33.
28. Bhagwagar Z, Hafizi S, Cowen PJ. Increased salivary cortisol after waking in depression. Psychopharmacology (Berl). 2005;182(1):54-7.
29. Messaoudi M, Lalonde R, Violle N, et al. Assessment of psychotropic-like properties of a probiotic formulation (Lactobacillus helveticus R0052 and Bifidobacterium longum R0175) in rats and human subjects. Br J Nutr. 2011;105(5):755-64.
30. Galland L. The gut microbiome and the brain. J Med Food. 2014;17(12):1261-72.
31. Schmidt K, Cowen PJ, Harmer CJ, et al. Prebiotic intake reduces the waking cortisol response and alters emotional bias in healthy volunteers. Psychopharmacology (Berl). 2015;232(10):1793-801.
32. Greenblatt JM. The brain on fire: inflammation and depression. [online] Available from https://www.psychologytoday.com/us/blog/the-breakthrough-depression-solution/201111/the-brain-fire-inflammation-and-depression [Last accessed December, 2019].
33. Khairova RA, Machado-Vieira R, Du J, et al. A potential role for pro-inflammatory cytokines in regulating synaptic plasticity in major depressive disorder. Int J Neuropsychopharmacol. 2009;12(4):561-78.
34. McCusker RH, Kelley KW. Immune-neural connections: How the immune system's response to infectious agents influences behavior. J Exp Biol. 2013;216(Pt 1):84-98.
35. Miller AH, Haroon E, Raison CL, et al. Cytokine targets in the brain: impact on neurotransmitters and neurocircuits. Depress Anxiety. 2013;30(4):297-306.
36. Udina M, Castellví P, Moreno-España J, et al. Interferon-induced depression in chronic hepatitis C: a systematic review and meta-analysis. J Clin Psychiatry. 2012;73(8):1128-38.
37. Kali A. Psychobiotics: an emerging probiotic in psychiatric practice. Biomed J. 2016;39(3):223-4.

38. Hakansson A, Molin G. Gut microbiota and inflammation. Nutrients. 2011; 3(6):637-82.
39. Martinowich K, Lu B. Interaction between BDNF and serotonin: Role in mood disorders. Neuropsychopharmacology. 2008;33(1):73-83.
40. Mitew S, Kirkcaldie MT, Dickson TC, et al. Altered synapses and gliotransmission in Alzheimer's disease and AD model mice. Neurobiol Aging. 2013;34(10): 2341-51.
41. Carlino D, De Vanna M, Tongiorgi E. Is altered BDNF biosynthesis a general feature in patients with cognitive dysfunctions? Neuroscientist. 2013;19(4): 345-53.
42. Lu B, Nagappan G, Guan X, et al. BDNF-based synaptic repair as a disease-modifying strategy for neurodegenerative diseases. Nat Rev Neurosci. 2013;14(6): 401-6.
43. Amaretti A, di Nunzio M, Pompei A, et al. Antioxidant properties of potentially probiotic bacteria: In vitro and in vivo activities. Appl Microbiol Biotechnol. 2013;97(2):809-17.
44. [online] Available from http://www.microbialinfluence.com/Brain.html [Last accessed December, 2019].
45. Tillisch K, Labus J, Kilpatrick L, et al. Consumption of fermented milk product with probiotic modulates brain activity. Gastroenterology. 2013;144(7):1394-401.
46. Borovikova LV, Ivanova S, Zhang M, et al. Vagus nerve stimulation attenuates the systemic inflammatory response to endotoxin. Nature. 2000;405(6785):458-62.
47. Kirchner A, Birklein F, Stefan H, et al. Left vagus nerve stimulation suppresses experimentally induced pain. Neurology. 2000;55(8):1167-71.
48. Morris GL 3rd, Mueller WM. Long-term treatment with vagus nerve stimulation in patients with refractory epilepsy. The Vagus Nerve Stimulation Study Group E01-E05. Neurology. 1999;53(8):1731-5.
49. Sackeim HA, Rush AJ, George MS, et al. Vagus nerve stimulation (VNS) for treatment-resistant depression: Efficacy, side effects, and predictors of outcome. Neuropsychopharmacology. 2001;25(5):713-28.
50. Rush AJ, Marangell LB, Sackeim HA, et al. Vagus nerve stimulation for treatment-resistant depression: a randomized, controlled acute phase trial. Biol Psychiatry. 2005;58(5):347-54.
51. Adinoff B, Mefford I, Waxman R, et al. Vagal tone decreases following intravenous diazepam. Psychiatry Res. 1992;41(2):89-97.
52. Abdel Salam OM. Fluoxetine and sertraline stimulate gastric acid secretion via a vagal pathway in anaesthetised rats. Pharmacol Res. 2004;50(3):309-16.
53. Smith R, Allen JJ, Thayer JF, et al. Increased association over time between regional frontal lobe BOLD change magnitude and cardiac vagal control with sertraline treatment for major depression. Psychiatry Res. 2014;224(3):225-33.
54. Davidson J (2014). Nature's Bounty: The Psychobiotic Revolution. [online] Available from https://www.psychologytoday.com/us/articles/201403/natures-bounty-the-psychobiotic-revolution. [Last accessed December, 2019].
55. Aziz Q, Doré J, Emmanuel A, et al. Gut microbiota and gastrointestinal health: Current concepts and future directions. Neurogastroenterol Motil. 2013;25(1): 4-15.

56. Hornig M. The role of microbes and autoimmunity in the pathogenesis of neuropsychiatric illness. Curr Opin Rheumatol. 2013;25(4):488-795.
57. Messaoudi M, Violle N, Bisson JF, et al. Beneficial psychological effects of a probiotic formulation (Lactobacillus helveticus R0052 and Bifidobacterium longum R0175) in healthy human volunteers. Gut Microbes. 2011;2(4):256-61.
58. Brenner SR. Blue-green algae or cyanobacteria in the intestinal micro-flora may produce neurotoxins such as Beta-N-Methylamino-L-Alanine (BMAA) which may be related to development of amyotrophic lateral sclerosis, Alzheimer's disease and Parkinson-Dementia-Complex in humans and Equine Motor Neuron Disease in horses. Med Hypotheses. 2013;80(1):103.
59. Carrasco-Pozo C, Mizgier ML, Speisky H, et al. Differential protective effects of quercetin, resveratrol, rutin and epigallocatechin gallate against mitochondrial dysfunction induced by indomethacin in Caco-2 cells. Chem Biol Interact. 2012;195(3):199-205.
60. Douglas-Escobar M, Elliott E, Neu J. Effect of intestinal microbial ecology on the developing brain. JAMA Pediatr. 2013;167(4):374-9.
61. Hayashi M. Anti-basal ganglia antibody. Brain Nerve. 2013;65(4):377-84.
62. Adams JB, Johansen LJ, Powell LD, et al. Gastrointestinal flora and gastrointestinal status in children with autism—Comparisons to typical children and correlation with autism severity. BMC Gastroenterol. 2011;11:22.
63. Finegold SM, Dowd SE, Gontcharova V, et al. Pyrosequencing study of faecal microflora of autistic and control children. Anaerobe. 2010;16(4):444-53.
64. Parracho HM, Bingham MO, Gibson GR, et al. Differences between the gut microflora of children with autistic spectrum disorders and that of healthy children. J Med Microbiol. 2005;54(Pt 10):987-91.
65. Sandler RH, Finegold SM, Bolte ER, et al. Short-term benefit from oral vancomycin treatment of regressive-onset autism. J Child Neurol. 2000;15(7):429-35.
66. Wang H, Lee IS, Braun C, et al. Effect of probiotics on central nervous system functions in animals and humans: A systematic review. J Neurogastroenterol Motil. 2016;22(4):589-605.
67. [online] Available from: https//www.discovermagazine.com/2007/jul/raw-data-is-dirt-the-new-prozac. [Last accessed December, 2019].
68. Sarkar A, Lehto SM, Harty S, et al. Psychobiotics and the manipulation of bacteria-gut-brain signals. Trends Neurosci. 2016;39(11):763-81.

CHAPTER 20

Advances in Brain Stimulation Therapies

Nand Kumar, Saurabh Kumar

INTRODUCTION

The field of neuromodulation in general and noninvasive brain stimulation in particular has witnessed exponential growth in last few decades. There are different types of brain stimulation techniques, each with varied application and evidence base for different psychiatric disorders. Amongst all the noninvasive brain stimulation techniques, the most evidence base exists for the use of repetitive transcranial magnetic stimulation (rTMS), with growing evidence base for other techniques. Researchers have also developed newer treatment paradigms for use of rTMS, which offers promise in reducing the treatment duration as well as improve treatment outcome in various neuropsychiatric disorders.

DEFINITION

Brain stimulation is use of electric or electromagnetic field to modulate the neuronal activity or neural circuitry of specific cortical regions. The various brain stimulation techniques can be broadly classified as invasive [e.g. deep brain stimulation (DBS)] or noninvasive (e.g. TMS). Recent neuroimaging techniques have enhanced the knowledge of various physiological and aberrant neural circuitries with potential of leading to development of symptoms of various psychiatric and neuropsychiatric disorders. The different brain stimulation techniques focally stimulate the desirable neural circuits leaving the nearby brain regions unaffected. This approach offers mechanistic focality beyond that offered by different pharmacological agents. Hence, minimizing the possible side effects as well as providing alternative therapeutic intervention in patients who have failed to respond to conventional pharmacotherapy.

The last two decades have seen remarkable advancement in the field of brain stimulation resulting in several regulatory agencies approving use of these modalities in various psychiatric disorders. In this chapter, we will focus on various brain stimulation techniques and their use in various psychiatric disorders. The major focus would be on noninvasive brain stimulation techniques, which has definite evidence for its use in various psychiatric disorders as per available literature.

NONINVASIVE BRAIN STIMULATION TECHNIQUES

Transcranial Magnetic Stimulation

Basic Principle of Use

Transcranial magnetic stimulation (TMS) is noninvasive brain stimulation technique. It involves application of alternating magnetic fields by stimulating coil placed directly above the cortical area resulting in induction of electric currents in the underlying area. Hence magnetic brain stimulation is misnomer; it is actually electrical stimulation of the brain cortical region through magnetic stimulator. The electric field alters the electrical charge of cell membrane resulting in neuronal depolarization or hyperpolarization depending upon the frequency of TMS. It can be administered as a single pulse or as repeated pulses at regular intervals known as rTMS. The effect of single pulse TMS usually last up to few milliseconds whereas repetitively pulses can have long-lasting effect on cortical function by mechanisms similar to long-term potentiation (LTP) and long-term depression (LTD).[1] The frequency of repetition of pulses in rTMS varies between 1 Hz and 25 Hz as per currently available magnetic stimulators. These frequencies have been classified as low frequency (≤1 Hz) or as high frequency (usually between 5 Hz and 20 Hz). The use of low frequency stimulation results in a significant reduction in underlying local cortical activity through LTD[2] whereas high-frequency results in increase in local cortical excitability through LTP.[3] Studies have also shown that treatment with high-frequency rTMS increased and low-frequency rTMS decreased regional cerebral blood flow (rCBF) in underlying cortical areas.[4] The therapeutic role of rTMS is based on the above-mentioned changes. For example, the use of rTMS to improve symptoms of depression is based on improving prefrontal area hypometabolism and imbalances in the cortical connectivity between the prefrontal cortex and limbic regions.[5]

Use of rTMS in Psychiatric Disorders

The most robust evidence for the clinical application of rTMS is in depressive disorders, the indication for which it has been approved by US Food and Drug Administration (FDA). Most of the studies have targeted left dorsolateral prefrontal cortex (DLPFC) using high-frequency rTMS. Different stimulation paradigms like using low-frequency rTMS over right DLPFC or bilateral rTMS has also been evaluated (e.g. sequential protocol). Various meta-analyses have observed the efficacy of both high-frequency rTMS of the left DLPFC and low-frequency rTMS of the right DLPFC, with no difference in treatment outcome between the protocols.[6,7] Several guidelines recommend both the treatment protocols as first-line protocols for administration of rTMS in management of patients with depression.[8] Bilateral rTMS involves combined application of high-frequency rTMS over left DLPFC and low-frequency rTMS over right DLPFC. The existing studies have failed to find any advantage of bilateral rTMS over unilateral rTMS in terms of efficacy and acceptability.[9] Therefore, in view of insufficient evidence base, it may be considered as second-line rTMS protocol.[8]

The current focus in TMS therapy is to develop optimal stimulation parameters and treatment schedules to improve outcome of patients with depression. Several studies have shown longer treatment duration and it was observed that more number of stimuli were associated with better treatment outcome.[10] Researchers have emphasized on the need to develop individualized treatment protocol as studies have shown there is not a one-size fit all dosing strategy.[11] Most of the studies have been able to establish the acute efficacy of rTMS but the durability of these effects has always been a matter of debate. A recent meta-analysis found the initial improvement sustained for 1 year in around 50% of the patients and recommended use of maintenance treatment to enhance the durability of the antidepressant effect of rTMS.[12] There are limited number of studies which have tried to explore the role of maintenance rTMS. The existing studies are heterogeneous in terms of study design, stimulation parameter, and duration of observation period.[13] Some authors recommend gradual tapering of rTMS giving one or two sessions of it every 2 weeks or 3 weeks for several months or years depending on the individual clinical picture.

Theta burst stimulation (TBS) is a newer form of rTMS protocol, which has generated a lot of excitement in field of brain stimulation and recently approved by the US FDA for use in depressive disorders. TBS administers magnetic pulses by using 50 bursts per second of 3 pulses each, delivered at the theta frequency of 5 Hz.[14] It has been postulated that it has greater ability to promote synaptic plasticity as these patterns of stimulation are more likely to occur naturally within the cortex. Theta burst exists in two different forms. The intermittent TBS (iTBS) delivers theta burst for 2 seconds with inter-train duration of 8 seconds whereas continuous TBS (cTBS) generates TBS without inter-train interval.[11] The advantages of this form of stimulation are that it requires lesser time (e.g. ≤6 vs. 20–40 minutes per session) and lower stimulation intensity (e.g. usually 80% of the active motor threshold vs. 120% of the resting motor threshold) compared to conventional rTMS.[15] Studies have shown, iTBS given over left DLPFC has potential for improving symptoms of patients with depressive disorder.[16] A recent randomized controlled multicenter trial compared the clinical effectiveness of TBS compared with standard rTMS in adults with treatment-resistant depression and it was observed that both the treatments were equally effective.[17] The side-effects, safety, and tolerability profiles were also found to be similar. The future studies should investigate more clinically relevant stimulation parameters as well as neurobiological predictors of treatment outcome with preferably larger sample sizes and long-term follow-up[16].

Another effort toward reducing the duration of treatment has been to develop accelerated TMS (aTMS) protocols. Fitzgerald et al. (2018) evaluated a schedule of accelerated rTMS compared to standard rTMS. Patients in the accelerated rTMS group received 63,000 high-frequency rTMS pulses delivered as three treatments per day over 3 days in week 1, 3 treatments over 2 days in week, 2 and 3 treatments on a single day in 3rd week. The authors found no significant differences in remission or response rates between the accelerated group and those who received standard rTMS.[17] The field of TMS for managing patients with depression is growing rapidly with development of new treatment protocols which can considerably reduce treatment duration. Efforts are also being made to identify neuroimaging and neurophysiological markers which could help in guiding TMS application for depression.

The role of rTMS has been evaluated in several neuropsychiatric disorders. In schizophrenia, the target symptoms have been medication resistant auditory verbal hallucinations (AVH) and negative symptoms. For AVH, the main site of stimulation has been either temporal cortex or temporoparietal (TP) junction which is based on the assumption that AVH manifestations are caused by hyperactivity of the temporal lobe.[18] Most of the studies have used low frequency rTMS to target these areas. However, the findings from different studies have been contradictory. Several meta-analyses have found rTMS as an effective treatment for AVH but called for methodologically more robust large-scale randomized controlled trials (RCTs) before recommending its use in clinical practice.[19,20] The negative symptoms of schizophrenia are often difficult to treat. There have been several studies of rTMS combined with antipsychotics in the treatment of the negative symptoms of schizophrenia, showing a relatively weak effect on the improvement of these symptoms.[21] Future research should focus on establishing moderator variables and optimal stimulation parameters to improve the outcome.[22]

More recently, there have been several studies which have suggested that TMS holds potential to effectively complement existing therapeutic modalities in the patients with obsessive compulsive disorders (OCD). In a meta-analysis, which included 18 RCTs on rTMS in the treatment of OCD, found rTMS interventions to be moderately effective.[23] Low-frequency rTMS when given over supplementary motor area showed the best results as compared to stimulation of other cortical areas. One of the interesting findings was the effectiveness of rTMS was also greater at 12 weeks follow-up than at 4 weeks follow-up suggesting that the therapeutic effect of rTMS might be visible after the stimulation period and longer follow-up studies are required to better understand these findings. In a naturalistic study, which included 79 patients, low-frequency rTMS was given over either supplementary motor area or orbitofrontal cortex (OFC) indicated rTMS as an effective treatment modality in ameliorating the OCD symptoms but there was no significant difference in outcome between different cortical areas.[24]

A growing body of literature is demonstrating possible therapeutic role of rTMS in various substance use disorders, anxiety disorders, and myriad of other disorders. However, most of these findings are still preliminary and require more number of studies which are methodologically sound and well-designed before rTMS can be recommended for clinical use in these disorders.

Safety of rTMS

Over the last few decade of its use, rTMS has been shown to be very safe and well-tolerated treatment with generally mild side effects and only rare serious adverse effects. The most common reported side effects of TMS are localized pain at site of stimulation, headache, and neck pain. The most serious adverse effect of TMS is possibility of seizures but the overall incidence is very low (0.1–0.6%) and almost equivalent to antidepressant treatment.[25] The risk of seizure is maximum with high-frequency stimulations and more intensive treatment protocols.[26] Some case reports have reported possibility of manic or hypomanic switch with the treatment.[27] There is no statistical difference between the rates of treatment emergent mania between the active and sham TMS groups. TMS appears to be a safe device to be used in special populations such as adolescents and pregnant females but more number of studies would be required with larger sample size to further establish its safety.

Transcranial Direct Current Stimulation

Basic Principle of Use

Transcranial direct current stimulation (tDCS) is a noninvasive brain stimulation technique, which has recently seen exponential rise in its use in both research and clinical practice. It offers certain advantages compared to other brain stimulation techniques—benign side effects, portability of device, relatively inexpensive, and possibility of domiciliary treatment by patient themselves.[18] It involves application of low intensity (typically between 1 mA and 2.5 mA) electric current to the underlying brain tissue through scalp electrodes. This results in neuronal depolarization in the region of anode and hyperpolarization in the region of cathode resulting in shift in the spontaneous rate of neuronal firing hence, modulating the cortical excitability.[18] The effect of tDCS on cortical excitability is dependent on the polarity of the electrodes as well as on the direction of the current flow. Anodal stimulation induces an increase of cortical excitability, whereas cathodal stimulation decreases cortical excitability.[28,29] The inward flow of current toward the cortex (anodal tDCS) results in hyperpolarization of apical dendritic regions of pyramidal cortical neurons and depolarization of somatic regions whereas the outward flow (cathodal tDCS) has exactly opposite action resulting in somatic hyperpolarization and apical dendrite depolarization of pyramidal cortical neuron.[30] The stimulation of target cortical area depends upon placement of the electrodes which is usually determined using the international electroencephalogram (EEG) 10-20 system.

Use of tDCS in Psychiatric Disorders

Till date most of the studies of tDCS have been on depression. The stimulation is usually carried out by placing the anode over the left DLPFC/F3 whereas cathode can be placed over another cephalic location (right DLPFC/F4, right supraorbital/Fp2, or frontotemporal area/F8) or in an extracephalic position. The ELECT-tDCS trial, which is one largest trial to date, compared the efficacy of tDCS with the maximum effective dose of escitalopram. Although the study found tDCS to be superior to sham stimulation but was not as effective as escitalopram.[31] In another study called SELECT-tDCS, the researchers evaluated the combined efficacy of tDCS and sertraline compared to sertraline or tDCS alone.[32] The combined effects of tDCS and sertraline were found to be superior to sertraline alone or sham stimulation. It was hypothesized that tDCS can accelerate and enhance the effect of sertraline. In a meta-analysis of individual patient data of 289 patients which were recruited in six randomized sham-controlled trials, active tDCS was found to be superior to sham tDCS in ameliorating the symptoms of depression.[33] The authors measured tDCS dose by measuring charge density which is dependent on current, duration, and number of sessions. The study failed to find any independent association of current intensity or number of sessions with treatment outcome but a longer session duration was directly associated with improvement in depressive symptoms. Several guidelines recommend the use of tDCS in depression but specify the need for further data to assess its effectiveness.[34]

Similar to TMS the studies evaluating the role of tDCS in schizophrenia has also focused on AVH and negative symptom domains. A systematic review which included six RCTs evaluated the efficacy of tDCS on auditory hallucinations in schizophrenia.[35] The findings of these studies were contradictory with only three studies showing superiority of real tDCS over sham tDCS. The authors concluded that although there is promising results for use of tDCS in AVH but due to the lack of studies with large sample size and heterogeneous nature of existing literature tDCS cannot be seen as therapeutic alternative. Systematic reviews assessing the effect of tDCS on negative symptoms also failed to find any conclusive evidence due to mixed results in different studies.[36]

In OCD, the most common montage placement has been placement of active electrode over the presupplementary motor area and the reference electrode in extracephalic position. The other areas of target have been left DLPFC and OFC. Brunelin et al. (2018) carried out a systematic review of existing literature and included eight case reports, three open-label studies, and one RCT with two active conditions. Although there was great deal of heterogeneity in terms of montage placement and stimulation parameters, it was noted tDCS has a possible efficacy in OCD but further sham-controlled studies are needed to confirm these preliminary results.[37]

Based on current findings, tDCS has failed to find level A recommendation for any clinical condition and the most promising results are for depression, with a level B recommendation. The advantages of tDCS over other brain stimulation techniques make this field promising for further research.

Side Effects

The side effect profile of tDCS is relatively benign including slight tingling at the site of stimulation, skin irritation, headache, fatigue, and nausea.[38]

INVASIVE BRAIN STIMULATION TECHNIQUES

Vagal nerve stimulation (VNS) and DBS are two major invasive brain stimulation techniques which has gained renewed interest in psychiatry for management of treatment refractory clinical conditions.

Vagus Nerve Stimulation

This technique was approved by FDA in 2005 for the treatment of patients suffering from major depressive disorders who have failed adequate trial of at least four antidepressants.[39] Contrary to noninvasive brain stimulation techniques, VNS works on "bottom up" model. Bilateral stimulation of afferent fibers of vagus nerve in nucleus tractus solitarii results in alteration of firing rate of noradrenergic neurons in the locus ceruleus and serotonergic neurons in dorsal raphe resulting in alteration of activities in different cortical structures.[40] It requires surgical insertion of watch-size generator consisting of a titanium-encased lithium battery. The generator is placed in the left chest or the left axillary region and a bipolar lead is anchored to the left vagus nerve. The stimulator is operated externally and the protocol for stimulation can be changed by computer signaling and can be switched on and off telemetrically by handheld device.[41]

The existing literature for its use in treatment refractory depression is mainly based on open noncontrolled trials with only one randomized sham-controlled trial. There is a wide discrepancy in the response rates between initial open label studies and the randomized double-blind trial. The initial studies showed significant response rates whereas the randomized trial failed to find superiority of VNS over the control group in achieving response in patients with depression. A meta-analysis of six trials found that addition of VNS in patients with medication refractory depression improves the response and remission rates.[42] Those patients who were receiving VNS were three times more likely to improve than those who were on treatment as usual. Researchers are making efforts to make the intervention minimally invasive by targeting transcutaneous stimulation of the vagus nerve through its auricular branch in the tragus. Preliminary findings from a nonblinded study in China have demonstrated promising result for this approach.[43]

Deep Brain Stimulation

Deep brain stimulation is a novel brain stimulation technique which targets specific brain areas. The stimulation occurs through stereotactically guided, deep surgical implantation of quadripolar electrodes which are connected to a pacemaker-like device through subcutaneous wires. These stimulators are implanted subcutaneously usually in the subclavicular region. Researchers have proposed several mechanisms through which DBS works. These include alteration in neuronal firing pattern, disruption of oscillatory dynamics, and by change in synaptic plasticity.[44]

The FDA provided licensing approval for DBS in the management of refractory OCD, with electrodes applied to the anterior limb of the internal capsule. Several studies have reported promising role of DBS in medication refractory OCD and have highlighted two main targets—the striatal region (including the anterior limb of internal capsule, the nucleus accumbens, the ventral caudate nucleus, and the ventral capsule/ventral striatum) and the subthalamic nuclei.[45-47] A meta-analysis which included 31 studies involving 116 patients found that DBS leads to a global decrease of about 45% of OCD symptom severity with 60% of patients considered responders. The study failed to find any difference in effectiveness of treatment between different targets.[48] The role of DBS has also been enquired in treatment-resistant depression with promising results in initial open label studies. There have been only three RCTs to evaluate the efficacy of DBS in major depressive disorders. The first two trials failed to find any statistical difference between the stimulated and the nonstimulated groups.[49,50] The recent RCT which stimulated anterior limb of internal capsule showed a significant effect of DBS on depression (with 40% responders).[51] The search for an optimal target in depression is ongoing with recent studies targeting superolateral medial forebrain bundle. 75% of the initial responders have maintained improvement even after 1 year of follow-up.[52]

CONCLUSION

There has been growing evidence which provides support to the hypothesis that various neuropsychiatric and psychiatric disorders results are produced by aberrant function within neural circuits of the cortical and subcortical regions. Brain stimulation techniques have shown promise in specifically modulating these circuits without affecting adjoining areas preventing systemic side-effects which are often seen with pharmacotherapy. Substantial literature is available for the effectiveness of these therapies in multiple psychiatric disorders. The future research is focused toward developing optimal stimulation parameters and newer techniques which can improve treatment outcome.

REFERENCES

1. Hallett M. Transcranial magnetic stimulation and the human brain. Nature. 2000;406(6792):147-50.
2. Chen RM, Classen J, Gerloff C, et al. Depression of motor cortex excitability by low-frequency transcranial magnetic stimulation. Neurology. 1997;48(5):1398-403.
3. Pascual-Leone A, Valls-Solé J, Wassermann EM, et al. Responses to rapid-rate transcranial magnetic stimulation of the human motor cortex. Brain. 1994;117(4):847-58.
4. Speer AM, Kimbrell TA, Wassermann EM, et al. Opposite effects of high and low frequency rTMS on regional brain activity in depressed patients. Biol Psychiatry. 2000;48(12):1133-41.
5. George MS, Lisanby SH, Avery D, et al. Daily left prefrontal transcranial magnetic stimulation therapy for major depressive disorder: a sham-controlled randomized trial. Arch Gen Psychiatry. 2010;67(5):507-16.
6. Kedzior KK, Azorina V, Reitz SK. More female patients and fewer stimuli per session are associated with the short-term antidepressant properties of repetitive transcranial magnetic stimulation (rTMS): a meta-analysis of 54 sham-controlled studies published between 1997–2013. Neuropsychiatr Dis Treat. 2014;10:727-56.
7. Leggett LE, Soril LJ, Coward S, et al. Repetitive transcranial magnetic stimulation for treatment-resistant depression in adult and youth populations: a systematic literature review and meta-analysis. The primary care companion for CNS disorders. 2015;17(6).
8. Milev RV, Giacobbe P, Kennedy SH, et al. Canadian Network for Mood and Anxiety Treatments (CANMAT) 2016 clinical guidelines for the management of adults with major depressive disorder: section 4. Neurostimulation treatments. Can J Psychiatry. 2016;61(9):561-75.
9. Chen JJ, Liu Z, Zhu D, et al. Bilateral vs. unilateral repetitive transcranial magnetic stimulation in treating major depression: a meta-analysis of randomized controlled trials. Psychiatry Res. 2014;219(1):51-7.
10. Schutter DJ. Antidepressant efficacy of high-frequency transcranial magnetic stimulation over the left dorsolateral prefrontal cortex in double-blind sham-controlled designs: a meta-analysis. Psychol Med. 2009;39(1):65-75.
11. Garnaat SL, Yuan S, Wang H, et al. Updates on transcranial magnetic stimulation therapy for major depressive disorder. Psychiatr Clin. 2018;41(3):419-31.
12. Senova S, Cotovio G, Pascual-Leone A, et al. Durability of antidepressant response to repetitive transcranial magnetic stimulation: systematic review and meta-analysis. Brain Stimulation. 2019; 12(1):119-28.
13. Rachid F. Maintenance repetitive transcranial magnetic stimulation (rTMS) for relapse prevention in with depression: a review. Psychiatr Res. 2018;262:363-72.
14. Huang YZ, Edwards MJ, Rounis E, et al. Theta burst stimulation of the human motor cortex. Neuron. 2005;45(2):201-6.

15. Chung SW, Hoy KE, Fitzgerald PB. Theta-burst stimulation: a new form of TMS treatment for depression?. Depress Anxiety. 2015;32(3):182-92.
16. Berlim MT, McGirr A, dos Santos NR, et al. Efficacy of theta burst stimulation (TBS) for major depression: an exploratory meta-analysis of randomized and sham-controlled trials. J Psychiatr Res. 2017;90:102-9.
17. Fitzgerald PB, Hoy KE, Elliot D, et al. Accelerated repetitive transcranial magnetic stimulation in the treatment of depression. Neuropsychopharmacology. 2018;43(7):1565-72.
18. Moffa AH, Brunoni AR, Nikolin S, et al. Transcranial direct current stimulation in psychiatric disorders: A Comprehensive review. Psychiatr Clin. 2018;41(3):447-63.
19. Otani VH, Shiozawa P, Cordeiro Q, et al. A systematic review and meta-analysis of the use of repetitive transcranial magnetic stimulation for auditory hallucinations treatment in refractory schizophrenic patients. International journal of psychiatry in clinical practice. 2015;19(4):228-32.
20. He H, Lu J, Yang L, et al. Repetitive transcranial magnetic stimulation for treating the symptoms of schizophrenia: a PRISMA compliant meta-analysis. Clin Neurophysiol. 2017;128(5):716-24.
21. Wang J, Zhou Y, Gan H, et al. Efficacy towards negative symptoms and safety of repetitive transcranial magnetic stimulation treatment for patients with schizophrenia: a systematic review. Shanghai Arch Psychiatry. 2017;29(2):61-76.
22. Aleman A, Enriquez-Geppert S, Knegtering H, et al. Moderate effects of noninvasive brain stimulation of the frontal cortex for improving negative symptoms in schizophrenia: Meta-analysis of controlled trials. Neuroscience & Biobehavioral Reviews. 2018;89:111-8.
23. Rehn S, Eslick GD, Brakoulias V. A Meta-analysis of the effectiveness of different cortical targets used in repetitive transcranial magnetic stimulation (rTMS) for the treatment of obsessive-compulsive disorder (OCD). Psychiatr Q. 2018;89(3):645-65.
24. Singh S, Kumar S, Gupta A, et al. Effectiveness and predictors of response to 1-hz repetitive transcranial magnetic stimulation in patients with obsessive-compulsive disorder. J ECT. 2019;35(1):61-6.
25. Taylor R, Galvez V, Loo C. Transcranial magnetic stimulation (TMS) safety: a practical guide for psychiatrists. Australas Psychiatry. 2018;26(2):189-92.
26. Loo CK, McFarquhar TF, Mitchell PB. A review of the safety of repetitive transcranial magnetic stimulation as a clinical treatment for depression. Int J Neuropsychopharmacology. 2008;11(1):131-47.
27. Xia G, Gajwani P, Muzina DJ, et al. Treatment-emergent mania in unipolar and bipolar depression: focus on repetitive transcranial magnetic stimulation. Int J Neuropsychopharmacology. 2008;11(1):119-30.
28. Nitsche MA, Paulus W. Excitability changes induced in the human motor cortex by weak transcranial direct current stimulation. J Physiol. 2000;527(3):633-9.
29. Nitsche MA, Paulus W. Sustained excitability elevations induced by transcranial DC motor cortex stimulation in humans. Neurology. 2001;57(10):1899-901.
30. Zaghi S, Acar M, Hultgren B, et al. Noninvasive brain stimulation with low-intensity electrical currents: putative mechanisms of action for direct and alternating current stimulation. Neuroscientist. 2010;16(3):285-307.
31. Brunoni AR, Moffa AH, Sampaio-Junior B, et al. Trial of electrical direct-current therapy versus escitalopram for depression. New Eng J Med. 2017;376(26):2523-33.

32. Brunoni AR, Valiengo L, Baccaro A, et al. The sertraline vs electrical current therapy for treating depression clinical study: results from a factorial, randomized, controlled trial. JAMA Psychiatry. 2013;70(4):383-91.
33. Brunoni AR, Moffa AH, Fregni F, et al. Transcranial direct current stimulation for acute major depressive episodes: meta-analysis of individual patient data. Br J Psychiatry. 2016;208(6):522-31.
34. Lefaucheur JP, Antal A, Ayache SS, et al. Evidence-based guidelines on the therapeutic use of transcranial direct current stimulation (tDCS). Clin Neurophysiol. 2017;128(1):56-92.
35. Pondé PH, De Sena EP, Camprodon JA, et al. Use of transcranial direct current stimulation for the treatment of auditory hallucinations of schizophrenia–a systematic review. Neuropsychiatr Dis Treat. 2017;13:347-55.
36. Pontillo M, Costanzo F, Menghini D, et al. Use of transcranial direct stimulation in the treatment of negative symptoms of schizophrenia. Clin EEG Neurosci. 2018;49(1):18-26.
37. Brunelin J, Mondino M, Bation R, et al. Transcranial direct current stimulation for obsessive-compulsive disorder: a systematic review. Brain Sci. 2018;8(2):37.
38. Rosa MA, Lisanby SH. Somatic treatments for mood disorders. Neuropsychopharmacology. 2012;37(1):102.
39. Aaronson ST, Conway CR. Vagus nerve stimulation: Changing the paradigm for chronic severe depression?. Psychiatr Clin. 2018;41(3):409-18.
40. Nemeroff CB, Mayberg HS, Krahl SE, et al. VNS therapy in treatment-resistant depression: clinical evidence and putative neurobiological mechanisms. Neuropsychopharmacology. 2006;31(7):1345.
41. Tracy DK, David AS. Clinical neuromodulation in psychiatry: the state of the art or an art in a state?. BJPsych Advances. 2015;21(6):396-404.
42. Berry SM, Broglio K, Bunker M, et al. A patient-level meta-analysis of studies evaluating vagus nerve stimulation therapy for treatment-resistant depression. Medical Devices (Auckl). 2013;6:17-35.
43. Rong P, Liu J, Wang L, et al. Effect of transcutaneous auricular vagus nerve stimulation on major depressive disorder: a nonrandomized controlled pilot study. J Affect Disord. 2016;195:172-9.
44. Bilge MT, Gosai AK, Widge AS. Deep brain stimulation in psychiatry: mechanisms, models, and next- generation therapies. Psychiatr Clin. 2018;41(3):373-83.
45. Greenberg BD, Malone DA, Friehs GM, et al. Three-year outcomes in deep brain stimulation for highly resistant obsessive–compulsive disorder. Neuropsychopharmacology. 2006;31(11):2384.
46. Denys D, Mantione M, Figee M, et al. Deep brain stimulation of the nucleus accumbens for treatment-refractory obsessive-compulsive disorder. Arch Gen Psychiatry. 2010;67(10):1061-8.
47. Mallet L, Polosan M, Jaafari N, et al. Subthalamic nucleus stimulation in severe obsessive-compulsive disorder. New England Journal of Medicine. 2008;359(20):2121-34.
48. Alonso P, Cuadras D, Gabriëls L, et al. Deep brain stimulation for obsessive-compulsive disorder: a meta- analysis of treatment outcome and predictors of response. PloS One. 2015;10(7):e0133591.

49. Dougherty DD, Rezai AR, Carpenter LL, et al. A randomized sham-controlled trial of deep brain stimulation of the ventral capsule/ventral striatum for chronic treatment-resistant depression. Biol Psychiatry. 2015;78(4):240-8.
50. Holtzheimer PE, Husain MM, Lisanby SH, et al. Subcallosal cingulate deep brain stimulation for treatment- resistant depression: a multisite, randomised, sham-controlled trial. Lancet Psychiatry. 2017;4(11):839-49.
51. Bergfeld IO, Mantione M, Hoogendoorn ML, et al. Deep brain stimulation of the ventral anterior limb of the internal capsule for treatment-resistant depression: a randomized clinical trial. JAMA Psychiatry. 2016;73(5):456-64.
52. Bewernick BH, Kayser S, Gippert SM, et al. Deep brain stimulation to the medial forebrain bundle for depression-long-term outcomes and a novel data analysis strategy. Brain Stimul. 2017;10(3):664-71.

CHAPTER 21
Surgical Interventions for Neuropsychiatric Disorders

Bikash R Behera, Paresh K Doshi

INTRODUCTION

Neuropsychiatric disorders (NPDs) are now one of the most important causes of disability accounting for in excess of 37%[1] of healthy life year lost, among which depression is leading the list affecting 10–15%[2] of the population worldwide. Majority of NPDs can be effectively managed by alone or in combinations of pharmacotherapy, psychotherapy, and electroconvulsive therapy (ECT). However, 10–30% patients discontinue treatment either due to the nonresponsiveness or due to the side effects of the above-mentioned therapies.[1] It is for these helpless patients, neurosurgical procedures in form of either ablation or deep brain stimulation (DBS) may be considered. Even if DBS has been approved by United States Food and Drug Administration (US FDA) for various movement disorders such as advanced Parkinson's disease (PD), its use in NPD is still in infancy but showing promising results in obsessive-compulsive disorder (OCD), major depressive disorder (MDD), and Tourette syndrome (TS), etc.

HISTORY

History of psychosurgery can be traced from way back to 5000 BC, when trephinations have been performed in order to make an escape route for evil spirits controlling brain by the tribe shaman on persons displaying psychiatric or epileptic symptoms.[3] The accidental left frontal lobe injury followed by permanent personality changes in Phineas Gage in 1848[3,4] captured the enthusiasm of contemporary medical community, which was further consolidated by experiences of Paul Broca[5] and Carl Warnicke[6] in formulating an informal association between brain and mental function. Swiss psychiatrist Gottlieb Burckhardt first attempted bilateral cerebral excisions based on his observational studies from animal model in 1888 and published his results in 1891, which was subsequently rejected by contemporary Swiss psychiatrists.[7]

Neurosurgery for psychiatric disorders has one of the most wobbling histories in the time frame of functional neurosurgery. In order to understand the present context of NPD, it is important to divide these ups and downs phases of psychosurgery into three distinct eras:[8]

1. Era of prestereotactic psychosurgery (1930-1960)
2. Era of stereotactic psychosurgery (1960-1990)
3. Era of neuromodulative psychosurgery (1990-2018).

Era of prestereotactic psychosurgery was dominated by frontal leucotomy, cingulotomy, and cortical undercutting.[8] In 1935, a Portuguese neurologist named Egas Moniz (awarded Nobel prize for his work in psychosurgery in 1949) along with Almeida Lima, a contemporary neurosurgeon, started doing prefrontal leucotomy for several psychiatric conditions like anxiety, schizophrenia, and depression.[9-12] Further popularized by Walter Freeman and James Watts, in USA, the number of prefrontal leukotomies raised to 60,000 by the year1956.[10] Large number of these surgeries were lacking any scientific basis with follow-up; and moreover were done for personality disorders rather than mood disorders. There was a huge rebuff from the society and the surgery was banned in several countries, which still continues in countries like Germany and Japan.[8]

In the second phase, even though the advent of chlorpromazine was marked by the severe backlash towards frontal lobotomy,[10] landmark neuroanatomical descriptions depicting the structural connections between limbic lobe, frontal lobe and sub cortical structures by James Papez and Paul Maclean, revived the dying psychiatric neurosurgery.[13,14] Subsequent developments in stereotactic techniques by Spiegel and Wycis opened up ways to more precise and focused lesions mitigating unwanted side effects of open surgery.[15] Several ablative procedures like subcaudate tractotomy (SCT),[16] anterior capsulotomy, and limbic leucotomy have been performed for OCD, MDD, and bipolar disorders.[17,18] Even if the number of psychosurgical procedures have decreased significantly and performed only in few centers in USA, Canada, England, Australia, and India, now the indications have swung from personality disorders towards mood disorders, laying foundation for the current surgical targets.[19]

During this period of neuromodulative psychosurgery, the ablative surgery was still practiced in very few centers around the world, namely in USA, UK, Sweden, New Zealand, Australia, and Netherlands.[20] In 1999, Bart Nuttin and his colleagues, introduced bilateral high-frequency DBS of the anterior limb of the internal capsule as a replacement for ablative psychosurgery in OCDs.[21] Despite several ups and downs, psychiatric surgery survived,[22-25] and the emergence of target specific DBS has laid the foundation of enthusiasm among psychiatrists, neurologists, and functional neurosurgeons.

Well before the world body taking any call for a consensus guideline in the field of psychosurgery, Doshi PK, took an initiative to bring eminent psychiatrists, neurologists, and functional neurosurgeons of India to form a first ever Core group meeting for surgical management of psychiatric disorder in 2009.[20] In order to have a more regulatory oversee and avoid the mistakes of the past, the World Society for Stereotactic and Functional

Neurosurgery setup a task force in 2011 in Shanghai, China (Doshi PK, the senior author being one of the members) to draw the guidelines for NPDs which was subsequently published in 2014.[26] In 2018, eminent psychiatrists and functional neurosurgeons representing the Indian Psychiatric Society (IPS), The Neuromodulation Society (TNS) of India, and Indian Society of Stereotactic and Functional Neurosurgery (ISSFN) came together to discuss on the current status, need, and legal aspects of surgery for NPD and came up with a consensus guidelines in accordance with the 2017, Mental Healthcare Act of India (Guidelines accepted to be published in Indian Journal of Psychiatry).

LEGAL PERSPECTIVE OF PSYCHOSURGERY IN INDIA

Even though the earlier versions of mental health legislations in India were silent about the surgical aspects of psychiatric disorders, Mental Healthcare Act, 2017 (section 96) has put forth some regulations towards psychosurgery as a treatment modality for mental illness.[27]

Mental Health Review Board

The Mental Healthcare Act (MHA), 2017 (Section 73) recommends the formation and functions of the Mental Health Review Board (MHRB), to oversee and regulate each and every case of psychosurgery to be performed in India. As per MHA 2017 (effective from 29th May, 2018) guidelines, MHRB enjoy the following privileges on receiving any applications for psychiatric surgery:
- The MHRB may ask for additional information and documents as necessary.
- The MHRB may ask the psychiatrist to attend in person and give evidence to the Board.
- The MHRB may examine the person on whom the psychosurgery is proposed to be performed and any other concerned person before arriving at its decision.
- As per section 80 subsection (4) of the Act, the Board shall dispose of the application by granting or denying permission for psychosurgery within a period of 90 days from the date of filing of the application.

Scope of Surgery in Neuropsychiatric Disorders

Surgical procedures can be grossly divided into lesional/ablation surgeries and stimulation surgeries.[28]

In lesional/ablation surgeries mechanical destruction of the target or a pathway of neuromodulative circuit is done. These surgeries can be invasive or noninvasive. Invasive ablative surgeries can be performed by stereotactic placement of radioactive yttrium (^{90}Y) seeds[16] or by placement of radiofrequency thermistor electrodes[29] or by placement of a cryogenic electrode tip[30,31] in the prespecified targets. Innovations such as Gamma Knife Radiation Surgery (GKRS)[32,33] and magnetic resonance-guided focused ultrasound (MRgFUS)[34,35] have come up as noninvasive ablative procedures to further enhance the safety of psychosurgery. Using ionizing radiations in a precise way to cause neuronal cell damage, GKRS can obviate the open neurosurgical procedures.[36] GKRS has few disadvantages like radiation exposure, long latency, and needs several sessions.[37] Multisource ultrasound is used under MRI guidance in MRgFUS to produce specific discrete lesions in brain.[34,37]

The DBS system consists of an electrode placed in the specific brain area connected to a pacemaker via a connecting wire which can modulate (stimulate/inhibit) the nucleus or the signal pathway. The beauty of DBS lies in its reversibility of side effects of the current.[38]

Advancements in stereotactic and functional neurosurgery have led to an expanding array of clinical and research indications for psychosurgery. Stringent ethical patient selection with strict adherence to the laid consensus guidelines along with subsequent extensive research in neurobiology of target specific psychosurgery has improved confidence among the psychiatrists, neurosurgeons as well as the society, regarding the therapy.[20,26]

Even if, treatment resistant OCD,[21,39-41] MDD,[42-44] and TS[45,46] are the most commonly performed surgery among several NPDs, obesity[47]/anorexia nervosa,[48,49] addictions,[50] and post-traumatic stress disorders (PTSDs)[51] are recently being evaluated with encouraging results.

Preoperative Evaluation for Psychosurgery

Surgical management of NPD needs to be approached in a collaborative manner by a senior psychiatrist, neurologist, and an experienced functional neurosurgeon. Thorough psychiatric evaluation by a psychiatrist is the cornerstone of evaluation to confirm the diagnosis along with history of pharmacotherapy, cognitive behavioral therapy (CBT), and ECT should be carried out to stamp the patient as treatment resistant psychiatric disorder suitable for psychosurgery.

Various preoperative assessment scoring systems such as Yale–Brown Obsessive Compulsive Score (Y-BOCS) for OCD, Hamilton Rating Scale for Depression (HAM-D), Hamilton Rating Scale for Anxiety (HAM-A), Montgomery–Asberg Depression Rating Scale (MADRS) for depression, Beck Depression Inventory (BDI) for depression, and OCD are necessary to compare with the postoperative improvements. Treatment response for MDD is defined as a ≥50% reduction in HAM-D-17 or MADRS, while remission is defined as HAM-D-17 ≤7 or MADRS ≤10 while treatment response for OCD is defined as ≥35% decrease in Y-BOCS score. Modified Rush Video Rating Scale (MRVRS) of the activities in TS patients are recorded to compare with the postoperative results.

Magnetic resonance imaging (MRI) of brain is essential to rule out any organic cerebral pathology as well as to locate and plan the targets for lesioning or DBS as per standard protocols. Preoperative contrast-enhanced computed tomography (CECT) brain with head ring and localizer is needed to be fused with the preoperative MRI on a work station to plan the target and trajectory for both lesional as well as DBS procedures. Routine blood investigations and cardiac evaluations are essential to rule out any contraindications for surgery under general anesthesia.

OBSESSIVE-COMPULSIVE DISORDER

Obsessive-compulsive disorder is defined as a psychiatric condition where repeated undesired thoughts, feelings, and ideas take over a person and forces him to do something unnecessary over and again. OCD has a worldwide prevalence of 2–3%[52] with 0.6% among Indian population.[53]

Pathophysiology of Obsessive-compulsive Disorder

The neurobiology of OCD revolves around the cortico-striato-thalamo-cortical (CSTC) loop where orbitofrontal cortex (OFC), anterior cingulate gyrus (ACG), and basal ganglia play the central role.[54,55] There are two postulated pathways—(1) direct and (2) indirect pathways. Direct pathway projects from cortex-striatum, internal globus pallidus (GPi), substantia nigra-thalamus then back to cortex. Indirect pathway is similar to direct pathway with relay from striatum going to external globus pallidus-subthalamic nucleus (GPe-STN) before joining to GPi and further.[54] It is presumed that OCD is caused by some primary striatal pathological process causing striato-thalamic inhibition resulting in hyperactivity in OFC, ACG, thalamus, and caudate nucleus.[38] The above regions in brain may be targeted for surgery in OCD.[38]

Indications for Surgery in Obsessive-compulsive Disorder[56]

Through patient evaluation, reviews of records, clinical assessments, and communication with treating clinician along with Y-BOCS scoring are meticulously performed to reconfirm the diagnosis of resistant OCD requiring surgical intervention. Some essential criteria for surgical candidature of OCD are depicted in **Box 1**.

Commonly used Surgical Targets for Obsessive-compulsive Disorder

Following anatomical targets are currently being investigated and used for OCD either for ablative surgery or for DBS surgery.
- Anterior capsule (AC)[21,57]
- Ventral capsule/ventral striatum (VC/VS)[58]

> **Box 1:** Selection criteria for surgery for obsessive-compulsive disorders (OCD).
> - Severe (Y-BOCS score ≥28 or ≥14 in case of illness with predominant obsessions or compulsions) and chronic unremitting OCD
> - The disorder is causing substantial distress and impairment in functioning (GAF ≤ 45)
> - The following treatment options tried systematically without appreciable effect on the symptoms:
>   - Adequate trial with at least two of the SSRI antidepressants for at least 3 months each
>   - Treatment with clomipramine at optimum therapeutic for at least 3 months unless poorly tolerated
>   - Augmentation with at least two agents, each for a period of at least 8 weeks, one of them being an atypical antipsychotic—atypical antipsychotics (risperidone and aripiprazole), clomipramine, memantine, N-acetyl cysteine, and ondansetron/granisetron commonly employed augmenting agents
>   - At least one adequate trial of cognitive behavior therapy (at least 20 sessions) or demonstrated inability to tolerate the anxiety due to therapy
>   - Previous treatment trials have not been abandoned prematurely due to solely mild side effects
> - Patient gives informed consent for surgery and willing to participate in the postoperative follow-up.
>
> *Relative contraindications*:
> - Comorbid intellectual disability, psychosis, bipolar disorder, and severe personality disorders
> - Clinically significant and unstable neurologic illnesses.

(GAF: Global Assessment of Functioning; SSRI: selective serotonin reuptake inhibitor; Y-BOCS: Yale–Brown Obsessive Compulsive Score)

- Bed nucleus of stria terminalis (BNST)[59]
- Anterior cingulate cortex (ACC)[60]
- Nucleus accumbens (NA)[61]
- Subcaudate tractotomy[62]
- Limbic leucotomy.[63]

Ablative Procedures

Cingulotomy, anterior capsulotomy, and limbic leucotomy are few of the commonly performed ablative procedures for treatment resistant OCD.[38]

Cingulotomy

In 1940s, Freeman and Watts performed cingulotomies for anxiety-related disorders with good results.[64] Cingulate gyrus plays a pivotal role in CSTC pathway transferring information from ACC to OFC and limbic system.[65] Cingulotomy procedure interrupts the tracts between cingulate gyrus and frontal lobe thus helps in controlling symptoms of OCD.[64] In a retrospective analysis of cingulotomy procedures in 198 patients, Ballantine observed improvement in 56% patients with OCD.[38] Several studies in literature find approximately 30–45% patients to be responders to cingulotomy.[66-68] Common side effect profile after cingulotomy procedure span from memory deficit, apathy, urinary incontinence to few reports of seizures and suicides.[68]

Capsulotomy

First described by Jean Talairach in the 1949 and popularized by Lars Leksell, the anterior capsulotomy has been in use for treatment refractory OCD and depression for over five decades.[64] Here anterior limb of the internal capsule is basically blocked from serving as a relay route between cortical structures and the thalamus and hence forming the basis of OCD surgery. A prospective study of bilateral anterior capsulotomy for refractory OCD by Oliver B et al. showed a 33% reduction in symptoms in 53% patients, 50% reduction in symptoms in 29% patients, and 66% reduction in 17% patients.[69] Liu et al. series of bilateral stereotactic capsulotomy for treatment refractory OCD with a 3-year follow-up results were encouraging as 57% became symptom free, 29% were having significant improvement.[70] Postcapsulotomy transient cognitive and affective dysfunction, were presented in form of lack of initiative and arousal in few patients.[71]

Subcaudate Tractotomy

Knight G[16] in 1965 first performed SCT in London. Traditionally this surgery is more commonly performed for resistant depression than OCD. A small lesion is created in the white mater tracts below the head of caudate nucleus targeting the CSTC pathway.[72,73] Most of the literatures show about 65% of symptom reduction with few adverse effects such as transient disorientation (10%), seizures (1.6%), and suicide (1%).[74]

Limbic Leucotomy

This procedure developed by Kelly and Richardson in the 1970s was essentially a combination of SCT and cingulotomy.[30,75] Limited outcome data available for limbic leucotomy showing improvement in approximately 36–62%[76,77] of treatment resistant OCD patients. Adverse effects commonly reported after limbic leucotomy include headache, laziness, stereotyped perseverative behavior, inadequate sphincter control, and transient memory loss.[31]

Deep Brain Stimulation in Obsessive-compulsive Disorder

In 1999, Nuttin et al. found that chronic electrical stimulation instead of bilateral capsulotomy in long-standing treatment-resistant OCD was beneficial in three out of four patients.[21] Subsequent modification of target from AC to VC/VS was proposed by Greenberg et al. in 2010.[58] They reported a full response of 28% patients at 1 month which increased to 61.5% at 2 year follow-up along with significant improvement in depression and anxiety.[58]

The gradual movement of the target in a posterior direction has resulted in the discovery of a new target for OCD known as BNST.[59] In 2010, Denys et al. presented a study of 16 patients with NA DBS for resistant OCD with a Y-BOCS reduction of 47% after 12 months and 52% after 21 months. Nine patients went into remission with a mean Y-BOCS reduction of 72%.[61]

A systemic review of DBS in OCD by Matilda N et al. found NA as one of the most common target used for OCD in 36 patients followed by VC/VS in 26 patients and STN in 16 patients.[78] Limbic part of STN has also been explored by a French multicenter study group in 2008 for resistant OCD with a 3-month results of mean Y-BOCS of 19.7 in stimulation group in comparison to 28.7 in nonstimulation group.[79] Side effects such as seizures, paresis, confusion, anxiety, and hypomania are reported in several study groups.[58,78,79] Doshi PK reported a case of mania following DBS of BNST for OCD contrary to hypomania reported by several groups.[80] Recently US FDA has also approved the use of DBS for OCD.[81]

DEPRESSION

Major depressive disorder is a heterogeneous and complex psychiatric illness with about 30% patients nonrespondents to currently available treatments (antidepressants, psychotherapies, and ECT) due to either lack of efficacy or tolerance to drugs.[82,83]

Neurobiology of Major Depressive Disorder[84]

Three important components of neurobiological aspect of MDD are cortical, subcortical/limbic, and modulatory.

Cortical Component

Major components being prefrontal cortex, premotor cortex, and dorsal portion of ACG, this is responsible for the psychomotor and cognitive aspects of depressive symptoms. This cortical component relays to striatum creating a feedback loop via thalamus.

Subcortical Component

Subgenual ACG, OFC, limbic structures, and NA constitute the subcortical component. This forms a functional loop with striatum and thalamus involving affective symptoms of depression like sadness and anhedonia.[85]

Modulatory Component

This pathway consists of amygdala, pregenual ACC, and the hypothalamic-pituitary-adrenal axis. This regulates the neuroendocrine aspects of depressive symptoms via inhibitory projections to cortical and limbic circuits.[64]

> **Box 2:** Selection criteria for surgical interventions in major depressive disorder (MDD).
> - Diagnosis of MDD or recurrent depressive disorder, current episode severe as per standard diagnostic criteria
> - Chronic unremitting illness or the presence of multiple recurrent episodes, with ≥1-year duration
> - Severe illness, with a (HAM-D-17) of ≥24
> - The disorder is causing severe distress or functional impairment (GAF ≤ 45)
> - The illness did not show substantive response after treatment with the following:
>   - Adequate trials of at least four antidepressant medications, belonging to three different classes, one of which should have been a tricyclic antidepressant or serotonin-norepinephrine reuptake inhibitor
>   - Trial of at least one evidence-based pharmacological augmenting such as lithium, triiodothyronine or atypical antipsychotic
>   - Trial of bilateral ECT
>   - At least 12 sessions of psychotherapy
> - Provides informed consent and is willing to comply with the preoperative evaluation and periodic postoperative follow-up

(ECT: electroconvulsive therapy; GAF: Global Assessment of Functioning; HAM-D-17: Hamilton Rating Scale for Depression)

Indications for Surgery in Depression

As per the consensus guidelines by Doshi PK et al.,[86] criteria listed in **Box 2** are essential for surgical interventions in MDD.

Common Surgical Targets for Major Depressive Disorder

Targets for Lesional Surgery

- Anterior cingulate cortex[87,88]
- Anterior capsule[89-91]
- Subcaudate tractotomy[29,73]
- Limbic leucotomy.[30,31,65]

Targets for Deep Brain Stimulation[78]

- Subcallosal cingulate gyrus (SCG)
- Ventral capsule/ventral striatum
- Nucleus accumbens
- Median forebrain bundle (MFB)
- Inferior thalamic peduncle (ITP).

Ablative Procedures for Major Depressive Disorder

Anterior Cingulotomy

Initial results of bilateral anterior cingulotomy by Ballantine et al. resulted in improvement of 90% patients with 20% being completely recovered.[92]

In a later study, by Ballantine et al. of 118 patients, considerable improvement was seen in 77 (65.3%) patients with few reported cases of suicides, seizures, and hemiplegia due to intracerebral hemorrhage (ICH).[93]

More recently, a series of anterior cingulotomy in 33 patients by Shields et al. resulted in 21.2% responders with 18.2% partial responders, and 60.6% nonresponders. They also reported few complications such as seizure, memory loss, urinary incontinence, and speech difficulty.[87] Steele et al. performed anterior cingulotomy on eight patients with an encouraging results of five (62.5%) responders (with three of these patients meeting the criteria for remission) 12 months postoperatively.[88]

Subcaudate Tractotomy

In a series of SCT in 23 patients suffering from MDD, Knight G observed positive clinical outcomes in 20 (87.0%) cases.[16] Initial use of radioactive yttrium (^{90}Y) by Knight G in substantia inominata was replaced by radiofrequency thermal lesions with better outcome and lesser side effects.[29] Hodgkiss et al. reported results from a cohort of 183 patients who underwent stereotactic SCT for MDD, of which, 63 (34.4%) recovered, 58 (31.7%) improved, and 57 (31.1%) remain unchanged.[73]

Kim et al. performed SCT in seven patients with MDD with a response rate of 71.4% and having no adverse effects.[94]

Limbic Leucotomy

Kelly et al. performed cryogenic limbic leucotomy on nine patients with MDD. At the 6-week follow-up, they found three patients (33.3%) were "symptom-free," three patients (33.3%) were "much improved," and three (33.3%) were "improved" with few adverse effects such as headache, severe laziness, urinary incontinence, and stereotyped perseverative behavior.[30,31] Montoya et al. reported six limbic leucotomy procedures for MDD with a response rate of 50%.[76]

Anterior Capsulotomy

Anterior capsulotomy has only recently been utilized to treat treatment-resistant depression (TRD). Christmas et al. performed anterior capsulotomy on 20 patients with MDD and at the mean follow-up of 7 years, 10 patients responded to treatment among which 8 patients met criteria for remission.[89] Few adverse effects such as urinary incontinence, headache, and confusion are seen postoperatively.[89,90]

Hurwitz et al. of the Vancouver Limbic Surgery Group (VLSG) reported eight patients with MDD who underwent bilateral anterior capsulotomy using radiofrequency lesions. Overall, four out of eight patients (50%) were classified as responders between 24 months and 36 months postoperatively. One patient suffered from akinetic mutism postoperatively.[91]

Deep Brain Stimulation for Depression

Matilda et al. reviewed various articles from 2005 to 2015 and concluded that a total of 67 patients underwent SCG DBS for MDD with a response rate of 50-58% and remission rate of 17% at 6-12 months.[78]

Two large multicenter randomized sham-controlled trials, one targeting SCG and the other targeting VC/VS, have raised several questions regarding the efficacy of DBS in MDD as these trials were unable to replicate the previously reported significant antidepressant effect.[95,96]

In contrast to the above-mentioned studies, a multicenter pilot study of SCG DBS by Lozano et al. in 2012 found 50% reduction of HAM-D-17 score in 57% patients at 1 month, 48% patients at 6 months, and 29% patients at 12 months.[97] Another randomized double-blind crossover trial of SCG DBS for TRD by Puigdemont et al., showed remission in five out of eight patients with four out of these five patients retained the remission for 3 months in "ON" phase compared to two-fifths patients during the "OFF" phase.[98] In a clinical study targeting ventral anterior limb of internal capsule (ALIC), Bergfeld et al. found 40% (10/25) patients as responders after 52 weeks of optimization in stimulation parameters before entering into a randomized crossover trial of stimulation "ON/OFF" phase. Here again patients had a significant lower score [Hamilton Depression Rating Scale (HDRS) 13.6 vs. 23.1] during ON as compared to OFF condition.[99]

The VC/VS DBS in 15 patients by Malone et al. resulted in six responders and three remitters after 6 months.[43] Another study of NA DBS in 10 patients by Bewernick et al., reported five responders and three remitters at 1 year evaluation.[42] Schlaepfer et al. presented seven patients with MFB DBS with two responders and four remitters after 3-6 months.[100] Two case reports also described remission after DBS in lateral habenula (LH) and ITP.[101,102]

Other than infection and hardware malfunctions, transient hypomania, agitation, psychosis, and confusion were common stimulation-related side-effects.[78]

TOURETTE SYNDROME

Tourette syndrome is a complex, chronic NPD of childhood characterized by motor and vocal tics along with several behavioral comorbidities such as attention deficit hyperactive disorder and OCD.[103] Surgical intervention may be considered in a small subset of pharmacobehavioral-resistant TS patients inflicted with self-injurious behavior (malignant TS).[103-105]

Neurobiology of Tourette Syndrome

Pathophysiology of TS revolves around the imbalance of CSTC relay circuits.[106] Centromedian-parafascicular (CM-Pf) nuclei has been used as a surgical target in treatment of TS due to its ability to modulate both the limbic and sensorimotor circuitry.[103]

As one of the proposed hypotheses suggests the role of altered signal output to GPi and substantia nigra from aberrant striatal neurons, GPi can rightly be modulated to get desired benefit in TS.[107]

Indications for Surgery in Tourette Syndrome

Tourette Syndrome Association International DBS Database/Registry recommendation proposed that age should no longer be a strict criteria along with compulsory approval from local ethical committee for a patient below 18 years for DBS in TS.[108]

Box 3 presents the criteria laid by the Indian authorities as consensus guidelines for surgery in TS.[86]

Common Surgical Targets for Tourette Syndrome

- Thalamus [centromedian nucleus-substantia periventricularis-nucleus ventro-oralis-internus complex (CM-Spv-Voi) and CM-Pf][109-112]
- GPi (posteroventral and anteromedial)[113-119]
- GPe[120]
- STN[121]
- ALIC/NA.[122,123]

Ablative Procedures

In past several ablative procedures such as prefrontal lobotomy, limbic leucotomy, anterior cingulotomy, thalamotomy, cerebellectomy, etc. have been attempted with unsatisfactory results and major side-effects for treatment refractory TS.[124]

Box 3: Indian expert consensus selection criteria for surgery for Tourette syndrome (TS).

- Primary diagnosis of TS as per standard diagnostic criteria
- Chronic and severe illness, preferably assessed with standardized scales such as Yale Global Tic Severity Scale (YGTSS), where the total tic severity score of >35/50
- The disorder is causing severe distress or functional impairment [Global Assessment of Functioning (GAF) ≤45]
- Resistant to standard available treatment strategies including the following:
    - Poor/unstable response or intolerable adverse effects after adequate trials (≥6 weeks at maximum tolerated dose) of treatment with at least (1) one alpha-adrenergic agonist, (2) one typical and an atypical antipsychotic medication, and (3) a drug another class of medication (benzodiazepine, tetrabenazine, topiramate, and baclofen)
    - Poor response/inability to adhere to behavioral therapy, which was tried for ≥10 sessions
- Provides informed consent and is willing to comply with the preoperative evaluation and periodic postoperative follow-up.

Deep Brain Stimulation for Tourette Syndrome

Vandewalle et al. published the first case of thalamic DBS for TS in 1999 with a 60.5% reduction in Yale Global Tic Severity Scale (YGTSS) at 1 year. The initial surgical target was 5 mm lateral to the anterior commissure-posterior commissure (PC) line, 4 mm posterior to the midcommissural point, and at the level of the anterior commissure-PC plane, targeting (CM-Spv-Voi).[109]

Porta et al. have reported the 2-year clinical follow-up results for 15 of their patients with thalamic DBS featuring significant improvement the YGTSS from 76.5 to 36.6. A clinically significant improvement was also seen on the Y-BOCS, the BDI scores.[111] Ackermans et al. presented their series of six patients targeting the CM-Spv-Voi complex. Their series had a statistically significant improvement in YGTSS compared to off stimulation phase which was maintained at 49% at 1-year follow-up.[45] Savica et al. in year 2012 reported a mean reduction of 70% YGTSS at 1-year follow-up in three patients who underwent CM-Pf DBS.[112]

Ten out of eleven patients undergoing anteromedial GPi (amGPi) DBS in Sachdev et al. series, improved after surgery with six patients scoring more than 50% improvement in YGTSS. Along with a 49% mean reduction in YGTSS, the Y-BOCS scores also improved from a mean of 15.82 to 6.55.[46] Similarly various reports showing GPi (posteroventral/anteromedial) stimulation for treatment refractory TS found significant improvements in YGTSS scores (70–93%) along with improvement in Y-BOCS scores.[113-118] However, a recent double blind randomized controlled trial (RCT) of anterior GPi (aGPi) DBS found no significant difference in YGTSS scores between active versus sham stimulation groups in 3 months. But subsequent open label stimulation for a period of 6 months revealed significant improvement in YGTSS score, suggesting longer stimulation may be required for eliciting the therapeutic effects of DBS in TS.[119] Few sporadic reports of chronic ALIC/NA stimulations also resulted in decrease in YGTSS score though not as effective as previous mentioned targets.[122-124]

International registry of TS patients created by Michael Okun, serves as a repository and data bank for all TS patients being operated worldwide.[125] This International Registry performed a prospective trial of DBS implantation for treatment resistant TS in 185 patients from 10 countries worldwide from 2012 to 2016 with a mean YGTSS score improvement from 75.01 to 41.19 at 1-year follow-up ($p < 0.001$). Mean motor/phonic tic score improved from 21.00/16.82 to 12.91/9.63 ($p < 0.001$) with an overall adverse effect in 35.4% patients.[125]

Complications[103]

Other than hardware-related issues, few cases of hematoma, infection, and neurological deficits are seen. Most of the stimulation-related side-effects were reversible and restricted to drowsiness, visual blurring, depression, bradykinesia, anxiety, and hypomania.

OBESITY/ANOREXIA NERVOSA

The neurobiology of obesity circuitry includes the lateral hypothalamus (LH), ventromedial hypothalamus, and NA and thus each of these areas form potential targets for chronic stimulation. Bilateral stimulation of the LH has been shown to cause weight loss in a rat model.[47] A 35-month post LH DBS follow-up of three patients by Whiting et al., reported encouraging results of 1%, 12%, and 16% increase in the metabolic rate.[126]

Only few case reports available in literature citing improvement of body mass index (BMI) along with associated improvement in mood, anxiety, and quality of life following chronic stimulation of SCG and NA.[48,49]

ADDICTION

Addiction is a type of strong psychological and physical substance dependence within a person along with withdrawal symptoms whenever stopped.[127] Various targets such as hypothalamus, cingulate gyrus, and substantia inominata have been tried in the past for treating addiction.[50] Muller et al. reported successful abstinence in two patients and improvement in one patient following DBS of NA.[128] Overall, DBS for addiction is in an investigational state and NA may prove to be a promising target in future.

POST-TRAUMATIC STRESS DISORDER

The neurobiology of PTSD revolves around the basolateral nucleus of amygdala (BLn) containing "fear cells" that are active during fear acquisition and "extinction cells" that are active during fear extinction. PTSD may alter the modulation in BLn from getting conditioned to ignore fear, by altering the neuroplasticity of the extinction cells.[129] Langevin et al. described a single case of BLn DBS in an American war veteran suffering from PTSD with considerable improvement.[129] Even if a pilot randomized blinded-controlled study has shown efficacy and safety of BLn DBS, this therapy is still in an investigational stage.[51]

STIMULATION OR ABLATION?

A comparative study between anterior capsulotomy and DBS of NA, VC/VS by Peeper J et al. in 2014 revealed a better reduction in Y-BOCS score (51%) in anterior capsulotomy group with a 9% more likely to go to remission in comparison to DBS group (40%) and found that the acceptability of DBS is more among most of the clinicians over anterior capsulotomy as a treatment modality for OCD.[130] The clinical effects of stimulation and ablation are similar. The advantage of DBS is the titratibility of the stimulation to control the clinical effect as well as limit the side effects. Ablative surgery obviates many of the risks and expense associated with a life-long implant. However, any potential negative therapeutic outcomes are permanent. So both procedures have their own existence in modern day functional neurosurgery depending upon the expertise of surgeon and the socioeconomic status of the patient.

OUR EXPERIENCE IN PSYCHOSURGERY

- Doshi and his team have operated eight patients of OCD, three patients of MDD and two cases of TS.
- For OCD, three patients have underwent capsulotomy,[131] three have underwent NA lesioning, With one NA DBS and one BST DBS. The mean Y-BOCS improved to 12.6 from 35.5 after 1 year.
- Three patients of major depression who underwent SCG DBS had a mean improvement of HAM-D/A score from 27/26 to 4/4 till last follow-up. (Unpublished data.)
- We have offered GPi DBS for TS in two patients with an 18-month YGTSS score improvement from 80/70 to 22/34, respectively.[132]

CONCLUSION

Deep brain stimulation has certainly more advantages in comparison to the lesional surgeries due to its titratibility and reversibility. Functional neurosurgery is a fast growing field with gradual encroachment of several treatment refractory NPD. Proper collaboration with psychiatric community along with futuristic oversight and strict ethical considerations via approved regulatory bodies will facilitate the ongoing research and development in this neglected area of medical science.

REFERENCES

1. Lopez AD, Mathers CD, Ezzati M, et al. Measuring the global burden of disease and risk factors, 1990–2001. In: Lopez AD, Mathers CD, Ezzati M (Eds). Global Burden of Disease and Risk Factors. Washington, DC: World Bank Group; 2006. pp. 1-14.
2. Al-Harbi KS. Treatment-resistant depression: therapeutic trends, challenges, and future directions. Patient Prefer Adherence. 2012;6:369-88.
3. Feldman RP, Goodrich JT. Psychosurgery: a historical overview. Neurosurgery. 2001;48:647-59.
4. Ratiu P, Talos IF, Haker S, et al. The tale of Phineas Gage, digitally remastered. J Neurotrauma. 2004;21(5):637-43.
5. Broca PP. Remarques sur le siége de la faculté du langage articulé; suivies d'une observation d'aphémie (perte de la parole). Bulletins de la Société Anatomique (Paris), 2e série 6. 1861;6:330-57.

6. Wernicke C. Der aphasische symptomen complex. Breslau: Max Cohn & Weigert; 1874.
7. Burckhardt G. Uber rindexcisionen, als beitrag zur operative therapie der psychosen. Allg Z Psychiatr Psych Med. 1891;47:463-548.
8. Neumaier F, Paterno M, Alpdogan S, et al. Surgical approaches in psychiatry: a survey of the world literature on psychosurgery. World Neurosurg. 2017;97:603-34.e8.
9. Moniz E. Tentatives Operatoires dans le Traitement de Certaines Psychoses. Paris: Masson; 1936.
10. Robison RA, Taghva A, Liu CY, et al. Surgery of the mind, mood, and conscious state: an idea in evolution. World Neurosurg. 2013;80:S2-S26.
11. Gross D, Schäfer G. Egas Moniz (1874–1955) and the "invention" of modern psychosurgery: a historical and ethical reanalysis under special consideration of Portuguese original sources. Neurosurg Focus. 2011;30(2):E8.
12. Hoffman JL. Clinical observations concerning schizophrenic patients treated by prefrontal leukotomy. N Engl J Med. 1949;241:233-6.
13. MacLean PD. Psychosomatic disease and the "visceral brain". Recent developments bearing on the Papez theory of emotion. Psychosom Med. 1949;11:338-53.
14. Papez JW. A proposed mechanism of emotion. Arch Neurol Psychiatry. 1937;38:725-43.
15. Spiegel EA, Wycis HT, Marks M, et al. Stereotaxic Apparatus for Operations on the Human Brain. Science. 1947;106:349-50.
16. Knight G. Stereotactic tractotomy in the surgical treatment of mental illness. J Neurol Neurosurg Psychiatry. 1965;28:304-10.
17. Leksell L. A stereotaxic apparatus for intracerebral surgery. Acta Chir Scand. 1949;99:229-33.
18. Talairach J, Hecaen H, David M. Lobotomie prefrontale limitee par electrocoagulation des fibres thalamo- frontalis leur emergence du bras anterior de la capsule interne, in Proceedings of the 4th Congress Neurologique Internationale. Paris: Masson; 1949. p. 141.
19. Valenstein ES. Brain stimulation and behaviour control. Nebr Symp Motiv. 1975;22:251-92.
20. Doshi PK. Neurosurgery for psychiatric disorders. Neurol India. 2017;65:777-8.
21. Nuttin B, Cosyns P, Demeulemeester H, et al. Electrical stimulation in anterior limbs of internal capsules in patients with obsessive-compulsive disorder. Lancet. 1999;354:1526.
22. Bridges P. Psychosurgery revisited. J Neuropsychiatry Clin Neurosci. 1990;2:326-31.
23. O'Doherty M, Bridges PK. Contemporary psychosurgery: indications, outcome and the Irish experience. Ir J Psychol Med. 1998;15:119-23.
24. Poynton AM. Current state of psychosurgery. Br J Hosp Med. 1993;50:408-11.
25. Lapidus KAB, Kopell BH, Ben-Haim S, et al. History of psychosurgery: a psychiatrist's perspective. World Neurosurg. 2013;80:S27.e1-S27.e16.
26. Nuttin B, Wu H, Mayberg H, et al. Consensus on guidelines for stereotactic neurosurgery for psychiatric disorders. J Neurol Neurosurg Psychiatry. 2014;85:1003-8.

27. Ministry of Law and Justice (2017). The Mental Healthcare Act, 2017. [online] Available from http://prsindia.org/uploads/media/Mental%20Health/Mental%20Healthcare%20Act,%202017.pdf. [Last accessed December, 2019].
28. Volpini M, Giacobbe P, Cosgrove GR, et al. The History and Future of Ablative Neurosurgery for Major Depressive Disorder. Stereotact Funct Neurosurg. 2017;95:216-28.
29. Malhi GS, Bartlett JR. A new lesion for the psychosurgical operation of stereotactic subcaudate tractotomy (SST). Br J Neurosurg. 1998;12:335-9.
30. Kelly D, Mitchell-Heggs N. Stereotactic limbic leucotomy—a follow-up study of thirty patients. Postgrad Med J. 1973;49:865-82.
31. Mitchell-Heggs N, Kelly D, Richardson A. Stereotactic limbic leucotomy—a follow-up at 16 months. Br J Psychiatry. 1976;128:226-40.
32. Ruck C, Karlsson A, Steele JD, et al. Capsulotomy for obsessive compulsive disorder: long-term follow-up of 25 patients. Arch Gen Psychiatry. 2008;65:914-21.
33. Lopes AC, Greenberg BD, Canteras MM, et al. Gamma ventral capsulotomy for obsessive- compulsive disorder: a randomized clinical trial. JAMA Psychiatry. 2014;71:1066-76.
34. Martin E, Jeanmonod D, Morel A, et al. High-intensity focused ultrasound for noninvasive functional neurosurgery. Ann Neurol. 2009;66:858-61.
35. Jung HH, Kim SJ, Roh D, et al. Bilateral thermal capsulotomy with MR-guided focused ultrasound for patients with treatment refractory obsessive-compulsive disorder: a proof-of-concept study. Mol Psychiatry. 2015;20:1205-11.
36. Kondziolka D, Ong JG, Lee JY, et al. Gamma knife thalamotomy for essential tremor. J Neurosurg. 2008;108:111-7.
37. Lipsman N, Mainprize TG, Schwartz ML, et al. Intracranial applications of magnetic resonance-guided focused ultrasound. Neurotherapeutics. 2014;11:593-605.
38. Doshi PK. Surgical treatment of obsessive compulsive disorder: current status. Indian J Psychiatry. 2009;51(3):216-21.
39. Nuttin BJ, Gabriëls LA, Cosyns PR, et al. Long-term electrical capsular stimulation in patients with obsessive-compulsive disorder. Neurosurgery. 2003;52:1263-72
40. Tsai HC, Chang CH, Pan JI, et al. Acute stimulation effect of the ventral capsule/ventral striatum in patients with refractory obsessive-compulsive disorder—a double-blinded trial. Neuropsychiatr Dis Treat. 2014;10:63-9.
41. Goodman WK, Alterman RL. Deep brain stimulation for intractable psychiatric disorders. Annu Rev Med. 2012;63:511-24.
42. Bewernick BH, Hurlemann R, Matusch A, et al. Nucleus accumbens deep brain stimulation decreases ratings of depression and anxiety in treatment-resistant depression. Biol Psychiatry. 2010;67:110-6.
43. Malone DA Jr, Dougherty DD, Rezai AR, et al. Deep brain stimulation of the ventral capsule/ventral striatum for treatment-resistant depression. Biol Psychiatry. 2009;65:267-75.
44. Kennedy SH, Giacobbe P, Rizvi SJ, et al. Deep brain stimulation for treatment-resistant depression: Follow-up after 3 to 6 years. Am J Psychiatry. 2011;168:502-10.

45. Ackermans L, Duits A, van der Linden C, et al. Double-blind clinical trial of thalamic stimulation in patients with Tourette syndrome. Brain. 2011;134:832-44.
46. Sachdev PS, Mohan A, Cannon E, et al. Deep brain stimulation of the anteromedial globus pallidus interna for Tourette syndrome. PLoS One. 2014;9:e104926.
47. Sani S, Jobe K, Smith A, et al. Deep brain stimulation for treatment of obesity in rats. J Neurosurg. 2007;107:809-13.
48. Lipsman N, Woodside DB, Giacobbe P, et al. Subcallosal cingulate deep brain stimulation for treatment-refractory anorexia nervosa: a phase 1 pilot trial. Lancet. 2013;381:1361-70.
49. Wu H, Van Dyck-Lippens PJ, Santegoeds R, et al. Deep-brain stimulation for anorexia nervosa. World Neurosurg. 2013;80:S29.e1-10.
50. Stelten BM, Noblesse LH, Ackermans L, et al. The neurosurgical treatment of addiction. Neurosurg Focus. 2008;25:E5.
51. Koek RJ, Langevin JP, Krahl SE, et al. Deep brain stimulation of the basolateral amygdala for treatment-refractory combat post-traumatic stress disorder (PTSD): Study protocol for a pilot randomized controlled trial with blinded, staggered onset of stimulation. Trials. 2014;15:356.
52. Stein DJ. Obsessive-compulsive disorder. Lancet. 2002;360:397-405.
53. Khanna S, Gururaj G, Sriram TG. Epidemiology of the obsessive-compulsive disorder in India presented at the first international obsessive-compulsive disorder congress. Capri; 1993.
54. Rauch SL, Jenike MA. Neurobiological models of obsessive-compulsive disorder. Psychosomatics. 1993;34:20-32.
55. Saxena S, Brody AL, Schwartz JM, et al. Neuroimaging and frontal subcortical circuitry in obsessive-compulsive disorder. Br J Psychiatry. 1998;172:26-37.
56. Janardhan Reddy YC, Sundar AS, Narayanaswamy JC, et al. Clinical practice guidelines for obsessive-compulsive disorder. Indian J Psychiatry. 2017;59(Suppl 1):S74-90.
57. D'Astous M, Cottin S, Roy M, et al. Bilateral stereotactic anterior capsulotomy for obsessive-compulsive disorder: long-term follow-up. J Neurol Neurosurg Psychiatry. 2013;84:1208-13.
58. Greenberg BD, Gabriels LA, Malone DA Jr, et al. Deep brain stimulation of the ventral internal capsule/ventral striatum for obsessive-compulsive disorder: worldwide experience. Mole Psychiatry. 2010;15(1):64-79.
59. Luyten L, Hendrickx S, Raymaekers S, et al. Electrical stimulation in the bed nucleus of the stria terminalis alleviates severe obsessive-compulsive disorder. Mol Psychiatry. 2016;21:1272-80.
60. Bourne SK, Sheth SA, Neal J, et al. Beneficial effect of subsequent lesion procedures after nonresponse of initial cingulotomy for severe treatment refractory obsessive compulsive disorder. Neurosurgery. 2013;72:196-202.
61. Denys D, Mantione M, Figee M, et al. Deep brain stimulation of the nucleus accumbens for treatment-refractory obsessive-compulsive disorder. Arch Gen Psychiatry. 2010;67:1061-8.
62. Malhi GS, Sachdev P. Novel physical treatments for the management of neuropsychiatric disorders. J Psychosom Res. 2000;53:709-19.

63. Lippitz BE, Mindus P, Meyerson BA, et al. Lesion topography and outcome after thermocapsulotomy or gamma knife capsulotomy for obsessive-compulsive disorder: Relevance of the right hemisphere. Neurosurgery. 1999;44:452-60.
64. Kopell BH, Greenberg B, Rezai AR. Deep brain stimulation for psychiatric disorders. J Clin Neurophysiol. 2004;21(1):51-67.
65. Lipsman N, Neimat JS, Lozano AM. Deep brain stimulation for treatment-refractory obsessive-compulsive disorder: the search for a valid target. Neurosurgery. 2007;61(1):1-11.
66. Baer L, Rauch SL, Ballantine HT Jr, et al. Cingulotomy for intractable obsessive-compulsive disorder: Prospective long-term follow-up of 18 patients. Arch Gen Psychiatry. 1995;52:384-92.
67. Spangler WJ, Cosgrove GR, Ballantine HT Jr, et al. Magnetic resonance image-guided stereotactic cingulotomy for intractable psychiatric disease. Neurosurgery. 1996;38:1071-6.
68. Dougherty DD, Baer L, Cogrove GR, et al. Prospective long- term follow-up of 44 patients who received cingulotomy for treatment refractory obsessive-compulsive disorder. Am J Psychiatry. 2002;15:269-75.
69. Oliver B, Gascón J, Aparicio A, et al. Bilateral anterior capsulotomy for refractory obsessive-compulsive disorders. Stereotac Function Neurosurg. 2003;81(1-4):90-5.
70. Liu K, Zhang H, Liu C, et al. Stereotactic treatment of refractory obsessive compulsive disorder by bilateral capsulotomy with 3 years follow-up. J Clin Neurosci. 2008;15(6):622-9.
71. Mindus P, Jenike MA. Neurosurgical treatment of malignant obsessive compulsive disorder. Psychiatr Clin North Am. 1992;15:921-38.
72. Bridges PK, Bartlett JR, Hale AS, et al. Psychosurgery: stereotactic subcaudate tractomy. An indispensable treatment. Br J Psychiatry. 1994;165:599-613.
73. Hodgkiss AD, Malizia AL, Bartlett JR, et al. Outcome after the psychosurgical operation of stereotactic subcaudate tractotomy, 1979–1991. J Neuropsychiatry Clin Neurosci. 1995;7:230-4.
74. Binder DK, Iskandar BJ, Kelly PJ. Modern neurosurgery for psychiatric disorders. Neurosurgery. 2000;47:9-23.
75. Kelly D, Richardson A, Mitchell-Heggs N. Stereotactic limbic leucotomy: neurophysiological aspects and operative technique. Br J Psychiatry. 1973;123:133-40.
76. Montoya A, Weiss AP, Price BH, et al. Magnetic resonance imaging-guided stereotactic limbic leukotomy for treatment of intractable psychiatric disease. Neurosurgery. 2002;50:1043-52.
77. Hay P, Sachdev P, Cumming S, et al. Treatment of obsessive-compulsive disorder by psychosurgery. Acta Psychiatr Scand. 1993;87:197-207.
78. Naesström M, Blomstedt p, Bodlund O. A systematic review of psychiatric indications for deep brain stimulation, with focus on major depressive and obsessive-compulsive disorder. Nord J Psychiatry. 2016;70:483-91.
79. Mallet L, Polosan M, Jaafari N, et al. Subthalamic nucleus stimulation in severe obsessive-compulsive disorder. N Engl J Med. 2008;359:2121-34.
80. Doshi PK. Mania induced by stimulation following DBS of the Bed Nucleus of Stria Terminalis for obsessive compulsive disorder. Stereotact Funct Neurosurg. 2016;94:326.

81. https://www.psychiatrictimes.com/obsessive-compulsive-disorder/deep-brain-stimulation-surgery-ocd-safety-efficacyand-financial-incentivesc.
82. Rush AJ, Trivedi MH, Wisniewski SR, et al. Acute and longer-term outcomes in depressed outpatients requiring one or several treatment steps: A STAR*D report. Am J Psychiatry. 2006;163:1905-17.
83. Rush AJ. STAR*D: what have we learned? Am J Psychiatry. 2007;164:201-4.
84. Shah DB, Pesiridou A, Baltuch GH, et al. Functional neurosurgery in the treatment of severe obsessive compulsive disorder and major depression: overview of disease circuits and therapeutic targeting for the clinician. Psychiatry (Edgmont). 2008;5(9):24-33.
85. Panksepp J. Textbook of Biological Psychiatry. Hoboken, NJ: Wiley-Liss, Inc.; 2004.
86. Doshi PK, Arumugham SS, Bhide A, et al. Indian guidelines on neurosurgical interventions in psychiatric disorders. Indian J Psychiatry. 2019;61(1):13-21.
87. Shields DC, Asaad W, Eskandar EN, et al. Prospective assessment of stereotactic ablative surgery for intractable major depression. Biol Psychiatry. 2008;64:449-54.
88. Steele JD, Christmas D, Eljamel MS, et al. Anterior cingulotomy for major depression: clinical outcome and relationship to lesion characteristics. Biol Psychiatry. 2008;63:670-7.
89. Christmas D, Eljamel MS, Butler S, et al. Long term outcome of thermal anterior capsulotomy for chronic, treatment refractory depression. J Neurol Neurosurg Psychiatry. 2011;82:594-600.
90. Riestra AR, Aguilar J, Zambito G, et al. Unilateral right anterior capsulotomy for refractory major depression with comorbid obsessive-compulsive disorder. Neurocase. 2011;17:491-500.
91. Hurwitz TA, Honey CR, Allen J, et al. Bilateral anterior capsulotomy for intractable depression. J Neuropsychiatry Clin Neurosci. 2012;24:176-82.
92. Ballantine HT Jr, Cassidy WL, Flanagan NB, et al. Stereotaxic anterior cingulotomy for neuropsychiatric illness and intractable pain. J Neurosurg. 1967;26:488-95.
93. Ballantine HT Jr, Bouckoms AJ, Thomas EK, et al. Treatment of psychiatric illness by stereotactic cingulotomy. Biol Psychiatry. 1987;22:807-19.
94. Kim MC, Lee TK, Choi CR. Review of long-term results of stereotactic psychosurgery. Neurol Med Chir (Tokyo). 2002;42:365-71.
95. Holtzheimer PE, Husain MM, Lisanby SH, et al. Subcallosal cingulate deep brain stimulation for treatment-resistant depression: a multisite, randomised, sham-controlled trial. Lancet Psychiatry. 2017;4(11):839-49.
96. Dougherty DD, Rezai AR, Carpenter LL, et al. A randomized sham-controlled trial of deep brain stimulation of the ventral capsule/ventral striatum for chronic treatment-resistant depression. Biological psychiatry. 2015;78(4):240-8.
97. Lozano AM, Giacobbe P, Hamani C, et al. A multicenter pilot study of subcallosal cingulate area deep brain stimulation for treatment-resistant depression. J Neurosurg. 2012;116:315-22.
98. Puigdemont D, Portella M, Perez-Egea R, et al. A randomized double-blind crossover trial of deep brain stimulation of the subcallosal cingulate gyrus in patients with treatment-resistant depression: a pilot study of relapse prevention. J Psychiatry Neurosci. 2015;40(4):224-31.

99. Bergfeld IO, Mantione M, Hoogendoorn ML, et al. Deep Brain Stimulation of the Ventral Anterior Limb of the Internal Capsule for Treatment-Resistant Depression: A Randomized Clinical Trial. JAMA Psychiatry. 2016;73(5):456-64.
100. Schlaepfer TE, Bewernick BH, Kayser S, et al. Rapid effects of deep brain stimulation for treatment-resistant major depression. Biol Psychiatry. 2013;73: 1204-12.
101. Jimenez F, Velasco F, Salin-Pascual R, et al. A patient with a resistant major depression disorder treated with deep brain stimulation in the inferior thalamic peduncle. Neurosurgery. 2005;57:585-93.
102. Sartorius A, Kiening KL, Kirsch P, et al. Remission of major depression under deep brain stimulation of the lateral habenula in a therapy-refractory patient. Biol Psychiatry. 2010;67:9-11.
103. Viswanathan A, Jimenez-Shahed J, Carvallo JFB, et al. Deep brain stimulation for Tourette syndrome: target selection. Stereotact Funct Neurosurg. 2012;90: 213-24.
104. Jankovic J. Treatment of hyperkinetic movement disorders. Lancet Neurol. 2009;8:844-56.
105. Cheung MY, Shahed J, Jankovic J. Malignant Tourette syndrome. Mov Disord. 2007;22:1743-50.
106. Mink JW. Basal ganglia dysfunction in Tourette's syndrome: a new hypothesis. Pediatr Neurol. 2001;25:190-8.
107. Albin RL, Mink JW. Recent advances in Tourette syndrome research. Trends Neurosci. 2006;29:175-82.
108. Schrock LE, Mink JW, Woods DW, et al. Tourette syndrome deep brain stimulation: a review and updated recommendations. Mov Disord. 2015;30(4):448-71.
109. Visser-Vandewalle V, Temel Y, Boon P, et al. Chronic bilateral thalamic stimulation: a new therapeutic approach in intractable Tourette syndrome. J Neurosurg. 2003;99:1094-100.
110. Maciunas RJ, Maddux BN, Riley DE, et al. Prospective randomized double-blind trial of bilateral thalamic deep brain stimulation in adults with Tourette syndrome. J Neurosurg. 2007;107:1004-14.
111. Porta M, Brambilla A, Cavanna AE, et al. Thalamic deep brain stimulation for treatment-refractory Tourette syndrome: two-year outcome. Neurology. 2009;73:1375-80.
112. Savica R, Stead M, Mack KJ, et al. Deep brain stimulation in Tourette syndrome: a description of 3 patients with excellent outcome. Mayo Clin Proc. 2012;87:59-62.
113. Diederich NJ, Kalteis K, Stamenkovic M, et al. Efficient internal pallidal stimulation in Gilles de la Tourette syndrome: a case report. Mov Disord. 2005;20:1496-520.
114. Shahed J, Poysky J, Kenney C, et al. GPi deep brain stimulation for Tourette syndrome improves tics and psychiatric comorbidities. Neurology. 2007;68: 159-60.
115. Ackermans L, Temel Y, Cath D, et al. Deep brain stimulation in Tourette's syndrome: Two targets? Mov Disord. 2006;21:709-13.
116. Dueck A, Wolters A, Wunsch K, et al. Deep brain stimulation of globus pallidus internus in a 16-year old boy with severe Tourette syndrome and mental retardation. Neuropediatrics. 2009;40:239-42.

117. Welter ML, Mallet L, Houeto JL, et al. Internal pallidal and thalamic stimulation in patients with Tourette syndrome. Acta Neurol. 2008;65:952-7.
118. Martinez-Fernandez R, Zrinzo L, Aviles-Olmos I, et al. Deep brain stimulation for Gilles de la Tourette syndrome: a case series targeting subregions of the globus pallidus internus. Mov Disord. 2011;26:1922-30.
119. Welter ML, Houeto JL, Thobois S, et al. Anterior pallidal deep brain stimulation for Tourette's syndrome: a randomised, double-blind, controlled trial. Lancet Neurol. 2017;16(8):610-9.
120. Filho OV, Ragazzo PC, Silva DJ, et al. Bilateral globus pallidus externus deep brain stimulation for the treatment of Tourette syndrome: an ongoing prospective controlled study. Stereotact Funct Neurosurg. 2007;85:42-3.
121. Martinez-Torres I, Hariz MI, Zrinzo L, et al. Improvement of tics after subthalamic nucleus deep brain stimulation. Neurology. 2009;72:1787-9.
122. Kuhn J, Lenartz D, Mai JK, et al. Deep brain stimulation of the nucleus accumbens and the internal capsule in therapeutically refractory Tourette syndrome. J Neurol. 2007;254:963-5.
123. Neuner I, Podoll K, Lenartz D, et al. Deep brain stimulation in the nucleus accumbens for intractable Tourette's syndrome: follow-up report of 36 months. Biol Psychiatry. 2009;65:e5-e6.
124. Temel Y, Vandewalle V. Surgery in Tourette syndrome. Mov Disord. 2004;19:3-14.
125. Martinez-Ramirez D, Jimenez-Shahed J, Leckman JF, et al. Efficacy and safety of deep brain stimulation in tourette syndrome: the International Tourette Syndrome Deep Brain Stimulation Public Database and Registry. JAMA Neurol. 2018;75(3):353-9.
126. Whiting DM, Tomycz ND, Bailes J, et al. Lateral hypothalamic area deep brain stimulation for refractory obesity: A pilot study with preliminary data on safety, body weight, and energy metabolism. J Neurosurg. 2013;119:56-63.
127. Le Moal M, Koob GF. Drug addiction: pathways to the disease and pathophysiological perspectives. Eur Neuropsychopharmacol 2007;17:377-93.
128. Müller UJ, Sturm V, Voges J, et al. Successful treatment of chronic resistant alcoholism by deep brain stimulation of nucleus accumbens: First experience with three cases. Pharmacopsychiatry. 2009;42:288-91.
129. Langevin JP, Chen JW, Koek RJ, et al. Deep brain stimulation of the basolateral amygdala: targeting technique and electrodiagnostic findings. Brain Sci. 2016;6:E28.
130. Pepper J, Hariz M, Zrinzo L. Deep brain stimulation versus anterior capsulotomy for obsessive- compulsive disorder: a review of the literature. J Neurosurg. 2015;122:1028-37.
131. Doshi PK. Anterior capsulotomy for refractory OCD: First case as per the core group guidelines. Indian J Psychiatry. 2011;53(3):270-3.
132. Doshi PK, Ramdasi R, Thorve S. Deep brain stimulation of anteromedial globus pallidus internus for severe Tourette syndrome. Indian J Psychiatry. 2018;60(1):138-40.

Index

Page numbers followed by *b* refer to box, *f* refer to figure,
fc refer to flowchart, and *t* refer to table.

A

Ablation 237
Ablative procedures 229, 235
Abnormal involuntary movements scale 71, 74
Acetylcholine 202
Acetylcholinesterase
   enzyme 172
   inhibitors 170, 172
Acyclovir 75
   dose of 70
   treatment 70
Addiction 147, 149, 237
Adjunctive valacyclovir 73
Adjuvant antiviral agents, clinical trials of 71*t*
Akathisia 28
Alcohol
   abuse 171
   intolerance 200
   use disorders 114, 117
Alzheimer's dementia 205
Alzheimer's disease 169, 170
   early-stage 31
American Academy of Child and Adolescent Psychiatry 115
American Psychiatric Association 134
   guideline 110, 156, 158
American Psychological Association 158
Aminothiazole 174
Amnestic mild cognitive impairment 174
Amobarbital 53, 54
Ampakines 128
Amphetamines 128
Amygdala, basolateral nucleus of 237
Amyloid deposition 174*t*
   modulation of 173
Amyotrophic lateral sclerosis 205
Angelman syndrome 192
Anorexia nervosa 237
Anti-amyloid aggregation agents 174
Antidepressants 5, 113, 128, 155, 157, 159, 164
   molecules 160
   tricyclic 110, 113, 117, 156
Antioxidant drugs 170, 174
Antipsychotic 29, 61, 102, 110, 192
   atypical 156, 192
   drugs 63, 69
Antiviral agents, effect of 72
Antiviral therapy 69
Anxiety 15, 200
   disorders 44, 113, 135, 203

neurosis 53
   related disorders 23
Aripiprazole 192
Arrhythmias 15
Artificial intelligence 6, 9, 12
   based therapies 8
   personalized treatment 11
   requirements of 8
   types of 9
Assertive community treatment 82, 86
Asthma 15
Attention deficit hyperactivity disorder 10, 19, 115, 117, 124
Attenuated positive symptom syndrome 87
Auditory hallucinations 65
Auditory verbal hallucinations 215
   psychological interventions for 64*b*
Autism spectrum disorder 10, 189, 192, 193, 205
Autoimmune neuropsychiatric disorders, pediatric 205
Autonomic nervous system 32
Avatar therapy 64, 65, 81, 89

B

Bacillus 202
Bacopa monniera 136
Bacteria 202
Bad breath 200
Barbiturates 48, 49, 50, 53, 54
Barnes akathisia scale 71
Basal ganglia 228
Beck depression inventory 24, 227
Benzodiazepine 41, 48-50, 54, 57, 58, 102, 113
   assisted psychotherapy 50
Beta-N-methylamino-l-alanine 205
Bhastrika pranayama 26
Bhujangasana 26
Bifidobacterium 202, 205
   animalis 204
   infantis 206
   longum 203
Biofeedback
   recent advances in 16
   therapy, recent advances in 14
Bipolar depression 112, 112*t*
Bipolar disorder 43, 111, 116, 171, 190-192
Bleeding 3
Bloating 200
Blood
   brain barrier 203

hemoglobin concentrations 19
oxygen level dependent 17
Bloodletting 4
Body mass index 237
Body odors 200
Bonferroni corrections 75
Borderline personality disorder 53
Brain
   activity 17
   contrast-enhanced computed
      tomography of 228
   derived neurotrophic factor synthesis
      148, 163, 203
   functions of 6
   gut
      axis 144
      connection 201
   heart axis 144
   magnetic resonance imaging of 228
   scans 6
   stimulation 212
      technique 219
      therapies 3, 212
   waves 14, 16
British Association of Psychopharmacology
      guidelines 157, 158
Bupropion 112, 156
B-vitamins, synthesis of 200

C

Canadian Network for Mood and Anxiety
      Treatment 157, 158
Candida 200
Canmat guidelines 158
Capsulotomy 230
   anterior 229
Cardiovascular disorders 15, 134
Catatonia 54, 55
Catechol-O-methyltransferase 132
Cathartic abreaction 49
Central nervous system 135, 199, 202
Cerebrolysin 174
Childhood autism rating scale scores 194
Chlorpromazine 5, 61, 192
Cholinesterase inhibitors 115, 128
Chronic depression
   drug treatment of 155
   management of 159
Chronic obstructive pulmonary disease 15
Chronic pain syndromes 10
Cingulate cortex, anterior 229, 232
Cingulate gyrus, anterior 228
Cingulotomy 229, 230
   anterior 232
   procedure 230

Circulating proinflammatory cytokines, high
      levels of 203
Clinical global impression severity 30
Clozapine 63, 66, 111, 192
Cocaine 123
Cognitive behavior therapy 5, 12, 39, 40, 64,
      81-83, 87b, 103, 146, 227
   model of 84fc
   role of 88b
Cognitive disorders 23
   minor 203
Cognitive dysfunction 72, 75
Cognitive enhancement therapy 85
Cognitive enhancers, current status of 169
Cognitive impairment, diagnosis of mild 31
Cognitive realignment therapy 88
Cognitive remediation 81, 82, 85
   intervention 85
   therapy 85, 91
      computer-assisted 90
Cold sores 72
Collapsin response mediator protein-2 192
Colostrinin 174
Combinatorial gene testing 181
Committee on Research on Psychiatric
      Treatments of American
      Psychiatric Association 134
Communication skills 83
Computerized neurocognitive battery 74
Computer-web-based programs 90
Conducting group therapy 93
Consciousness 144
Constipation 200
   chronic 16
Continuous positive airway pressure
      therapy 146
Conversion disorder 55
   treatment for 56
Cortico-striato-thalamo-cortical loop 228
Cosmetic
   medications 128
   psychopharmacology 123, 124
Coumarin-Huperzine derivatives 172
Cravings, treatment of 102
Crisis management 83, 100
Crooked cells 6
Cybernetics theory 14
Cytokines 203
Cytomegalovirus 71, 72

D

Data search methodology 156
Deep brain stimulation 212, 219, 224, 230,
      232, 234, 236, 238
Dehydroepiandrosterone sulfate 25

Delusions 62t
  assessment of 62
  scales for 62
Dementia 117
Deoxyribonucleic acid 178
Dephosphorylation 162
Depression 19, 23, 30, 33, 42, 58, 110, 116, 117, 148, 155, 159, 169, 191, 200, 205, 227, 231, 234
  chronic major 155
  indications for surgery in 232
  long-term 213
  major 171
  severity of 157
  study, treatment for adolescents with 42
  treatment-resistant 117, 162, 233
Depressive disorder 134, 155
  neurobiology of major 231
Detoxification 114
Dexamethasone nonsuppression 202
Dhanurasana 26
Dialectical behavior therapy 103
Diarrhea 159, 200
Diazepam 49, 50, 54
Disability
  adjusted life years 155
  years lived with 155
Disease-modifying agents 170, 173
Dissociative disorder 55, 57
Distress tolerance 104
Docosahexaenoic acid 134
Donepezil 170-172
Dopamine 202, 203
  D_2 receptor 163
  lower levels of 204
Dorsolateral prefrontal cortex 213
Dysbiosis 200
  symptoms of 200t
Dysfunctional coping modes 106
Dysfunctional parent modes 106
Dystonia 28

E

Eczema 200
Eicosapentaenoic acid 134
Electrical stimulation, chronic 230
Electrocardiogram 15
Electroconvulsive therapy 3, 20, 65, 91, 156, 224, 232
Electrodermal activity 15
Electrodes, placement of 20
Electroencephalograph 16, 17
  quantitative 16
Electromyogram 15
Encephalitis 72

Endophenotypes 5
Enteric nervous system 200
Enterococcus 202
Enzyme acetylcholinesterase 170
Epigenetics 179
Episode
  medication 73
  psychosis, nonpharmacological therapies in first 87
Epstein-Barr virus 71
  infection 70
Equipment, types of 15
Escherichia 202
Euphoria 6
European Medicines Agency 170
Exercise 148, 149
External reward, role of 18

F

Facial emotion recognition deficits 26
Facial expression 12
Factitious disorder 55
Fatigue 133, 200
Federal Health Agency of Germany and British Herbal Compendium 136
Fetal stem cell 193
  transplantation 193
Ficus platyphylla 136
First episode psychosis 88
Flumazenil 114
Fluoxetine 112, 128
Food and Drug Administration 170, 181, 213, 224
Forward-backward bending 26
Fragile X syndrome 192
Free radicals 204
Frequent colds 200
Frequent urination 200

G

Gabapentin 112
Galantamine 115, 170-172
Gamma knife radiation surgery 227
Gamma-amino butyric acid 32, 132, 171, 202
Gas 200
Gastrointestinal bleeds 159
Gastrointestinal function 14
Gastrointestinal system 200
Gastrointestinal upset 133
Generation antidepressants 156
GeneSight psychotropic test 183, 185
Gestures 12
Ginkgo biloba 128, 137, 174
Glutamate 203
  system 163
Granulocyte-colony stimulating factor 193

H

Habenula, lateral 234
Hallucinations 62*t*
  assessment of 62
  focused integrative treatment 64
  scales for 62
  treatment strategies for 62
Hallucinogenic substances 48
Haloperidol 111, 192
Hamilton anxiety rating scale 227
Hamilton depression rating scale 30, 157, 227, 232, 234
Hand stretch breathing 26
Hatha yoga 24
  effect of 30
Headache 15, 230
Healing hand 2
Health, management of 144
Heart rate 14, 15
Hemoencephalography 19
Heroin 123
Herpes simplex virus 71, 72, 75
Histocompatibility complexes, major 73
Human deoxyribonucleic acid 70
Human erythropoietin 128
Human genome project 201
Human immunodeficiency virus 69
Human intelligence 6, 8, 13
Human microbiome 205
Human studies 149
Humanitarian movement 4
Hypericum perforatum 132
Hypersomnia 200
Hypertension 15
Hyponatremia 159
Hypothalamic-pituitary-adrenal axis 32, 202
Hypothalamus, lateral 237

I

Ibogaine 49
Iliac spine, anterior superior 193
Illnesses, psychological model of 37
Imipramine 112
Immunization
  active 174
  passive 174
Immunoglobulin
  G 72
  M 72
Immunotherapy 174
Impulse control, loss of 97
Inadequate sphincter control 230
Indian Psychiatric Society 226
  treatment guidelines 116*t*
Indian Scale for Assessment of Autism Scores 193
Indian Society of Stereotactic and Functional Neurosurgery 226
Individual-gene testing
  advantages of 182
  disadvantages of 182
Inflammation, chronic 203
Information and communication
  technology 89
  use of 89
Initial randomized controlled studies 25
Injectable antipsychotics, long-acting 63
Inositol 112
Insane 4
Insomnia 146, 200
Insulin-like growth factor 128, 146
Intelligent agents, design of 9
Intermittent psychotic symptom syndrome 87
Internal capsule, anterior limb of 234
International Electroencephalogram 10-20 System 217
International personality disorder examination 99
International Yoga Day 23
Intracerebral hemorrhage 233
Intravenous amobarbital 56
Invasive brain stimulation techniques 218
Irrational polypharmacy, reduction of 115*b*
Irritable bowel syndrome, management of 206
Itching 200

J

Jogging 26
Joint aches 200

K

Ketamine 49, 53-55, 162
Knowledge, power of 2

L

Lactobacillus 202, 205
  bulgaricus 204
  helveticus 203
  rhamnosus 204
Lactococcus lactis 204
Lamotrigine 112
Laziness 230
Levomilnacipran 161
Limbic leucotomy 229, 230, 233
Limbic system 201
Lipopolysaccharides 204
Lipoprotein, high-density 144
Lithium 112, 156, 192

Live microorganisms 199
Lorazepam 49, 50, 54
L-thyroxine 112
Lunatic asylums 6
Lysergic acid diethylamide 49, 51, 54, 57, 123

M

Magnetic resonance-guided focused ultrasound 227
Major depressive disorder 10, 25, 110, 155, 158t, 184, 224, 232, 232b
    ablative procedures for 232
Makarasana 26
Mammals, microbial colonization of 199
Mania 111
Maprotiline 156
Matsyasana 26
Maudsley guidelines 158
Median forebrain bundle 232
Memantine 172, 175
Memory, poor 200
Menstrual disorders 32
Mental derangements 2
Mental disorders 3, 37, 38, 98
    severe 25, 102
    statistical manual of 98
    treatment of 6
Mental faculties 1
Mental health 7, 8, 144
    disorders 138
    psychobiotic therapy for 6
    rejuvenation of 7
    review board 226
Mental Healthcare Act 226
Mental illness 3, 4
    active 100
    interventions for 5
    medical model of 37
    treatment of 37
Mental operations 6
Mental state 87
Mental tasks 6
Mentalization based therapy 104
Metabolic syndrome 145
Metabotropic glutamate 163
Metacognitive
    therapy 64
    training 84
Methylene blue 173
Methylenedioxymethamphetamine 54, 123
Methylphenidate 56, 110, 128
Mianserin 156
Microbiome, potential role of 201
Midazolam 49, 50
Milieu therapy 89

Mindfulness
    based interventions 65
    based therapy 64
Mirtazapine 156
Modafinil 112, 128
Modified rush video rating scale 227
Monoamine oxidase 117
    inhibitors 110, 159
Monoclonal antibodies 174
Mononuclear cells 193
Montgomery-Asberg depression rating scale 160, 227
Mood 146
    altering agents 128
    disorders 132, 134, 157
    stabilizer 102, 111
    swings 200
Multiple gene testing 182
    advantages of 182
    disadvantages of 182
Muscle 200
Musculoskeletal activity 14
Mycobacterium vaccae 206

N

N-acetylcysteine 112, 136
Nadanusandhana 26
Nadi Shuddhi Pranayama 26
Naloxone 114
Narcosuggestion 54
Natural language processing 10
Natural nootropics 170, 174
N-dimethyltryptamine 51
Near-infrared spectrography 16, 19
Neural circuitry 38
Neural progenitor cells 190
Neurocognitive enhancement therapy 85
Neurodevelopmental diseases 12
Neurofeedback 16, 20
    connectivity-based 18
    in disorders, use of 19
Neurogenesis 150
Neuroimaging biomarkers 10
Neuroinflammation 204
Neuroinflammatory hypothesis 203
Neuromodulation 204
    field of 212
    Society 226
Neuronal cells, types of 190
Neuropeptide
    agonists 128
    antagonists 128
Neuroplasticity 32
Neuropsychiatric disorders 212, 224
    recognition of emotions in 26
    scope of surgery in 226
    treatment of 49

Neurotherapy 16
Neurotic reactions 56
Neurotransmitter 93
	functioning of 37
	synthesis of 202
	systems 171
Newer theories 5
N-methyl D-aspartate 162, 205
	receptors antagonists 170, 172
Noninvasive brain stimulation 62
	techniques 65, 212, 213
Nonmentalizing modes 105
Nonpharmacological biological therapies 91
Nonpharmacological therapies 82*t*
	principles of 81
Nonpsychiatric population 73
Nonsteroidal anti-inflammatory drugs 117, 163
Norepinephrine 202
Nucleus accumbens 229, 232
Nutraceuticals 131
Nutrition 131

O

Obesity 144, 145, 237
Obsessive-compulsive disorder 10, 113, 133, 205, 215, 224, 228, 229*b*, 230
	indications for surgery in 228
	pathophysiology of 228
Obstructive sleep apnea 145
Olanzapine 111, 112
Omega-3 fatty acids 112, 134
Online counseling 90
Opioid use disorders 114, 117
Oral medication 63
Orbitofrontal cortex 215, 228
Organic delirium 55
Organic mutism 55
Organophosphorus compounds 170
Oryza sativa 201
Outpatient psychiatrist 100
Oxoisoaporphine 172

P

Pains 200
Palpitations 200
Panic disorder 113
Parkinson's disease 224
Paroxetine 112
Passiflora incarnata 136
Patient-therapist interaction 5
Persistent depression, management of 159
Persistent depressive disorder 159
Personal purity 3

Personality
	assessment schedule 99
	diagnostic questionnaire 99
	resist drug therapy 102
	standardized assessment of 99
Personality disorder 20, 97, 101*b*, 106, 107
	assessment of 98, 99
	classification 98
	development of 103
	diagnosis of 99
	interventions for 97
	management of 98, 100
	medication management 102
Pesticides 170
Pharmaceuticals 131
Pharmacogene, selection of 184
Pharmacogenetics 179, 180*f*
Pharmacogenomics 179, 180*f*, 185
	disadvantages of 183
Pharmacological agents 38
Pharmacotherapy 20, 63, 224, 227
	intervention 44
Phelan McDermid syndrome 192
Phenotype-behavior 5
Photodermatitis 133
Physical health 144
Physical pain 126
Physiological function 14
Piper methysticum 135
Placebo-controlled study 134
Pluripotent cells 6
Pluripotent stem cell 189
Pneumograph 15
Polypharmacy 109, 114
	debate 109
	rationalization of 115
Poor metabolizer 181
Positive and negative syndrome scale 26, 62
Positive placebo-controlled randomized controlled trials 112
Post-traumatic stress disorder 18, 40, 103, 113, 237
Posture 12
Potassium levels 192
Potent psychoactive substance 52
Potentiation, long-term 213
Pranayama 31
Preparatory psychotherapy 52
Probiotics 199
Prodrome 87
Promote neurotrophic growth 203
Prophylaxis 112
Propranolol 128
Pseudocholinesterase 178
Psilocybin 49, 51, 53-55
Psoriasis 200

Psychedelic 49, 50, 52, 54, 55
  mushrooms 49
  psychotherapy 52
Psychiatric classificatory systems 109
Psychiatric diagnosis 9
  artificial intelligence in 9
Psychiatric disorder 38, 58, 109, 127, 144, 189, 212, 213, 217
  chronic 169
  major 24
  neurosurgery for 224
Psychiatric illnesses 48, 61, 189, 190
  modeling of 190
  symptoms of 48
Psychiatric rating scale 70, 71
Psychiatric therapeutics 2, 6
  advancing frontiers of 2
Psychiatric treatment 39
  artificial intelligence in 11
Psychiatrists, self-care for 107
Psychiatry 8, 23, 178, 189
  artificial intelligence in 9
  literature 57
  nutraceuticals in 131
  pharmacogenomics in 178
  spiritual therapies in 23
Psychobiotic 199, 206, 207
  therapy 199
Psychodynamic model 42
Psychodynamic psychotherapy 4, 89
Psychoeducation 39, 82, 83
Psychogenic amnesia 55
Psychological interventions 64
Psychologically-based disorders 39
Psychometric testing 17
Psychoneurosis 56
Psychopathology 4, 32, 39
Psychopharmacological agents 38
Psychopharmacology 5, 40, 44
  interface of 37
Psychopharmacotherapeutic agents, development of 58
Psychosis 33, 55, 92, 117, 136
  cognitive behavioral therapy for 82, 83
  early 88
    detection 10
  psychotherapies for 82fc
  severity of 102
Psychosocial intervention 44, 87, 88
Psychosocial rehabilitation 39
Psychosocial skills 39
Psychosurgery 238
  history of 224
  legal perspective of 226
  preoperative evaluation for 227

Psychotherapeutic 57
  interventions 37, 41
    stage of 5
Psychotherapy 37, 40, 44, 52, 103, 224
  biological underpinnings of 39
  drug-assisted 49b, 52, 54t, 58
  interface of 37
  interventions 40
  plan 100
  process of drug-assisted 49f
  psychedelic assisted 52, 53, 58
  research evidence for drug-assisted 55
  transference-focused 106
  update on drug-assisted 48
  uses 11
Psychotic disorders 79, 81
  nonpharmacological therapies for 79, 80
Psychotic symptom 102
  rating scale 62
Psychotropic drug 5, 38
  clinical application of 54t
  modeling 192
Purging 3, 4
Pyrazolopyridines 174

Q

Quetiapine 111

R

Randomized controlled
  study 27
  trials 73, 159, 173, 215
Reciprocal emotional response 99
Recovery-oriented treatment 39
Refractory delusions, treatment strategies for 62
Regional cerebral blood flow 213
Rehabilitation back 7
Relapse prevention 83
  program for 42
Repetitive transcranial magnetic stimulation 92, 128, 212
Reptile brain 201
Residual and resistant auditory
  delusions, management for 61
  hallucinations, management for 61
Resistant anxiety disorders, treatment of 113t
Respiratory patterns 14
Restless legs syndrome 147
Rett syndrome 192
Ribonucleic acid 200
Risperidone 111, 192
Rivastigmine 170, 171
Rorschach test 100

S

S-adenosylmethionine 133
Schema-focused therapy 105
Schizoaffective disorder 79
Schizoid 102
Schizophrenia 10, 23, 27, 33, 42, 61, 69, 70,
    71t, 79, 81, 87, 92, 93, 110, 111, 116,
    149, 169, 171, 190, 203, 205
  antiviral
    medications in 69
    therapy in 69
  cytomegalovirus infection in 72
  diagnosis of 33
  infected 72
  international pilot study on 61
  interventions in 81
  management of 28, 79
  nonpharmacological therapies for 81
  outpatients of 27
  prevalence of 61
  rehabilitation center 28
  treatment of 79, 80, 92
    acute 91
  treatment-resistant 61, 91
Schizotypal 102
  personality disorder 79, 87
Second messenger systems 150
Seizures 230
Sensorimotor rhythm 16
Serotonin 202, 203
  lower levels of 204
  noradrenaline reuptake inhibitors 156
  reuptake inhibitors, selective 102, 113,
    117, 128, 132, 156, 159, 229
  transporte 164
Sertraline 112, 159
Sexual dysfunction 159
Shalabhasana 26
Shashankasana breathing 26
Sheehan disability scale 161
Short message service 89
Single-gene testing 185
Skin rash 200
Skull, trephining of 3
Sleep 144-147
  apnea 145
  disorders 145, 147
  disturbances 145
  quality 16
  restriction 144
  therapeutic role of 144

Smart devices use 90
Social anxiety 113
Social skills training 82, 86
Socio-occupational functioning scale 26
Socrates model 88
Sodium
  amobarbital 49
  thiopental 49
  valproate 174
Somatic hyperpolarization 216
Somatoform
  disorder 23, 53
  pain disorder, diagnosis of 32
  symptoms 32
Spiritual advancements, states of 32
Spiritual approaches 24
Spiritual dimensions 23
Spiritual therapies 23
Stem cell 189, 192, 194
  generation 190
  therapy 6, 189
Stigma avoidance 11
Stimulation 237
Streptococcal infections 205
Streptococcus 202
  thermophiles 204
Stress 131, 202
  hormone
    cortisol 204
    reduction of level of 202
  management 12
  reduction 15
Stria terminalis, bed nucleus of 229
Stroke 2
  rehabilitation 20
Subcallosal cingulate gyrus 232
Subcaudate tractotomy 225, 229, 230, 232,
    233
Subcortical component 231
Substance
  abuse 102
  use disorders 44, 114
  withdrawal, treatment for 102
Sudarshan kriya 31
Superintelligence, artificial 9
Supported Employment Programs 85
Supportive psychotherapy 86
Surya Namaskar 26
Synaptogenesis 150

T

Tacrine 172
Tau deposition, modulation of 173
Technological sophistication 3
Technology, use of 89t

Index

Telepsychiatry 89
Temporoparietal junction 215
Tenacious human curiosity 1
Texas medication algorithm 111
Thalamic peduncle, inferior 232
Thalamus 235
Thematic apperception test 100
Theoretical framework 103
Therapeutic loop 2
Therapeutic serious games 91
Therapy, principles of 103
Thermal biofeedback 15
Theta burst stimulation 214
Thyroid hormone 156
Tiger breathing 26
Timothy syndrome 192
Tolerate clozapine 63
Toll-like receptor 4 145
Topiramate 112
Tourette syndrome 224, 234, 235, 235b, 236
    indications for surgery in 235
    neurobiology of 234
    surgery for 235b
Toxic carbamates 170
Traditional path 5
Trait loci, quantitative 195
Tramiprosate 174
Transcranial direct current stimulation 66, 92, 216
Transcranial magnetic stimulation 20, 65, 213
    safety of repetitive 216
Transient memory loss 230
Tranylcypromine 112
Traumatic neurosis 53
Trazodone 156
Trihexyphenidyl 28
Trikonasana 26

U

Ultrarapid metabolizers 181
Urinary and fecal incontinence 15
Ushtrasana 26

V

Vaccination 174
Vagal modulation 204
Vagus nerve 204
    stimulation 92, 93, 204, 218
Vakrasana 26
Valacyclovir 70
    treatment 72
        trials 72
        trials 75
Valproate 112
Vancouver limbic surgery group 233
Venlafaxine 112
Ventral capsule 228
Ventral striatum 228, 232
Verbal memory 72
Videoconferencing gadgets 89
Vilazodone 162
Viparita karani 26
Virtual reality 90
Vitamin 174
    A 174
    B 133
        group 133
    B_{12} 133, 174
        deficiencies 133
    B_6 174
    B_8 133
    B_9 174
    C 174
    E 128
    K 200
Vocational rehabilitation 85
Vomiting 3, 4
Vortioxetine 160
Voxel patterns 18

W

Water
    boiling 3
    ice-cold 3
Weight gain 159
Working memory 74
World Federation of Societies of Biological Psychiatry 158
    guidelines 157

Y

Yale global tic severity scale 235, 236
Yale-brown obsessive compulsive score 227, 229
Yoga 23
    current status of 23
    for antipsychotic-induced side effects 28
    for caregivers with schizophrenia 29
    for cognitive disorders 30
    for somatoform disorders 32
    in anxiety-related disorders 30
    in depression 24
    in psychiatry, role of 32
    in psychosis 25
    in substance use disorders 31
    in therapy, role of 23
    large effects of 30
    programs, types of 31
    role of 24
    therapy 26, 33
    treated for psychosis 29
Yogic philosophy 23

Z

Zinc 192
Ziprasidone 63
Zonisamide 112